ДЕТИ-ОЛИГОФРЕНЫ

DETI-OLIGOFRENY

OLIGOPHRENIA
Mental Deficiency in Children

Other volumes in

The International Behavioral Sciences Series:

SLEEP THERAPY IN THE NEUROSES
by B. V. Andreev

Research on the ETIOLOGY OF SCHIZOPHRENIA
by Prof. G. Yu. Malis

ANIMAL BEHAVIOR — Its Normal and Abnormal Development
by Prof. L. V. Krushinskii

BIOPOTENTIALS OF CEREBRAL HEMISPHERES IN BRAIN TUMORS
by N. P. Bekhtereva

CEREBRAL FUNCTION IN INFANCY AND CHILDHOOD
by Prof. Albrecht Peiper

The

International Behavioral Sciences

Series

editor Joseph Wortis, M.D.

OLIGOPHRENIA

Mental Deficiency in Children

by

M. S. PEVZNER

With a Preface by J. Tizard

Authorized translation from the Russian

SPRINGER SCIENCE+BUSINESS MEDIA, LLC

The Russian text
was published by
the Publishing House of the Academy
of Pedagogical Sciences of the RSFSR
in Moscow in 1959.
The translation contains
revisions made by the author
subsequent to the publication
of the Russian original.

Мария Семеновна Певзнер

ДЕТИ-ОЛИГОФРЕНЫ

Library of Congress Catalog Card Number: 61-11207

Originally published by Consultants Bureau Enterprises, Inc. 1961

ISBN 978-1-4684-0657-3 *ISBN 978-1-4684-0655-9 (eBook)*
DOI 10.1007/978-1-4684-0655-9

CONTENTS

EDITOR'S NOTE

Considerable effort has been expended to bring this important book to the English speaking reader in a form that fully preserves the intent and thought of the author in language that is clear and comprehensible to the reader. Since the Soviet frame of reference and its terminology are different from our own, literal translation would often be misleading. The term oligophrenia connotes a type of mental retardation basically due to biological rather than social-psychological causes, or more specifically, as the author makes clear, to brain damage or defect. It is thus a narrow term within the wide area of mental retardation and is closer to the British concept of mental defect. The three broad categories of mild, moderate, and severe degree of defect, corresponding roughly to educable, trainable, and nontrainable (sometimes equated in this country with intelligence quotients of 74-50, 49-25, and 24-0) are accepted by the author under the terminology of feeble-minded (debile), imbecile, and idiot. We have sometimes taken the liberty of substituting "moron" or "mild" for "feeble-minded" to avoid confusion. Social-psychological types of retardation are described in the book as temporary or transitory (these have sometimes been translated as pseudoretardation) Intelligence quotients, the reader will soon realize, are of little interest to the author or her colleagues since they obscure the qualitative analysis which is the main interest of the book.

For elucidation of the Pavlovian terminology the reader is advised to acquaint himself with Pavlov's basic concepts through some of the source material so readily available.

The identification of Western names rendered phonetically in Cyrillic letters always presents a serious problem, and although every effort was made to verify the spelling of all names, the possibility of error in some of the more obscure citations cannot be excluded.

Readers are requested to call the editor's attention to any errors or obscurities remaining in the text, so that they may be corrected in subsequent editions.

Joseph Wortis

This book was edited during the tenure of a grant from the National Institute of Mental Health MY-2679 for the translation and interpretation of Russian psychiatric literature.

PREFACE

In 1958 I had the opportunity to visit the Soviet Union for three weeks, on behalf of the World Health Organization, to see what was being done for children with mental and physical handicaps. Two things in particular impressed me. One was the large number of staff, and the quality of care, in residential institutions for children; the second was the amount of research being done on problems of "higher nervous activity." The Institute of Defectology in Moscow, a research institute with close ties with the University, the medical schools, and the educational system, plays a leading part in this research. Here more than 50 scientists, drawn from different disciplines, undertake research on problems of deafness and blindness, cerebral palsy, and mental retardation, in children. It is here too that Dr. Pevzner works; she is the Senior Psychiatrist at the Institute of Defectology.

Until two or three years ago, little was known in the West about Soviet work in this field. But recent publications have done something to bridge the gap, and today it is becoming increasingly easy for those of us who speak no Russian to follow the work of our Soviet colleagues. Of those working in this field Professor A. R. Luriya, who heads the Department of Clinical and Physiological Studies at the Institute of Defectology, is the best known. He developed many of the methods of investigation which are used in the studies outlined in this present book; and for a fuller account of these methods the reader will wish to turn to Professor Luriya's own description of what he and his colleagues are doing.*

Luriya, Sokolov, and others at the Institute of Defectology and Moscow University are concerned primarily with theoretical and general problems. Dr. Pevzner, as a psychiatrist, has a more particular interest in individual children, and in the clinical application of methods of investigation which have been found illuminating. She has been studying problems of oligophrenia since 1938;

*In addition to the work by Professor Luriya cited in the Bibliography, the reader might also see the chapters by Luriya and Sokolov in "The Central Nervous System and Behavior," edited by Mary A. B. Brazier (New York: Josiah Macy Jr. Foundation 1960).

and in this book she gives the reader the fruits of her experience in diagnosing and studying educationally retarded children with disturbances of higher nervous activity.

The reader familiar with postwar advances in the study of mental deficiency outside the Soviet Union will undoubtedly find much to criticize in Dr. Pevzner's review of the literature on this subject. Though many of the references she cites date from the 1940's and 1950's there is little reference in the text to anything of importance published outside the U.S.S.R. since the 1937 edition of Tredgold's textbook. For this reason, and because the style of reporting follows a very different tradition from the one we are accustomed to, one can easily overlook the real contribution that Dr. Pevzner sets out to make. The problem she is concerned with is, briefly, to describe and characterize the mechanisms responsible for the dysfunction which characterizes all, or some, of the mentally retarded. This problem, of fundamental importance to our understanding of mental subnormality, has received very little attention here. From the time of Alfred Binet (a great psychologist whose contribution to our knowledge about individual differences I think most Soviet psychologists misjudge) we have been concerned more with measuring and classifying abilities than with studying the dynamics of function.

Dr. Pevzner's work is primarily qualitative and dynamic rather than quantitative and descriptive as is so much of our own work. Hence it is not surprising that two Western writers whom she cites with approval are Kurt Lewin and Kurt Goldstein. With Goldstein in particular she has obvious similarities and affinities, and many of the same strengths and weaknesses appear in her writing.

The decisive influence in Dr. Pevzner's work is however that of Pavlov. Pavlov created a new science; but owing to language and other barriers, too little is known in the West of the formidable amount of research—of varying quality—that the Pavlov school has carried out in the Soviet Union. An urgent and exciting task to which, fortunately, increasing numbers of neurophysiologists and psychologists both in the U.S.S.R. and in the West are turning their attention, is the synthesis of classical and Pavlovian theory. We can be grateful that publishers are now providing more translations of the work of our Soviet colleagues, since most of us are entirely dependent upon translation for first-hand knowledge of what is being written in other parts of the world.

J. Tizard

Social Psychiatry Research Unit
Institute of Psychiatry
Maudsley Hospital, London

INTRODUCTION

The study of oligophrenia has an important relationship both to our knowledge of inherited defects and to child psychiatry. No adequate scientific basis has yet been developed for the proper organization of special schools. Boys and girls are often inappropriately referred to these schools; children who are incapable of being educated there (deaf children, children with speech defects, children with a delay of development or with asthenic states).

The scientific approach to the solution of the problem of the organization of special schools requires a careful clinical study of oligophrenic children and their differentiation from children with only an external resemblance to an oligophrenic state.

The study of oligophrenia is equally important to child psychiatry, for little work has yet been done on the study of the etiology, pathogenesis, pathophysiology and symptomatology of this condition. Two points of view can be found in the literature dealing with the nature of oligophrenia. Some authorities include variants of the normal in the oligophrenic group (limited, dull, or backward children) on the assumption that the intellectual deficiency of all such children is inherited. Others, widening the definition of oligophrenia to the limit, include in it various forms of dementia (epileptic, traumatic, encephalitic, and schizophrenic).

In my definition of oligophrenia I include those forms of mental deficiency which arise as a result of intrauterine or early lesions of the central nervous system and which show no tendency to progress. All other forms of mental deficiency arising in consequence of organic lesions of the central nervous system in later stages of development are excluded from the category of oligophrenia.

It has been my object to analyze the fundamental pathogenetic nature of oligophrenic mental deficiency on the basis of the results of the comprehensive investigation of oligophrenic children. Most of the work which has been done on the study of mentally retarded children in general, as well as the work on oligophrenic children, is characterized by an absence of pathophysiological analysis. It has been my aim to study the pathophysiological mechanisms lying at the basis of the clinical picture of oligophrenic mental deficiency.

The study of the way in which disturbances of the various parameters of higher nervous activity are combined has been of considerable importance to the description of the different forms of oligophrenia. In some studies which have been made of mentally retarded children, the whole symptomatology has usually been described under a series of different headings. Most authorities have spoken of the loss of memory, the narrowness of perception, the poverty of the vocabulary, the limitation of judgment, and the extreme weakness of logical thought. In contrast to this, I have attempted to identify those fundamental symptoms of oligophrenic mental deficiency which would permit the establishment of meaningful relationships among the individual symptoms and facilitate the study of the defect as a whole.

In most researches oligophrenia is regarded as a static condition, in which all aspects of the clinical picture are not infrequently directly associated either with some hereditary defect or with a localized lesion of the central nervous system. In contrast to this view, I look upon oligophrenia as a special form of development anomaly. Development itself is a complex process in which the disturbance of a given function depends on the place which this function occupies in the general psychic development of the infant and on the stage of development at which this disturbance took place.

Until recently, the starting point for the classification of oligophrenia was the severity of the cerebral defect. In the present study I shall identify the various forms of oligophrenia on the basis of the qualitative analysis of the actual structure of the mental deficiency.

Through the study of the various forms of oligophrenia it is possible to develop a more rational and correct approach to the question of differential diagnosis, a matter of importance where the organization of special schools is concerned. The differentiation of the variants of mental deficiency in oligophrenia permits a truly scientific basis for the selection of corrective and educational measures for these children.

In the present study I have not attempted to fully discuss the whole complex problem of oligophrenia. My aim has been the relatively narrower one of studying the various forms of oligophrenia, attempting to understand them from the point of view of the interrelationship between their etiopathogenesis, pathophysiology and clinical pattern, and, on the basis of the individual characteristics of the structure of each type, indicating appropriate therapeutic and educational measures.

The clinical study of oligophrenia began in the Institute of Special Schools and Children's Homes in 1938. From 1943 until 1951 it continued at the Children's Psychiatric Clinic of the Central Institute of Psychiatry of the RSFSR, under the direction of Professor G. E. Sukhareva. During this same period I studied the various forms of mental deficiency caused by hydrocephalus at the Burdenko Institute of Neurosurgery. In 1951 I began a comprehensive study of oligophrenic children receiving their education at a special school at the Instute for the Study of Inherited Defects of the Academy of Pedagogic Sciences of the RSFSR. Clinical material, accumulated over many years, also provided information on some of the complex clinical and pathophysiological problems of oligophrenia.

Considerable help in the execution of this work was given by many of my colleagues, to whom I express my deep and sincere thanks. I should like to mention in particular the great assistance rendered in this study by my colleagues in the Department of Clinical and Pathophysiological Study of the Anomalous Child of the Institute for the Study of Inherited Defects of the Academy of Pedagogic Sciences of the RSFSR: A. R. Luriya, V. I. Lubovskii, L. A. Novikova, N. N. Zislina, and others. Valuable help was given by G. E. Sukhareva, by the teaching staff of the 30th Special School and the headmaster N. S. Sekun, and by the medical and teaching staff of the Sanatorium for Nervous Children and its director K. M. Kukhanov. I am very grateful to the directorate of the Institute for the Study of Inherited Defects of the Academy of Pedagogic Sciences of the RSFSR for granting good facilities for the work. I wish to convey my deep gratitude to my colleagues in the Children's Department of the Burdenko Institute of Neurosurgery. I must also express my appreciation to I. V. Zhukov, Editor of the Publishing House of the Academy of Pedagogic Sciences of the RSFSR, for his exceptional care in the editing of the text.

Institute of Defectology
Moscow, USSR

M. S. Pevzner

CHAPTER 1

THE CLINICAL PATTERN AND PATHOPHYSIOLOGY OF OLIGOPHRENIA

1. A Survey of the Literature

THE ETIOLOGY OF OLIGOPHRENIA

The residual phenomena following intrauterine or early infections of the brain often lead to a disturbance of the mental development of the child. The term "mentally retarded child," like the term "dementia," can encompass essentially very different clinical forms. Such terms are often applied to certain concurrent organic diseases where features of dementia can be observed (for example, amaurotic idiocy, tuberous sclerosis, epilepsy with mental deterioration, etc.).

The concept of oligophrenia is sometimes also extended to residual states following meningo-encephalitis and para-infectious encephalitis, where the signs of dementia develop during the later stages of development of the child.

Foreign psychiatrists often include mentally deficient and backward children in one group. This unjustifiable widening of the concept of oligophrenia leads to erroneous conclusions regarding its etiology, pathogenesis and clinical pattern. Our investigation is directed to the study of a narrower group of conditions – namely, to oligophrenia.

Oligophrenia may be defined as that type of maldevelopment of the complex forms of psychic activity which arises as a result of a lesion of the anlage or as an organic lesion of the central nervous system in the early stages of intrauterine development of the fetus or in the earliest period of life of the child.

In the past, in the first stages of the investigation of mental deficiency, all forms of psychic maldevelopment were designated by one common term "idiocy." We may dwell briefly on the history of this aspect of the problem. Esquirol (1838)* defined idiocy as a particular state in which the mental abilities have not developed. Soon, however, the less clearly marked form of mental retardation began to be distinguished from the group of the idiots. A still less marked degree of backwardness, namely debility, was subsequently distinguished. All these forms were combined in the general concept of "dementia," which has had different meanings at different times. Sometimes it has meant any state of psychic maldevelopment, at others, only its more severe degrees. Sometimes these states were regarded as progressive, in contrast to the idea of idiocy, which was considered to be a nonprogressive condition. Ireland (1880) employed two terms – "idiocy" and "dullness" – distinguishing them from dementia, which he regarded as a progressive condition. Kraepelin, who laid the foundations of the nosological trend in psychiatry, combined the various forms of psychic maldevelopment in the concept of "oligophrenia."

Fundamental problems remain unsolved, however, in the study of oligophrenia: its etiology, pathogenesis, symptomatology, and classification.

In the initial stages of the investigation mental deficiency was erroneously regarded as one form of devolution (Morel, 1857). In a special monograph devoted to the study of the genealogy of individual families, Morel (1857) endeavored to show that devolution takes place over several generations in accordance with the law of degeneration. The clinical manifestations of this devolution took different forms. In their first stages, for instance, they appeared as various changes of temperament (increased excitability, general irritability). In the progeny of this generation cases of hysteria and epilepsy were observed. In subsequent generations marked psychoses developed, and finally, in the last stage of degeneration gross forms of devolutive dementia appeared (imbeciles, idiots).

Like Morel, Magnan (1903) regarded all cases of congenital feeble-mindedness as manifestations of devolution. Claude (1932), one of the foremost French psychiatrists, also regarded the various forms of congenital feeble-mindedness as degenerative. The contemporary British geneticist Penrose, in several of his papers, regards several different forms of congenital feeble-mindedness as types of hereditary devolution. In this connection Karl Vogt's

*Here and subsequently we have indicated the year when a particular idea was first expressed by particular authors. The bibliography (page 399) sometimes cites later publications.

well known work "Microcephalics" (1873) must not be forgotten. In his study, Vogt elaborated his theory of atavism, relating microcephalic idiots to man's ape-like ancestors by comparing the anatomy of their brain and skull.

Several authorities (Weygandt, 1915; Strohmayer, 1928; Bürger-Prinz, 1936; Dubitscher, 1942; Penrose, 1938, 1944) have mistakenly regarded hereditary factors as dominant and decisive in the etiology of oligophrenia. These workers have tended to regard exogenous noxious agents as factors which merely excite an hereditary predisposition.

This point of view has been expressed most emphatically by certain American psychiatrists. In a paper by Baker (1947), Director of the Detroit Psychological Clinic, on the subject of exceptional children, he claims that heredity is one of the most potent and natural causes of mental deficiency. Heredity was apparently the cause of mental deficiency in 476 of 482 cases investigated. In the American journal "Heredity" in an article by Hunt (1945) on mental development and Mendel's law, the author claims that in accordance with the laws of heredity, a certain proportion of mentally deficient children must be born even to perfectly normal parents.

It must also be borne in mind that a purely psychoanalytical interpretation of mental retardation also exists. Clark (1933) claimed that mental retardation may represent an unconscious desire of the child to return to the mother's womb. This point of view has received no recognition, even among psychoanalysts.

In later research, excessive importance has been attached to the hereditary factor. Goldkuhl (1930) in a monograph on mild forms of oligophrenia points out that in most cases these forms are due to constitutional factors. Though Kraepelin (1913) for instance stated that oligophrenia is a collective group of conditions which subsequently must be studied and classified on the basis of etiology, the nature of the pathological process and the time of its development, he nevertheless did nothing to advance the positive aspects of his position and to all intents and purposes upheld the conventional point of view. He supported the established division of the oligophrenias into three groups (idiots, imbeciles, and morons) and considered that heredity is the dominant etiological factor in oligophrenia.

Thus Kraepelin, who began by criticizing the complex theoretical views held at that time on oligophrenia, was unable to advance beyond the bounds of the very views which he condemned.

In subsequent work foreign psychiatrists have been compelled to admit that exogenous noxious factors are of some significance. In a paper by Brander (1937) great importance is attached to "natural" trauma. This worker found cerebral hemorrhage present in 65% of his cases when he studied 500 instances of infants dying at birth or during the first month of life following "natural" trauma.

Even those authorities like Brander however who recognized the role of exogenous factors in their descriptions of the various forms of mental deficiency emphasized its endogenous origin, though the evidence which they cited clearly contradicted this claim.

As a result of their incorrect concept of the hereditary nature of mental retardation, several foreign psychiatrists have attempted to clinically differentiate inherited and acquired forms of oligophrenia. Hecker (1939), for instance, draws attention to the difficulty of such a distinction and tries to classify as exogenous only those cases where certain character traits are found together with the intellectual disturbances. In this worker's opinion such children display certain distinctive traits, such as general restlessness and destructiveness.

In other researches the criterion suggested for distinguishing exogenous forms of oligophrenia from inherited forms is the presence of central nervous system pathology. The exogenous forms are thus supposed to be characterized by marked changes in the central nervous system, while these changes are said to be usually absent in the hereditary forms. But this criterion also does not permit a differential diagnosis of these states and leads to obviously irreconcilable contradictions. In amaurotic idiocy, for instance, and in tuberous sclerosis, gross central nervous system pathology is found at autopsy – in spite of the fact that these are hereditary diseases.

Various foreign psychiatrists have attempted to develop a clinical diagnostic approach to the problem of mental deficiency or oligophrenia. Feuchtwanger (1926) for instance regarded mental deficiency as a symptom of brain disease comparable to aphasia, apraxia, and paralysis, and suggested that the condition be studied in relation to time of onset and localization of the lesion. This authority did not however put his views into practice when carrying out his clinical investigations.

A very similar point of view is found in the work of Stertz (1928), who stated that certain forms of mental deficiency may be due to systemic, focal, or diffuse lesions of the brain.

More recently the study of toxoplasmosis has helped a great deal in the elucidation of exogenous factors in oligophrenia. Two forms of toxoplasmosis are recognized, congenital and acquired. The main manifestations of congenital toxoplasmosis are chorioretinitis, which is considered to be a pathognomic sign, and retardation of psychophysical development. Since retardation of psychophysical development is a frequent manifestation of congenital toxoplasmosis, several workers have investigated the relationship between toxoplasmosis and mental retardation. Burkenshaw, Kirman, and Sorsby (1953) found a positive serological reaction in 55 of 698 oligophrenics examined. Kozar, Dluzhevskii, Dluzhevskaya, and Yaroshevskii (1954) consider that toxoplasmosis is a possible cause of oligophrenia. Declus*(1948) indicated the role of toxoplasmosis in the genesis of certain forms of oligophrenia.

In recent years a special form of oligophrenia has been distinguished abroad — "phenylpyruvic oligophrenia" — which is characterized by abnormalities in the metabolism of the amino acid phenylalanine in the body. Jervis believes that hereditary factors of recessive type play a decisive role in the development of this disease. In this form of oligophrenia epileptiform fits are often observed, beginning in early childhood and later becoming more frequent and polymorphic in character.

No less interesting is the finding that rubella in pregnant women can cause embryonic defects. The clinical abnormalities most frequently found were lesions of the eyes (cataracts, retinopathies), deaf-mutism, heart disease, and mental deficiency. No specific constant clinical picture of the mental deficiency following rubella in the mother during pregnancy has been observed. Gilmore and Cook (1944) attach etiological importance to the Rhesus factor in the genesis of certain forms of oligophrenia.

It should also be mentioned that in the work of certain prerevolutionary Russian psychiatrists confirmation of the importance of the exogenous factor in the etiology of oligophrenia may be found. Dyad'kovskii (1847) considered that internal hydrocephalus with consequent maldevelopment of the brain was an organic cause of idiocy. Malinovskii (1847) also emphasized the role of organic brain disease in the genesis of idiocy. Merzheevskii (1901) stated that development is disturbed in many cases of idiocy because of pathological processes occurring in embryonic life or during early childhood.

Of no less interest is the paper of Tomashevskii (1892) entitled "The pathology of idiocy." In it there is a definite statement that mental deficiency may be exogenous in origin. In Tomashevskii's opinion the pia mater in early childhood shows a particular susceptibility to acute and chronic inflammatory diseases. Since vessels from the pia enter the cerebral cortex, the inflammatory process in the pia mater may lead to atrophic changes in the cortex. As in Merzheevskii's work, in this investigation we find agreement between the clinical and anatomical findings. The author cites the results of his observations on a boy, 12 years old, who was incapable of education and irresponsible in his behavior. After a severe infectious disease the boy died. At autopsy the findings were as follows: the dura mater was hyperemic and edematous and separated with difficulty from the internal surface of the skull. In the subarachnoid spaces of the frontal region an accumulation of cerebral fluid was found. The pia mater was vascularized and adherent to the brain tissue in the region of the frontal and parietal lobes. The frontal gyri were atrophic, and a lesser degree of atrophy was observed in the parietal regions. The lateral ventricles were dilated and the ependyma was altered and strewn with small nodules. The cerebellum, brainstem, and spinal cord were normal. Microscopic examination of brain tissue taken from the frontal region of the cortex showed the following: an increase in the number of capillaries, thickening of the walls of the small arteries and, in places, areas of subadventitial extravasation. The connective tissue was considerably hypertrophied, the fibers being thickened and increased in number. The neuroglial tissue was more abundant than in the healthy cortex, and arachnoid cells were found in its entire thickness. In this anatomical research, remarkable in its time, Tomashevskii (1892) related the picture of mental deficiency to organic disease of the brain. He found support for his point of view, striking a blow against the teaching of genotypical forms of maldevelopment, among the more advanced scientists of his time. For instance, he cites Lallemand, who showed that residual traces of previous illnesses may lie at the root of atrophic processes in the cerebral cortex. Tomashevskii also cites the work of Cruveilhier (1845), "A general treatise on pathological anatomy," in which the author concludes that atrophy arises only as a result of exogenous diseases of the brain.

In support of his advanced views on the exogenous nature of mental deficiency, Tomashevskii quotes the work of Gotar (1868), who said that atrophy and dysgenesis cannot be sharply separated from each other: there is no basic difference between them – they merely occur at different stages. Whereas in adult life the ingestion of food merely maintains the equilibrium between the processes of assimilation and metabolic breakdown, in childhood and during gestation it ensures the predominance of the process of assimilation, to satisfy the demands of growth and development of the individual.

Tomashevskii's general conclusion – that idiocy most commonly arises as a consequence of inflammatory processes, sometimes taking the form of a chronic disease – was progressive for its time and to some extent retains its meaning even today.

Kovalevskii (1906) also put forward the hypothesis that external, exogenous noxious factors were of importance in the development of different forms of idiocy; although his work contains certain inaccuracies, these are by no means typical of the work as a whole. Kovalevskii attaches great importance to encephalitis when considering the etiology of idiocy. Korsakov pursued his investigations in an original manner. In 1901 he claimed that an exogenous factor was predominant in the etiology of oligophrenia. Serbskii (1912) considered that the principal causes of mental deficiency are severe traumatic lesions of the brain or inflammatory lesions caused by infectious diseases at an early age.

Soon afterwards (1914) Gilyarovskii published a paper on "The pathological anatomy and pathogenesis of porencephaly," a condition often associated with mental deficiency. In the first part of his paper the author presents an analysis of all the cases of porencephaly described in the world literature between 1812 and 1907, with detailed anatomical findings. In the second part of his paper, Gilyarovskii criticizes the existing explanations of the pathogenesis of porencephaly. Some authorities regarded hydrocephalus as the cause of porencephaly; others thought that this defect was due to premature fusion of the cranial bones; a third group was of the opinion that the developmental anomaly in porencephaly was due to maldevelopment of the brain itself. Most researchers relate the porencephalic defects to vascular disturbances. The theory of the inflammatory origin of this condition has been supported by very few authorities, and these have interpreted the inflammation itself differently, sometimes not without recognizing the genotypical predisposition to this inflammation.

On the basis of the analysis of his findings, Gilyarovskii emphasizes two fundamental causes of porencephaly: traumatic lesions and vascular-inflammatory lesions. These conclusions are supported by careful anatomical investigations. In particular, he demonstrated changes in the vessel walls not only in the region of the defect but also in other parts of the brain. As a counterpoise to the genotypical idea, Gilyarovskii showed convincingly in his researches that porencephaly arises as a result of inflammatory changes. In his subsequent investigations he elaborated this materialistic point of view. It served a progressive purpose, since it stood in opposition to the widely accepted theory of Karl Vogt, according to which the microgyria observed in cases of mental deficiency was regarded as a manifestation of atavism.

Geier noted that infectious diseases of the brain play a dominant role in the development of oligophrenia. Osipova (1925) emphasized the great variety of etiological factors lying at the basis of mental deficiency.

An obvious tendency has been observed in recent years abroad to admit the significance of exogenous factors in the etiology of oligophrenia. In one of their papers on mental deficiency, for instance, Hilliard and Kirman (1957) cite experimental findings which showed clearly that if animals were kept on vitamin-deficient diets or were irradiated during pregnancy, a variety of malformations occurred among their offspring (microcephaly, microphthalmia, anencephaly, etc.). Much more importance is attached to natural trauma, and greater attention is paid to postnatal trauma in the form of subdural hematomas and intracranial hemorrhage. These workers accept the concept of "blastophoria" as a disturbance of developmental capacity due to changes in the reproductive cells. This concept embraces a host of factors causing injury to the cell (the age of the mother at the time of pregnancy, or the presence of disease, starvation, alcoholism, and syphilis in the mother). They discriminate between the concept of "blastophoria" and true heredity, which is determined by genes.

THE CLASSIFICATION OF OLIGOPHRENIA

The classification of oligophrenia is in an even less advanced stage of development, although several attempts have been made in this direction. Ireland (1880) attempted to classify the various forms of psychic maldevelopment according to etiological factors. He distinguished between psychic maldevelopment of a traumatic or inflammatory character and maldevelopment due to dystrophic disturbances. Similar attempts were undertaken by other psychiatrists, but all were unsatisfactory because they did not try to establish a connection between the clinical pattern of the psychic maldevelopment and the responsible cause.

Meinert (1892), Bourneville (1900) and others attempted to utilize anatomical principles for the classification of oligophrenia. They differentiated forms of mental retardation associated with hydrocephalus, microcephaly, with agenesis of various parts of the brain and with hypotrophic and atrophic sclerosis of the whole brain or of individual parts of that organ.

This anatomical classification however had as little success as the etiological classification, because these authorities failed to relate their anatomical findings to any distinctive features of the clinical picture.

Other attempts were made to classify these conditions. Griesinger (1867), for example, divided all mentally retarded children into two large groups – apathetic and excited. Weygandt (1915) divided children with signs of intellectual backwardness into two large groups: (a) passive, dull, apathetic, torpid; (b) active, excited, vivacious, erethistic. This distinction between excitatory and torpid oligophrenias, which originated with Griesinger and with Weygandt, is still encountered even today.

Few attempts have been made to classify the oligophrenias in recent times. Even in the latest papers by Tredgold (1937, 1952), as in the work of Cook (1944), the classification of oligophrenia is nothing more than a list of the various diseases in which feeble-mindedness is observed. Tredgold, for instance, offers the following classification:

1. Primary amentia
   a) simple
   b) mongolism
   c) microcephaly
2. Secondary amentia
   a) traumatic lesions
   b) meningitis
   c) encephalitis
   d) hydrocephalus
   e) syphilis
   f) amaurotic idiocy
   g) epilepsy
   h) cretinism

There is no need to criticize this classification for it is patently obvious that it is not a classification at all.

Other attempts to discriminate between the various types of mentally deficient children may be mentioned. Paddle (1934) distinguishes the following types of mental deficiency: a sexual type, a pugnacious type, an acquisitive type, and a self-confident, assertive type. Paddle's attempt also cannot be regarded as a true classification. Equally unsuccessful attempts were made by Kurt Schneider, who distinguished the following types of oligophrenics: the boasting chatterbox, the inveterate hypocrite, the stupid and obstinate, and the inert and passive.

Goldkuhl distinguishes three groups of mental deficiency:

1) a mild maniacal type – extroverted, irresponsible, and superficial in judgment;

2) depressive defectives – with increased sensitivity, a tendency to tearfulness and anxiety reactions;

3) irritable, irascible.

Kohler divides oligophrenic children into two groups: harmonic and disharmonic. The disharmonic group, in turn, is subdivided into the stupid, the unstable, and the emotional. In their mental qualities the harmonic group of oligophrenics resemble infants.

In the article by the German teacher Ledemann, entitled "Living crutches" (Lebendige Krücken, 1925), the author criticizes earlier classifications in which all mentally retarded children were described by the single word "stupid." He also considers that it is not sufficient to use the long established division of the mentally retarded into idiots, imbeciles and morons. He points out that it is essential to discover not only the degree but also the type to which the mentally defective children belong, and suggests the following classification: 1) inhibited, 2) awkward, and 3) disinhibited. The whole paper is permeated with the idea that it is imperative to understand the qualitative differences between the various types of mental retardation and to take them into consideration when planning corrective training.

None of the attempts to subdivide the oligophrenics which we have given above can be regarded essentially as classifications. The difficulties encountered in the drawing up of a truly scientific classification of these conditions have led to the fact that in recent decades various authorities, among them Soviet psychiatrists (Ozeretskii, 1932; Gurevich, 1949; and others), have refrained from making any attempts to classify these conditions, and have differentiated the whole group of mentally retarded children purely in accordance with the degree of the disability. Corresponding to the severity of the disability, a distinction is drawn between idiots (the severest form of maldevelopment), imbeciles (children with severe mental retardation and incapable of education) and morons or feeble-minded (children with a less severe degree of mental retardation, with considerable maldevelopment of abstract forms of mental activity but capable of education under special conditions). The division of oligophrenics according to the severity of the disability is of theoretical importance, for the severity of the lesion influences the nature of the clinical picture. It is also of practical importance, for the severity of the disability often determines the type of institution the child requires. However, the criterion of the severity of the lesion by no means determines the qualitative structural pattern of the disability.

THE SYMPTOMATOLOGY OF OLIGOPHRENIA

In all of these investigations, clinical, psychological, and pathophysiological, the authors above have tried as a rule to describe only the general features of the oligophrenic. The symptomatology of oligophrenia has thus been studied without refined discrimination. Symptoms of oligophrenia that are always observed in clinical investigations are: stereotypy and poverty of objective ideas, weakness of judgment, and an extremely limited range of vocabulary and ideas.

Esquirol (1838), in describing the symptomatology of these conditions, attempted to use the level of speech development as a basis for appraisal. Séguin (1846) considered that the idiot is especially deficient in the "primitive will" to use his intellectual capacities. Sollier (1891), in describing imbeciles and idiots, thought that the disturbance of attentiveness represented a common clinical pattern in these conditions. Idiots, in Sollier's opinion, cannot voluntarily pay attention, while in imbeciles the capacity to pay attention is unstable. Ziehen (1918) considered that in a child at the level of idiocy very few concrete ideas are encountered. Imbeciles more frequently present objective ideas but can combine them only into simple associations. The feeble-minded, although possessing objective ideas and capable of forming them into associations, cannot form complex notions and in this respect are far behind normal children of their age. Bleuler (1920), discussing the symptomatology of oligophrenia, draws attention to the poverty of association which is present along with the deficiency of perception and of memory. This poverty of association makes the formation of ideas more difficult.

Strohmayer (1926) considers that weakness of attention is the main symptom of mental deficiency. Some mentally deficient children show an obvious depression of this psychic function, and are therefore apathetic and dull in response to impressions from the outside world. In complete contrast to these mental defectives are those children who suffer from pathological mobility of attention. Strohmayer considers that a no less characteristic symptom of mental deficiency is the poverty of ideas, and when investigating their mental capacity it is important to make a careful distinction between their stock of word-ideas and their stock of true ideas. In many mental defectives speech is not accompanied by thought, a state of affairs which "excludes any understanding of the mutual relationships between objects, cause and effect, quality and purpose, an article and its value, and also leads to the fact that an empty verbal ideal has absolutely no influence on their ego." *

Korsakov (1894), in describing severe types of mental retardation, observed that the psychic life of these patients is not sufficiently developed to create notions. Serbskii (1912) considered that in idiocy the ability to form abstract notions is absent; in the feeble-minded the formation of abstract notions is possible, but these do not attain that wealth and variety which characterizes the normal child. The most correct point of view on the nature of oligophrenia was put forward by Troshin (1915), who declared that imbeciles are capable only of mechanical abstraction, and that the impossibility of true abstraction and generalization distinguishes the moronic from the normally developing child. Gurevich (1949) describes the symptomatology of oligophrenia on the basis of the severity of the disability, and characterizes idiocy by the almost total absence of psychic functions, imbecility by poverty of ideas and inaccessibility to the formation of abstract notions, and feeble-mindedness by the maldevelopment only of abstract forms of thought.

The uniformity and poverty of the symptomatology were demonstrated particularly clearly during the study of oligophrenia in those clinical investigations which were devoted to the study of the psychoses associated with oligophrenia.

The absence of a sufficiently clear definition of the very concept of dementia was bound to have a hampering effect on the solution of problems connected with the classification and symptomatology of oligophrenia. Several psychological theories of in-

*W. Strohmayer, The Psychopathology of Childhood. Lectures for Doctors and Teachers (Moscow—Leningrad, 1926) p. 168.

telligence exist. According to Spearman's (1927) theory, intelligence is composed of two factors: general and special capabilities. This idea of Spearman has been widely accepted in work published abroad, and has been reflected in particular in the work of Burt on the study of the backward child (1953) and on the subnormal mind (1955). In both these works the developed theory of factors is presented in its application to the backward child. Following Spearman, for instance, Burt considers that intelligence is composed of two factors, a general factor (G) and a special factor (S). The factor G lies at the basis of the general intellectual endowment, and the special factor determines the musical, technical and other forms of intellectual attainment.

The characteristics of intelligence have been studied by Spearman and Burt by means of the correlation between the individual forms of ability for both the general and the special factor. Individual forms of activity related to the general factor give a high coefficient of correlation, which indicates their essential interconnection and mutual dependence. The coefficient of correlation between the individual forms of activity for the general and for the special factor is very low.

These studies present us with an analysis of a large number of statistical correlations, essentially involving purely quantitative relationships rather than a truly qualitative analysis of intelligence.

In Burt's opinion it is the general factor which is affected in mental retardation. The opposite point of view is expressed by Thorndike (1927), who regards intelligence as the sum of different abilities. From the point of view of the gestalt psychologists, an act is reasonable if the elements of the situation are combined into a rational structure.

Jaspers distinguishes between intelligence proper and its fundamental components. Among the latter he includes perception, attention, memory, speech and practice. Intelligence proper is thought. An attempt has been made to divide intelligence into practical, theoretical and gnostic components (Lipman-Bogen). Gruhle divides intelligence into higher and formal aspects.

Different definitions of mental deficiency have been current. Some workers, Gruhle for example (1932), regarded mental deficiency as an acquired and permanent psychic weakness. Others, for example Stertz, Fleck, and Bostrom, defined mental deficiency as a primary weakness of the intellectual functions. A common feature of the definitions of congenital and acquired mental deficiency, however, was the recognition of the presence of two fundamental characteristics: a loss or weakness of the intellectual functions, and its permanence or irreversibility. At the beginning of the present century both these features began to be re-examined.

The study of epidemic encephalitis, which could induce mental retardation even in the absence of primary intellectual disturbances, and with preservation of the formal intellectual functions, introduced a number of new clinical facts which apparently did not accord with the generally accepted concept of mental deficiency as a purely intellectual and irreversible disability. The reversal of certain symptoms in general paresis in response to malaria treatment led to similar considerations. As a result of these findings, such notions as "affective dementia (Minkovskaya), "motor dementia" (Hauptmann), "dementia of motives" (Bürger-Prinz), "subcortical dementia" (Stockert), and "brainstem dementia" (Stertz) began to be introduced into psychopathology. It can thus be seen that, as a result of the accumulation of clinical evidence, the old ideas of dementia as a purely intellectual and irreversible disability were shown to be clearly contrary to the facts.

The experimental psychological study of the problem went some distance toward meeting this new clinical trend. Of exceptional interest is the "dynamic theory of mental deficiency in children" enunciated and developed by Kurt Lewin. Lewin regards the concrete pattern of thought as the most significant feature distinguishing the intelligence of the mentally deficient child from that of the normal child. He infers the concrete pattern of thought directly from the inertia and the obliquity of the affective systems. This theory, however, still does not explain what is responsible for the obliquity of the affective systems in mental defectives. Vygotskii assumed a close connection between affect and intelligence and stressed their internal connection and their mutual influence on each other. In his paper "The problem of mental retardation," Vygotskii (1935) stated that concreteness in the field of thought and inertia in the field of the dynamic systems are connected internally and appear as a single feature, and not as a fortuitous combination, in the mentally deficient child.

THE PATHOGENESIS AND PATHOPHYSIOLOGY OF OLIGOPHRENIA

The slow advance of our knowledge of the etiology, classification and symptomatology of oligophrenia is largely the result of our ignorance of the nature of the disturbances and the lack of pathological, anatomical and pathophysiological data.

In most of the existing published work on the pathological anatomy of oligophrenia, only the severest forms of this maldevelopment are considered. Two different series of anatomical changes are described, depending on the time at which the central nervous system was affected. Merzheevskii (1901), Tomashevskii (1892), Korsakov (1901), Gilyarovskii (1914), Troshin (1915), Ziehen (1926), and Gurevich (1949) draw attention to the maldevelopment of the brain. These changes take the form of incomplete development of the cerebral hemispheres, inadequate development of the gyri (signs of agyria and microgyria), a decrease in the number of layers of the cortex, an irregular arrangement of the cells in the layers, a diminished number of nerve cells, maldevelopment of the white matter and the appearance of cells in the white matter, i.e., of heterotopia. Anatomical changes of this type are due to early intrauterine lesions of the central nervous system.

In organic lesions arising at later stages of development of the fetus or in the early period of life of the infant, the anatomical changes are somewhat different in character. In these cases thickening of the meninges and their adherence to the brain tissue may be observed, sometimes with empty, sclerotic areas, cysts, localized or diffuse atrophy, and complete absence of the corpora callosa. Most anatomical investigations have shown the presence of a residual hydrocephalus, manifesting itself as an accumulation of cerebrospinal fluid in the subarachnoid spaces, dilatation of the cerebral ventricles and changes in the ependyma.

It is natural that the pathological changes in the central nervous system should lead to considerable malfunction of the higher nervous activity. For this reason great attention has been paid to the study of the higher nervous activity in oligophrenia. This study however has been undertaken quite separately from clinical investigations. Our purpose in the present volume is to compare the clinical and experimental findings, and it is therefore deemed necessary to preface this with a short survey of the literature concerning the special features of the higher nervous activity in oligophrenia.

The investigation of the higher nervous activity of oligophrenic children began in 1926 with work by Lukina and Shnirman. These workers showed that conditioned reflexes are formed on the average more quickly in oligophrenic than in normal children. Automatization of the reflexes thus formed, however, is not so well marked. In the process of development of these reflexes a large number of intersignal reactions are observed. Differentiation is difficult to induce.

Panferov (1927) found that conditioned reflexes are formed with great difficulty in idiocy. Segal' (1929) observed the rapid formation of a grasp reflex. In mild degrees of idiocy differentiation could be induced. In severe idiocy the conditioned reflexes remained unconsolidated and no differentiation was developed. Attempts to induce differentiation caused inhibition of the conditioned reflex. The researches of Gartsshtein (1930) showed that the process of stimulation is defective in oligophrenics (this is shown by the instability of the conditioned reflexes). Many superfluous movements are observed in oligophrenics. In the attempt to induce conditioned inhibition, an acute inadequacy of inhibition was found. Mirolyubov (1935) pointed out the difficulty in producing a conditioned reaction to an attitude, and showed that in the more severe degrees of oligophrenia the development of such a reaction was generally impossible.

The work of Kaz'min and Fedorov (1951) showed that the formation of elementary conditioned connections in oligophrenics was not disturbed, and that it was also possible to induce simple differentiation reactions, but that the addition of new conditioned connections to a previously developed system was difficult because of negative induction. The presence of negative induction in the cases which they investigated was, in the opinion of these workers, "the main physiological basis of mental deficiency." Trofimov (1958) carried out an investigation of the higher nervous activity in different degrees of oligophrenia. In severe idiocy it was impossible to induce conditioned reflexes. In less severe degrees of idiocy and in imbeciles the process of stimulation was weakened and inert; extreme weakness of internal inhibition and the rapid development of states showing changing phases were observed. Cortical regulation of vegetative functions was disturbed. In less severe degrees of oligophrenia the process of stimulation was adequate in strength but inert. The conditioned reflexes remained for a long time in a stage of generalization and successive inhibition was well marked. Weakness and inertia of internal inhibition were found.

Molotkova (1954) studied the higher nervous activity in oligophrenics and noted difficulty in the formation of secondary conditioned reflexes and instability of the conditioned reflexes that were formed. The induction of differentiation was difficult. The translation of available conditioned reflexes into trace reflexes was an even more complicated task. Gakkel' (1953) made a comparative study of the higher nervous activity in oligophrenia and in senile dementia, and drew attention to the weakness of stimulation and, in particular, of inhibition in oligophrenics. Zhuravleva and Morgen (1954) observed difficulty in the formation of conditioned inhibition and impossibility of its consolidation in severe oligophrenics. The investigations of the authors cited above revealed a number of interesting features of the higher nervous activity of oligophrenics: weakening of the processes of stimulation and inhibition; disturbance of the mobility of the fundamental nervous processes, a tendency for them to irradiate and to be concentrated with difficulty; and a disturbance of complex synthetic activity.

It is apparent, however, that most investigations into the nature of the higher nervous activity suffer from a common inherent defect. Studies are frequently based on a vague, and sometimes incorrect, concept of the clinical picture of oligophrenia. Consequently they attempt to construct a system of differentiation between the members of this composite group of conditions based only on the degree of severity of the disability. Frequently they even misuse this criterion. Trofimov, for instance, groups grossly disabled cases among those with a mild degree of oligophrenia, for, as indicated in his paper, his patients could not master the rudiments of reading and writing, and some of them were even incapable of articulate speech.

In some sections of the same paper a clinical description of individual cases is given, and from the descriptions they cannot always be regarded as belonging to the oligophrenic group. In none of the researches devoted to the study of the higher nervous activity of oligophrenics is an attempt made to compare the experimental findings with the characteristic features of the clinical picture.

ANALYSIS OF THE INDIVIDUAL PSYCHIC FUNCTIONS IN MENTALLY RETARDED CHILDREN

Much research has been done into the individual aspects of the psychic activity of mentally retarded children. Perception in mentally retarded children has been studied by numerous investigators (Bappert, 1927; Sander, 1929; Schwab, 1929). They observed meagerness and lack of clarity in the perceptions of oligophrenic children. Experimental work by Soviet investigators (Zankov, 1939, 1941; Veresotskaya, 1940; Solov'ev, 1953; Nudel'man, 1953; Shif, 1940; etc.) has shown that the correct interpretation of the image of objects by mentally retarded school children required a much longer period of exposure and repeated presentations of the same object. As a result of these handicaps the mentally retarded school children failed to attain the necessary intensity of recognition of the objects and of their images.

In a series of experimental studies of memory in the mentally retarded child it is shown (Linder, 1925; Sterzinger, 1924; Troshin, 1915; Miller, 1918; etc.) that the memory of mentally retarded children is much weaker than that of the normally developed child. Of special interest is the investigation of the memory of mentally retarded children carried out by Leont'ev (1931) and by Zankov (1935). This research, based on Vygotskii's theory of the development of higher psychic functions, showed that at the end of preschool age there is a hiatus in the memory development of the normal child, and during the earliest period of school age a transition to a volitional and rational kind of memorizing begins. This transition is markedly delayed in mentally retarded children. Zankov's experiments clearly showed that, insofar as the development of the higher functions of memory is concerned, mentally retarded children showed an especially pronounced deviation from the normal. While the normally developed child of ten, for example, could completely master the operation of rational memorizing, in the mentally retarded child of the same age this ability is absent.

When we consider the pattern of the emotional life of oligophrenics, different points of view have been advanced. Some authorities have asserted that oligophrenia implies merely an intellectual deficiency, and that the emotional sphere in oligophrenia is intact. Others have stated that oligophrenia is characterized by profound primary changes in the emotional area. A third group believes that in oligophrenia we are dealing with a maldevelopment of the whole personality of the child.

Recently a certain shift of emphasis has been noted in psychological investigations of mental retardation, associated with an attempt to shift from the study of the discrete particular processes which characterize the intellectual deficiency of oligophrenic children, to the investigation of the personality of the mentally retarded child as a whole. Among such investigations may be mentioned the most recent work of Zankov and his associates, Dul'nev, Petrova, and Pinskii (1953).

This shift of interest among research psychologists was motivated by the very reasonable expectation that a study of the pattern of development of the personality of the mentally retarded child could furnish a great deal of new information which in turn could create a basis for appropriate educational and training techniques for these children.

THE EDUCATION AND TRAINING OF THE MENTALLY RETARDED CHILD

At the end of the eighteenth and beginning of the nineteenth centuries most psychiatrists regarded idiots and mentally deficient children as doomed, and the question of their training and education did not arise. These children grew up along with adults in poorhouses or lunatic asylums, and sometimes mentally retarded children were kept in institutions along with deaf-mutes and blind children.

During the first quarter of the nineteenth century, however, an increased social interest in the fate of idiots and defectives began to appear, associated with the humanistic attitude toward the problems of abnormal childhood engendered by the ideas of the French Revolution of 1789. These humanistic ideas were first taken up by Itard, Séguin, and Huguenbuhl. On the basis of his theory of sensualism, i.e., the theory that you must treat mental deficiency by trying to eliminate the defects of sensory perception, Itard was successful in the task of training the "Wild Boy of Aveyron." This success was followed by other attempts at individual training of idiots and by the organization of special institutions.

The greatest success in this work was achieved by Edouard Séguin, who described his method of training of severely retarded children in a paper entitled "Training, hygiene and moral treatment of mentally abnormal children."

Not long before the opening by Séguin in Paris of a special boarding school for severely retarded children, the psychiatrist Voisin organized in 1834 his "Orthophrenic Institute" for idiots and mental defectives, in which corrective medical and educational measures were carried out. In 1900 the Belgian, Professor Jean Demoor, of the medical faculty, again raised the problem of abnormal children and of their training in the family and at school.

Beginning with the first quarter of the nineteenth century and until the present time, the education and training of mentally retarded children has been essentially a joint medical and pedagogic problem. At the beginning of the twentieth century, at first in Germany and then in other countries, a network of schools was organized for the education of mentally retarded children.

The question of the correct organization of these schools soon became pressing. In 1905, for instance, at Decroly's initiative in Belgium observation classes were created, diagnostic in type, in the special schools, to which children presenting difficulties in diagnosis could be admitted.

As the network of special institutions for mentally retarded children developed, the question of the individual approach to the children was continually being clarified. The Italian psychiatrist de Sanctis organized a special institution for mentally retarded children for experimental research purposes and insisted upon the maximum of individualization in the approach to these children. In the period 1922 to 1930 congresses on remedial pedagogy were convened under the auspices of the Remedial Pedagogic Scientific Society.

In Russia at the end of the nineteenth and beginning of the twentieth centuries remedial pedagogic institutions began to appear. The earliest institution of this type was the hospital-school of Malyarevskii. Among the institutions which may also be mentioned was the "Medical Pedagogic Institute for Educationally Subnormal and Mentally Retarded Children" in Kiev (Sikorskii) and the Kashchenko Boarding School, opened in Moscow in 1908. A boarding school for mentally retarded children was organized by Troshin in 1911.

After the October Revolution a real development of the science of care of the handicapped began to emerge. A state system of special education was created. Special institutes were organized for the study of mentally retarded children, in which considerable work was done on the analysis of the character of the disability and the development of adequate methods of correction. Special faculties were created for the training of teachers of handicapped children.

An important place in the theory of education and training of mentally retarded children is occupied by the ideas put forward by Vygotskii and subsequently developed by his pupils. The study of mentally retarded children, subordinated to the task of finding the most effective methods of compensation for their disability, has proceeded in four directions: clinical, pedagogic, psychological, and physiological.

* * *

In spite of some success in the study of oligophrenic children, research in this field has had several inherent defects:

1) A vagueness of definition of the concept of mental deficiency.

2) A wrong methodological approach to the understanding of the development of the anomalous child.

3) A lack of a valid classification of oligophrenia.

2. Presentation of the Problem

THE THEORY OF DEVELOPMENT

A proper examination of the problem of oligophrenia in childhood, (in which we are concrened with a faulty development or, more accurately, with an anomaly of development of the psychic functions) cannot be achieved without a correct understanding of the process of development itself. The fact that development takes place is accepted by nearly all authorities: the point at issue is, what do we understand by development?

For a very long time the process of development was misunderstood. In their deliberations, some authorities have worked on a basis of the theory of preformation. The supporters of this theory believe that the anlage possesses a predisposition to the development of all the characteristic properties of the adult individual. Development is nothing more than the realization, maturation, and combination of these anlagen. This theory was reflected in a number of psychiatric investigations. Hoffmann, for example, understands the development of personality (1922) as the fruition of genotypical predispositions, brought to light or provoked by a more or less amorphous environment. From Hoffmann's point of view, nothing can appear in the personality which was not originally laid down there. A similar view is held by many other workers: Berkman (1899), Götz (1929), Brugger (1933, 1938, 1939, 1940), Benda (1941), Bassek (1942), Luxenburger (1932), etc.

In contrast to the above, Korsakov (1901) clearly recognizes the importance of the social factor to man's mental development. In support of his point of view he cites the case of the patient Laura Bridgman, in whom idiocy developed because from early childhood she was deprived of sight and hearing.

Even more valuable information in relation to an understanding of oligophrenia as a particular form of developmental anomaly may be found in Korsakov's special monograph "The psychopathology of microcephalia" (1894). In his description of the female microcephalic M., who lived in a psychiatric hospital for 23 years, Korsakov states that M.'s mental life had not developed sufficiently for her to be capable of having any concepts. M. had no words with a definite meaning, and her speech was useless for conversation with others. Although she had ideas and images, the manifestations of her mental life, writes Korsakov, were automatic acts. All M.'s organs of the senses were functioning, but they were not coupled productively with any form of understanding. "I regard the formation of rational products of coupling," writes Korsakov, "as a third act of development of man's psychic life, giving a completely new countenance to his mental manifestations, namely introducing into them an element of understanding, but such actions in M. were almost completely absent. She had almost no understanding, no ideas, no mentality, and there was no reason in all her sensations and actions. Any human quality that was dependent on understanding, awareness of purpose, or awareness of attitude was either absent in M., or, if present, was so only in a rudimentary state, and all her living psychic activity was irrational and all her actions automatic."* "Thus by the 'rational' coupling of ideas I have in mind their coupling in accordance with the principle of logical combination, their coupling by virtue of a predestined tendency to find simplicity in multiplicity. . . . The ability to form a large number of ideas and to amass a great store of them is an exclusive property of the human intellect." †

This interpretation of the formation of ideas as the result of a definite stage of development of the psychic life of man demonstrates Korsakov's materialistic approach to the problem of the development of the anomalous personality. The study of the development of the anomalous child also attracted a great deal of attention from Bekhterev. A group of Bekhterev's pupils (Shchelovanov, Povarnin, et al.) investigated the problem of child development by means of objective methods.

In her clinical lectures, Sukhareva (1955) pays very great attention to the study of the significance of the age characteristics of children and adolescents in the clinical pattern of mental diseases. She considers that the age characteristics of children and adolescents at different stages of development can only explain the greater or lesser susceptibility to various pathogenic agents. In her opinion, however, the role of age characteristics is thrown into much greater relief in the formation of the clinical pattern of the disease. Age characteristics influence both the course of a disease and its eventual outcome. Certain infectious diseases, for instance, are complicated by encephalitis much more often in young children than in adults. Schizophrenia, when it begins in early childhood, often leads

*S. S. Korsakov. "The psychopathology of microcephalia." Complete collected works (Moscow, Medgiz, 1954) p. 237.

†Ibid., p. 239

to considerable mental deficiency as a result of an acute disturbance of the process of development. Epilepsy leads to far more severe forms of mental deficiency in children than in adults. Following traumatic injury to the brain in early childhood, a severe mental deficiency may often ensue, quite out of proportion to the seriousness of the trauma. Syndromes of mental retardation or behavior disorders which may be observed in combination with the clinical picture of any mental disease commencing in early childhood are due not only to the special susceptibilities of the child but also to disturbances of the course of its development. Simson also attaches great importance to the age factor.

The work of foreign psychiatrists in recent years has reflected a greater appreciation of the role of age factors in the formation of the clinical picture of a disease. In a paper by Tramer (1952) dealing with the relationship between child psychiatry and pediatrics, the author stresses that the study of child psychiatry demands a knowledge of the normal stages of mental development of the child as well as its variations. He discusses in considerable detail the critical age periods and indicates the important role of different forms of partial and general infantilism in the psychopathology of childhood.

In an article entitled "The psychiatric problem in children's hospitals," Lutz (1953) attaches great importance to those diseases of childhood which are associated with a disturbance or retardation of the child's intellectual development. The specific nature of child psychiatry is principally due to the fact that any disease process in childhood impinges on the continuing process of the child's development. That is why it is so important to have a proper understanding of the process of development.

The analysis of various pathological states in childhood has confirmed the validity of Vygotskii's theory of the psychic development of the child. Vygotskii claimed that the chief and essential feature which distinguishes development from all other processes, was the fact that in its course new properties and new qualities appeared. The development of the child is characterized not by simple quantitative increases but by the appearance at each stage of development of new qualities and new properties. The development of the child takes place in the course of active interrelationship with the surrounding environment. Though each successive stage in the development of the child is connected with the preceding one, nevertheless the specific feature of each age milestone is the emergence of new properties, differing qualitatively from those occurring in previous stages. For example, the change by the child from crawling to walking, from babbling to speaking, and from direct to abstract thinking is not just a simple increase in the corresponding function but a qualitative conversion of one function into another.

Development is an elaborately organized process and its rhythm does not coincide with that of time. The tempo of development is not constant. The process of development is marked by cycles in which particular functions display a distinctive development. The development of the child can be divided into stages or phases. On the basis of numerous experiments and the analysis of different forms of anomalous development, Vygotskii showed clearly that complex forms of memory, perception, and abstract thinking are formed in the course of the child's development, and that these are based not so much on natural proclivities as on the ways and means of organization of the child's activity.

The development of the abnormal child is the result of a complex process in which the disturbance of a given function depends: (a) on the place occupied by this function in the general psychic development of the child, and (b) on the stage of development at which the disturbance takes place.

Only a proper materialistic understanding of the development of personality will enable an approach to be made to the truly scientific analysis of the different forms of anomalous development. By starting from such a correct understanding of anomalous development, in 1935 I was able to give an analysis of that peculiar type of anomaly which arises in the chronic stage of epidemic encephalitis in children. Clinicians have described changes arising in the affective-volitional life and behavior of the child who has suffered from epidemic encephalitis in early childhood. These children show antisocial tendencies, hypersexuality, fatiguability, compulsive behavior, unmotivated actions, and unawareness of their conduct. Bonhoeffer (1922), Wolfgang (1923), Kirschbaum (1922), Paterson (1921), Albrecht (1921), and others, have associated the principal features of the personality changes with a disturbance of the function of the diencephalon, which led them to the psychomorphological conclusion that the higher divisions of the brainstem are the central apparatus for the higher forms of psychic life of the personality.

Whereas 25 years ago attempts to localize the higher forms of specific human activity in the subcortical region were made in connection with behavioral changes following epidemic encephalitis in children, the problem is nowadays again posed from this point of view in connection with the introduction of new methods of investigation (neurosurgical and electroencephalographic techniques). According to Penfield, the upper divisions of the brainstem embody a special system of neurons connected symmetrically with the cortex, called the "diencephalic system." From the point of view of these American and British neurologists and neurophysiologists, this "diencephalic system" should be regarded as the basis of the highest level of integration, to which the level of the cortex is subordinated.

As long as 17 years ago (Pevzner, 1941), I showed on the basis of Vygotskii's theory that the personality changes in a child who had suffered from epidemic encephalitis could not be regarded as disturbances of the "ethical orientation of the personality" or as "amoral behavior," but must be looked upon as a maldevelopment of the complex specific human forms of activity and behavior, arising from a primary disturbance of the dynamics of the most elementary affective and psychomotor processes. A lesion of the diencephalic divisions of the brain initially disturbs the dynamics of psychomotor acts and primitive impulses, with the result that, in the process of development, the behavior of these patients is composed of uncontrolled, direct psychomotor acts.

Whereas in the adult patient epidemic encephalitis also leads directly to psychomotor outbursts, they are inhibited by the more complex cortical systems, and disturbances of the complex forms of behavior do not arise. With involvement of the subcortical ganglia at an early age, it is quite another matter.

Disturbances of the simpler affective processes, which are the primary result of a lesion of the subcortical ganglia, lead to acute changes in the whole mental development. The affective processes of children are only gradually incorporated in the most complex forms of their activity to become rational and deliberate in character. Only in the course of development do complex affective relationships towards the environment develop: assessment of the surroundings, emotional attachments to people, conscious relationships to situations, i.e., the complex psychic components of the human character are formed.

The abnormal postencephalitic development is characterized by the fact that these new functional formations generally fail to appear, and therefore the primitive impulsivity and direct psychomotor outbursts remain without any form of control by the complex cortical functional systems, for these fail to achieve their normal complexity. It is for this reason that the behavior of postencephalitic children is more like the behavior of adult patients with lesions of the anterior divisions of the frontal cortex than the behavior of the adult postencephalitic, in whom these complex systems are already firmly established and in whom a disease of the subcortical ganglia does not lead to such extensive systemic disturbances.

Hence we may postulate with some justification that in children who have suffered from epidemic encephalitis in early childhood, there is a faulty development of those connections which link the subcortical region to the frontal cortex of the brain. If the disturbance of coordination between the higher and lower divisions of the brain resulting from failure of the latter to develop manifests itself differently in children and in adults, this means that the normal connections between these parts are established in the course of maturation of the child.

This concept of the process of development of the human personality as an active process, the most characteristic feature of which is the appearance of new properties and qualities, is confirmed by the study of the structure of the cerebral cortex. The work of the Moscow Brain Institute is very pertinent to our investigation, for it does not merely provide a static description of the various cortical structures, but also considers their development in onto- and phylogenesis. Polyakov (1949) showed that in the initial stages of intrauterine development, when only a cortical plate can be observed, the future human cerebral cortex still has a simple, single-layered structure. In it is represented only the lower and most primitive layer of the cortex, evidently related to primitive functions. After a few weeks of intrauterine life we can gradually distinguish the middle layer of the cortex, whose cells are the potential receptive and motor centers. It is only after this that the upper layers of the cortex are formed, the functions of which are connected with synthetic cortical activity.

Of still greater interest are the findings which demonstrate the unequal tempo of development of the individual layers in different areas of the cortex. Filimonov and Preobrazhenskaya (1949), who studied the occipital area of the brain, showed that after birth the width of the cortex in the occipital area increased, the density of arrangement of the cells is reduced, and the area occupied by each field on the surface of the hemisphere is increased.

The width of the cortex in Area 17 reaches the adult width at the age of only two years, whereas the width of the cortex in Areas

18 and 19 increases much more slowly, and only at the age of seven years does it approximate the width of the adult occipital cortex. After birth the growth of the cells in all areas of the occipital region continues, and the surface area of the occipital region increases roughly threefold in the course of postnatal ontogenesis. This increase in the area of the cortex takes place most intensively during the first two years of life, when it reaches 75% of the surface area of the adult cortex. The field of Area 17 attains its maximal extension sooner than the other areas of the occipital region. By the fourth year it is equal to 86.7% of the area of the cortex in the adult, whereas at the same age, Area 18 reaches only 69.9% of its adult extent. The earlier maturation of the phylogenetically older Area 17 is in full agreement with the more elementary character of the function of this area. The later and less uniform development of the phylogenetically newer Areas 18 and 19 is in full agreement with their more complex functions.

The same pattern is apparent in the work of Stankevich (1949) on the inferior parietal region. The surface area of the cortex in this region undergoes a more than 37-fold increase in the course of ontogenesis. A rapid growth of the inferior parietal region is observed until the age of two years, when the area of this region corresponds to about 80% of the average adult figure.

The distinctive pattern of development of the frontal lobe is of particular interest (Kononova, 1949). In the postnatal period the growth in width of the cortex in each area has its own special character. In some areas the cortex widens gradually, while in others, gradual growth gives way to spurts of varying intensity, as a characteristic of the different ages. After birth the width of the cortex in Area 45 increases by 95%, that in Areas 44 and 46 by 75%, and that in Area 10 by 55%. The layers of the cortex are distinguished not only by their tempo of growth but also by changes in their structure. The width of Layers II and IV decreases in all areas in the course of development; the width of Layer III, however, increases gradually and very considerably. The increase in width of the cortex in the course of ontogenesis takes place mainly as a result of widening of Layer III. The surface area of the frontal region increases gradually with age. The increase begins in the prenatal period, and from the moment of differentiation of the cortex until birth it increases by 400%, and in the adult it increases by 350-360% compared to its size in the newborn. In nearly all areas a great increase in the surface area of the frontal region may be observed at the age of two years, again at seven years, and subsequently considerable changes are seen at the age of 13 years.

The development of Areas 44 and 45 takes place more slowly in the right hemisphere than in the left; the widening of the cortex and, in particular, of Layer III, does not reach the degree observed in the left. The study of the architectonics of the various divisions of the cerebral cortex has shown that in embryogenesis there is a particularly intensive development of the inferior parietal areas, connected with the specifically human functions of praxis and gnosis.

The researches of Soviet workers enumerated above (clinical, physiological, cytoarchitectonic, and psychological) show that development takes place in a series of steps, and that the process of development itself is characterized by the fact that new properties and qualities arise at each stage. The process of development goes from the elementary to the complex, from the automatic to the voluntary. The decisive factor in development is the relationship between the body and the external environment.

To return to the analysis of the state of scientific knowledge of oligophrenia, it must be pointed out that the defects in the investigations which we previously discussed (the absence of a precise definition of the concept of oligophrenia, defects in the existing classification of the forms of oligophrenia, failure to pay adequate attention to the factor of development) were the reasons for the lack of progress in the clinical study of oligophrenia, since it concerned itself with the description of only the most general features of oligophrenic children. The entire wealth of manifestations of variants of oligophrenia, differing in pathogenesis and clinical features, still awaits the necessary clinical study, but such a study is nevertheless extremely important. Mention of the urgency of the study of the various forms of oligophrenia in childhood can also be found in the writings of foreign authorities. In a survey of the problems of child psychiatry, Bittner (1952) stresses that the basic problem of child psychiatry is the study of the different forms of mental deficiency and of related states. He rightly draws attention to the frequency of misdiagnosis of oligophrenia in children with partial disturbances of hearing, vision, speech, or motor defects, which impair scholastic attainment in spite of normal intelligence.

Similar remarks may be found in the paper by Lutz (1953), in which he regards the group of diseases characterized by disturbance or retardation of the intellectual development of varied etiology as the most challenging problem of child psychiatry.

The importance of the study of oligophrenia in childhood is further underscored by the fact that inadequate knowledge of this maldevelopment leads from time to time to gross clinical errors in diagnosis and subsequent placement of children in special schools.

CLINICAL AND PATHOPHYSIOLOGICAL ANALYSIS OF THE MAIN SYMPTOM OF OLIGOPHRENIA

The purpose of our investigation was to undertake a careful study of the individual variants of the disability in oligophrenia. The investigation was based on a comprehensive clinical, experimental, and laboratory study of 158 children, aged from eight to 18 years duration of dynamic study from one to ten years). Of the total number of children investigated, 98 were boys and 60 girls. (See Table 1 below.)

We regard oligophrenia as a clinical entity embracing a variety of conditions, differing in their etiology but similar in their mani-

Table 1. Distribution of Clinical Findings According to the Form of Oligophrenia

Forms of oligophrenia	No. of children	Distribution of children by sex		Distribution of children by age	Etiology		
					A	B	C
					Disturbance of intra-uterine development	Abnormal labor	Post-natal disease
		Boys	Girls				
I. Principal variant of oligophrenia	43	27	16	8–17	22	6	15
II. Oligophrenic children with gross disturbance of cortical neurodynamics							
Mental deficiency complicated by hydrocephalus*	17	11	6	10–14	3	2	12
A. Excitable oligophrenics	48	30	18	8–16	12	15	21
B. Inhibited oligophrenics	18	11	7	10–16	5	7	6
C. Oligophrenics with weakness of both nervous processes	10	6	4	10–14	3	4	3
III. Oligophrenics with deficiency of the frontal systems	22	13	9	8–18	8	4	10
	158	98	60	8–18	53	38	67

*The clinical analysis of the gross forms of hydrocephalus with a syndrome of mental deficiency assisted in the understanding of the pathogenesis of oligophrenia with disturbance of the cortical neurodynamics.

festations, and expressed as a maldevelopment of the whole personality. The clinical unity of oligophrenia is determined by the fact that none of these conditions is progressive. Oligophrenia is a form of anomalous psychic development basically caused by defects of the anlage, or by the residual defects from an organic injury of the central nervous system, especially affecting the cerebral cortex, sustained during intrauterine life or in early childhood.

The investigations of Pravdina-Vinarskaya showed that in all the oligophrenic children whom she examined a residual, mainly cortical, neurological symptomatology could be found. These residual symptoms were expressed as central, differentiated palsies involving individual cerebrospinal nerves or the limbs. These paretic manifestations were not gross, and they were particularly prominent when the children carried out the more complicated and delicate voluntary movements. During the investigation of olfaction, vision, hearing, and the different forms of cutaneous, muscle-joint, and complex sensation, disturbances of the analysis of the respective stimuli were observed. No obvious local sensory disturbances were present in the majority of children.

These facts confirm the view that the lesion in the oligophrenic children we investigated was mainly cortical. In some chidren there was evidence of lesions of other parts of the brain (brainstem, subcortical diencephalic region, and meninges).

The presence of residual neurological symptomatology in the children we examined is proof that in the past they had suffered from an organic disease of the central nervous system.

Equally clear results were also obtained by the electroencephalographic method of investigation of oligophrenic children. Bertran and others attempted to establish a correlation between the changes in the electrical activity and the severity of the intellectual defect. Cook (1944) considered that the disturbance of function of the brain cells takes the form of dysrhythmia. Schütz and Müller-Limmroth (1952) investigated the cerebral action potentials in 50 children with different degrees of mental retardation. Marked abnormalities were found in 38 of the 50 children examined. In 13 patients the alpha-rhythm was absent and in 25 patients it was highly abnormal. A normal electroencephalogram was found in only 12 patients.

An investigation of the electrical activity of the brain carried out on oligophrenic children by Novikova (1956) showed that in the overwhelming majority of cases the electrical activity of the brain of the oligophrenic children whom we examined clinically differed from that of normal children of the same age.

The electroencephalogram of oligophrenics is characterized by depression of the alpha-rhythm. An alpha-rhythm in the occipital region of the cortex is found in 75% of normal children in the age group from 13 to 16 years, but in only 19% of oligophrenic children of the same age. Compared with normal children, in oligophrenics we find a greatly increased number of cases in which pathological slow waves are recorded. A fact of particular importance is that in many oligophrenics the electroencephalograms show typical "delta-waves" among the slow waves, characterized by their great amplitude and distinctive configuration. "Delta-waves" are an indication of a profound disturbance of the functional state of the cortical neurons and are usually found in organic lesions of the brain. A characteristic feature of the electroencephalogram of oligophrenic children is a change in the electrical activity of the brain in all regions of the cortex.

An electroencephalogram typical of oligophrenia is presented in Fig. 1. For purposes of comparison, Fig. 2 shows the curve of a normal child of the same age. It is clear from this curve that a well marked alpha-rhythm is recorded in all regions of the cortex. In the electroencephalogram of the oligophrenic of the same age (Fig. 1) an absence of the alpha-rhythm and increase of the slow waves can be observed. Attention is drawn to the disturbance of the electrical activity of the brain in all regions of the cortex.

Investigation of the electrical activity of the brain in oligophrenics revealed differences related to the degree of severity of the disability. These differences are illustrated in Table 2, which is taken from Novikova's paper.

Besides recording the electroencephalogram in a resting state, in the investigation we also used the method of recording action potentials during rhythmic stimulation with a light. These investigations, carried out in the electrophysiological laboratory of the Institute of Defectology of the Academy of Pedagogic Sciences of the RSFSR by Zislina (1956), showed that the cortex of the normally developing child can accommodate high frequency flashes of light, thus demonstrating its high functional mobility (Fig. 3, A, B).

Meanwhile, in the great majority of oligophrenic children,

Table 2. Comparative Characteristics of the Electroencephalograms of Children at Moron and Imbecile Levels

Type of electroencephalograms	Morons (%)	Imbeciles (%)
1. Normal type of curve	8	–
2. Slightly abnormal curve	51	23
3. Grossly abnormal curve	41	77

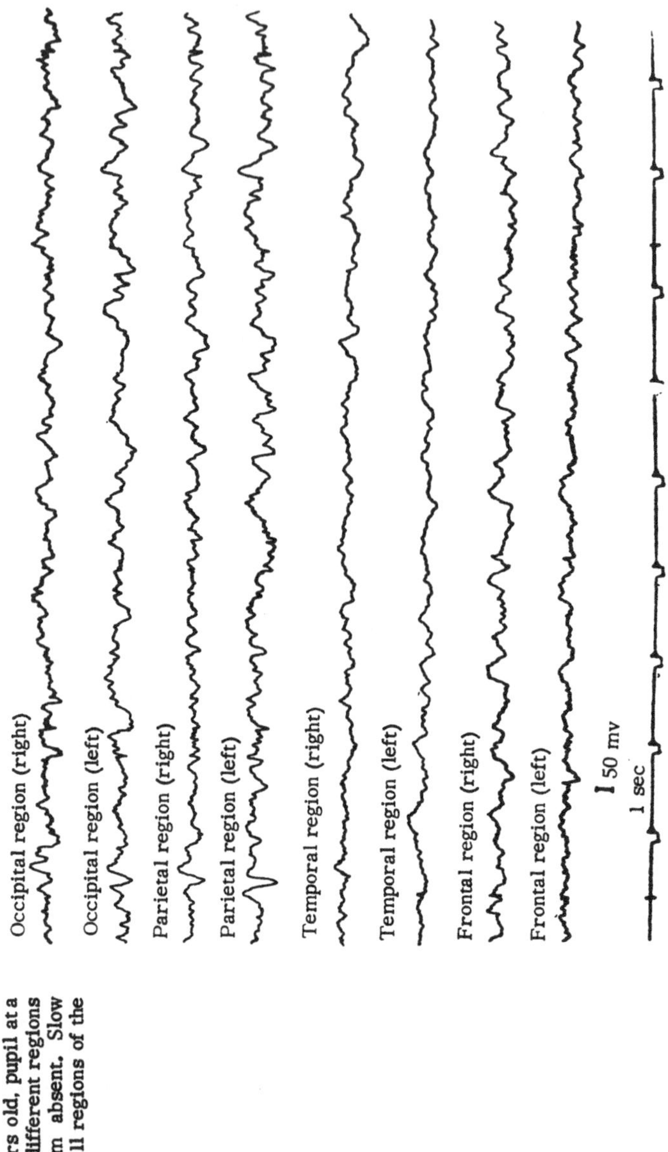

Fig. 1. Sasha, A., 9 years old, pupil at a special school. EEG of different regions of the brain. α-rhythm absent. Slow waves predominate in all regions of the cortex.

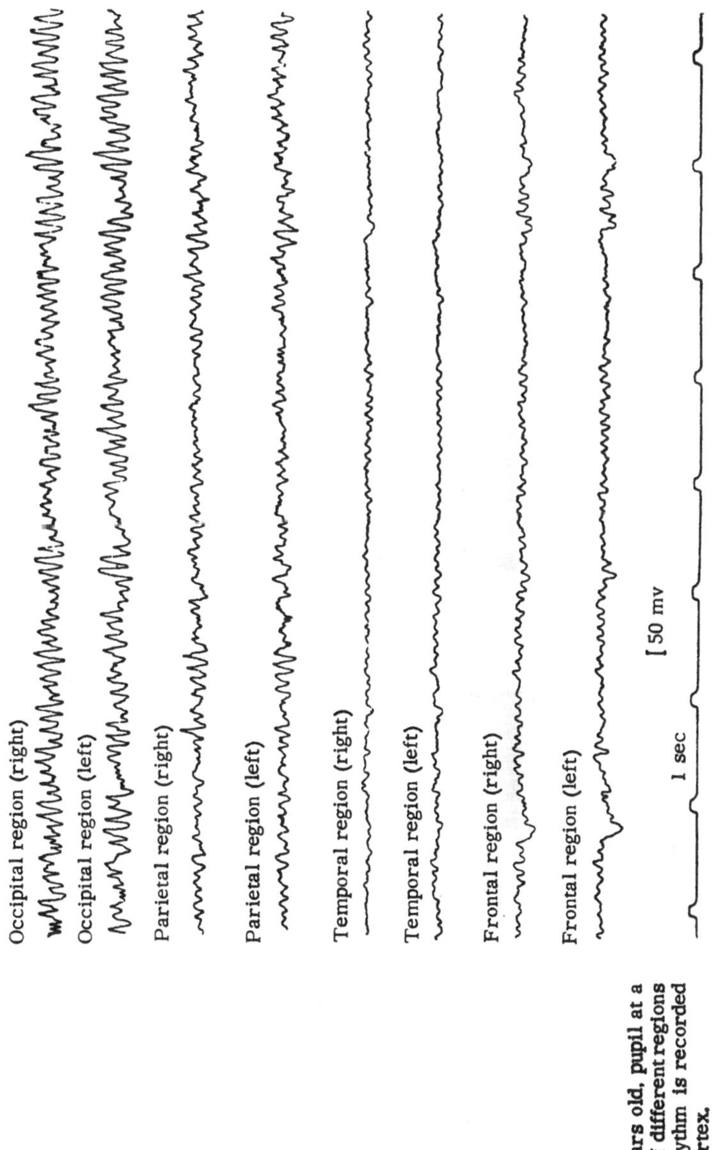

Fig. 2. Zina. N., 9 years old, pupil at a regular school. EEG of different regions of the brain. An α-rhythm is recorded in all regions of the cortex.

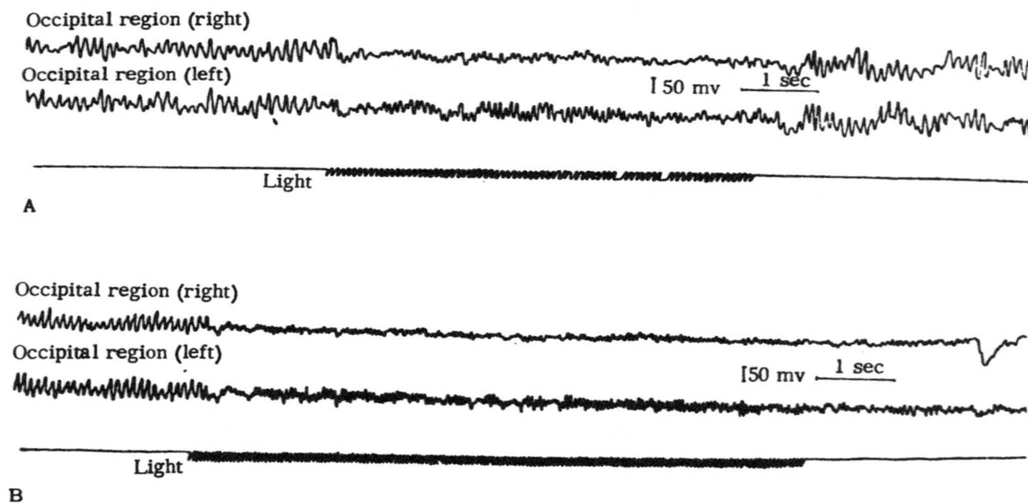

Fig. 3. A. Subject V., aged 14 years, pupil at a regular school. Modification of the electrical waves in the occipital region of the cortex in response to flashes of light at a frequency of 14 per second. Initial frequency of α-rhythm 9.5–10 cps. B. Subject I., aged 13 years, pupil in a regular school. Modification of the electrical waves in the occipital region of the cortex in response to flashes of light at a frequency of 20 per second. Initial frequency of α-rhythm 10 cps.

either a very ill-defined modification of the cortical rhythms in response to high-frequency light flashes or no modification whatsoever was observed (Fig. 4, A, B). In contrast to healthy children, it was possible to observe in the oligophrenics a modification to light flashes of low frequency (Fig. 5). The absence of modification in oligophrenics in response to high-frequency flashes of light and the presence of modification in response to low-frequency flashes of light are indicative of a reduced level of functional mobility of the brain in oligophrenic children.

The clinical findings were compared especially carefully with the results of the investigation of the higher nervous activity, for investigation of the higher nervous activity of these children must help in the understanding of the pathophysiological features responsible for the production of both the individual symptoms and the clinical picture as a whole.

The investigation of the higher nervous activity of these same oligophrenic children was undertaken by Lubovskii (1956). As a result of the investigations, in which a motor conditioned reflex technique with speech reinforcement was used, a series of pathological changes in the higher nervous activity could be established in the oligophrenic children. During the testing of connections formed in the course of the children's past experience, abnormal features were observed, which consisted mainly of inadequate concentration of the process of stimulation and the manifestation of some degree of inertia. During the formation of new conditioned connections these abnormal features were especially prominent, but differed in degree during the formation of simple and of complicated systems of connections.

In most of the oligophrenic children investigated, simple positive conditioned reflex connections were formed just as quickly and easily as in normal children; in most mild oligophrenics simple differentiation was also readily induced.

Essential difficulties are encountered in oligophrenics during the formation of relatively more complex systems of connections, in the induction of which the child must abstract from the total number of signs of the direct conditioned signal one particular sign which has little to distinguish it from the rest. This takes place for example when we first induce a positive response to a given signal, and then a differentiation to it based on the duration of action of the signal. If we use colored lamps as the conditioned stimulus, then the sign acting as the signal is not the previously repeated and most obvious sign – the light stimulus – but a supplementary one – its duration.

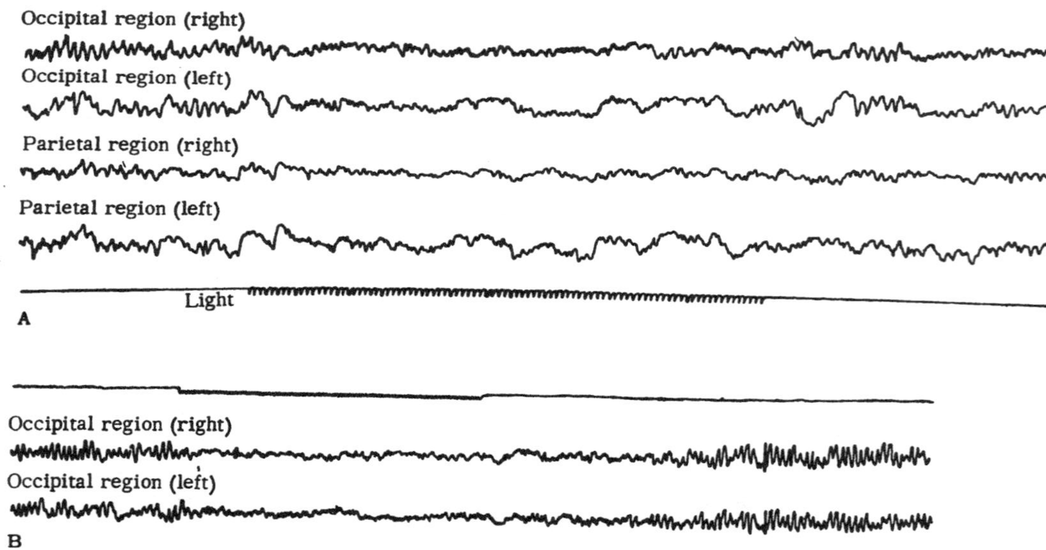

Fig. 4. A. Dima S., 13 years old, pupil at a special school (oligophrenia of a feeble-minded degree). In the occipital regions of the cortex an ill-defined modification is recorded in response to flashes of light with a frequency of 15 per second. B. Subject V., aged 14 years, pupil at a special school (oligophrenia of a feeble-minded degree). Modification of cortical rhythm in response to flashes of light of high frequency absent. Frequency of light flashes 18 per second. Initial background of α-rhythm of a frequency of 9 cycles per second in conjunction with waves of delta type.

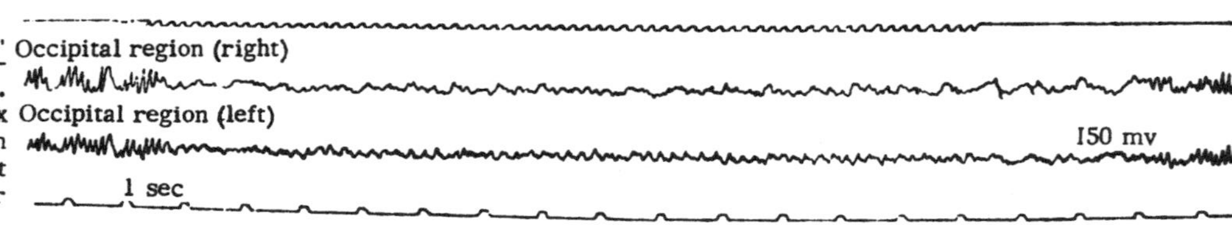

Fig. 5. Subject V., 14 years old, pupil at a special school (oligophrenia of a feeble-minded degree). In the occipital regions of the cortex a modification of the cortical rhythm is recorded in response to light flashes of low frequency (5 per second).

The abstracting and generalizing functions of speech do not take part in the identification of the signal sign, and the formation of this particular connection takes place as a rule in these children gradually and "mechanically," requiring a large number of combinations. The long period of "learning by routine" and the gradual concentration of the processes of stimulation and inhibition are also very clearly apparent during the formation of other complex systems of connections based on some abstract signal sign (as an example of such a connection may be given the formation of a reaction after two signals, i.e., a reaction in accordance with the principle of alternation).

The oligophrenic cannot distinguish the quantitative abstract sign from the basic, obvious properties of a signal, and the connection is formed not in a steplike manner, as is the case in normal children, but gradually, after a large number of combinations. The connection which is formed remains unstable and unconsolidated, it is dependent on concrete conditions of application of the signals, it is readily disturbed when slight changes are made in these conditions, and it is not formed into speech.

The slower and more difficult formation of relatively complex connections is based on disturbances of differential and delayed inhibition. Pathological inertia plays a role of special importance in these difficulties. Pathological inertia, which appears in its highest degree in verbal connections, is also found at more elementary levels of high nervous activity. In the motor sphere this inertia takes the form of tonic motor reactions, superfluous movements of a perseverative character, the incomplete or unstable alteration of the conditioned meaning of the stimuli, the restoration of old conditioned connections without reinforcement, the practical impossibility of alteration of nonverbalized systems of connections, etc.

Tonic movements are observed in most oligophrenic children when their simple motor reactions in response to a direct command are investigated. The strengthening of the tonic character of the movements during a prolonged investigation is shown in Fig. 6.

All oligophrenic children show marked superfluous movements of a perseverative character, which are persistently maintained throughout the experiment. In Fig. 7 the appearance of superfluous stereotyped movements is illustrated after the cessation of verbal commands. In normal children, even if such movements do appear, they are very easily inhibited.

The incomplete or unstable alteration of the conditioned meaning of the stimuli is another indication of the inertia of the nervous

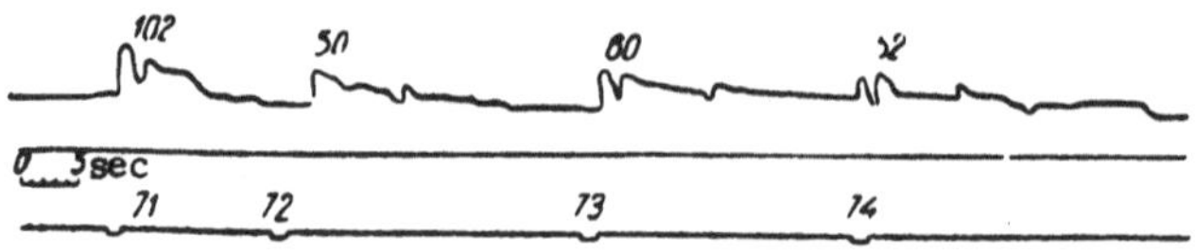

Fig. 6. Vova S., aged 11 years (oligophrenia). Tonic character of the motor reaction. Top line: tracing of motor reactions; bottom line: marker for the verbal command "press!"

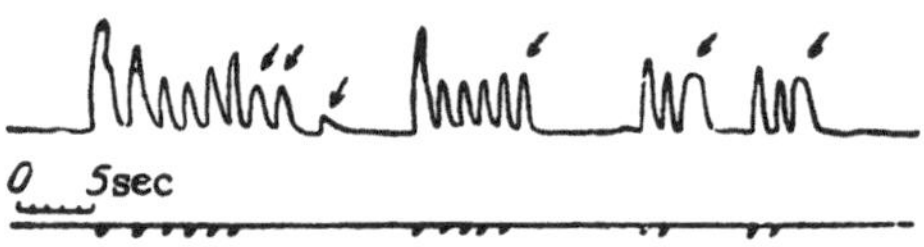

Fig. 7. Zina P., aged 13 years (oligophrenia). Superfluous movements of a perseverative character. Top line: tracing of motor reactions; bottom line: marker for the verbal command "press!" The superfluous movements are indicated by arrows.

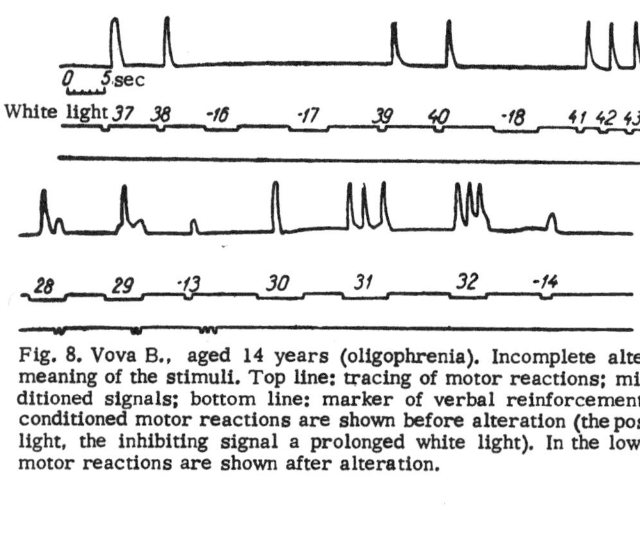

Fig. 8. Vova B., aged 14 years (oligophrenia). Incomplete alteration of the conditioned meaning of the stimuli. Top line: tracing of motor reactions; middle line: marker of conditioned signals; bottom line: marker of verbal reinforcement. In the upper curves the conditioned motor reactions are shown before alteration (the positive signal a short white light, the inhibiting signal a prolonged white light). In the lower curves the conditioned motor reactions are shown after alteration.

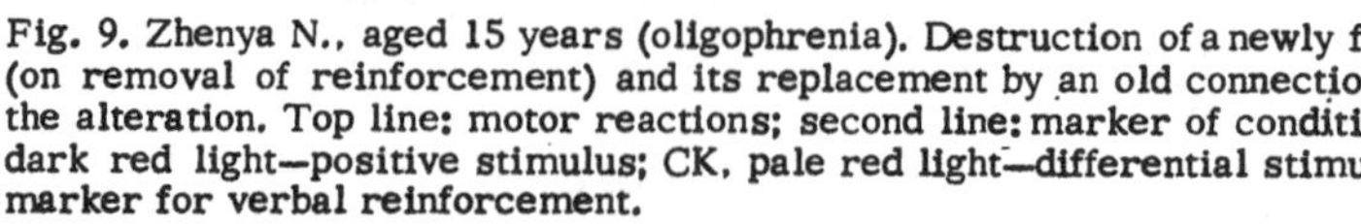

Fig. 9. Zhenya N., aged 15 years (oligophrenia). Destruction of a newly formed connection (on removal of reinforcement) and its replacement by an old connection, existing before the alteration. Top line: motor reactions; second line: marker of conditioned signals (TK, dark red light—positive stimulus; CK, pale red light—differential stimulus); bottom line: marker for verbal reinforcement.

processes. In Fig. 8 there is demonstrated the perseveration of small positive reactions to an inhibitory signal after its alteration from a positive, which indicates the incomplete alteration of the conditioned meaning of this stimulus.

The inertia of the nervous processes in oligophrenic children is evidence of restoration of the old connections when reinforcement is removed. In Fig. 9 are shown the curves from the investigation of Zenya N., aged 15 years. It may be seen from the curves that the newly created connection is extinguished after removal of the reinforcement and is replaced by the pre-existing, more firmly consolidated connection.

Clear proof of the inertia of the nervous processes is afforded by the much greater difficulty of alteration of the nonverbalized systems of connections. The difficulty of alteration of the conditioned meaning of the stimuli is demonstrated in Fig. 10.

At the level of the second signal system the following are found: gross inertia of the old verbal connections (in accounts), perseveration in speech reactions, ease of formation of verbal stereotypes (dissociating themselves from direct reactions), and inertia of the verbal connections after alteration of the direct conditioned reactions.

Perseveration in speech reactions was conspicuous in those cases when, besides motor reactions, the oligophrenic children gave verbal responses to stimuli. Inertia also appeared in these verbal responses. In the subject Vova B., aged 14 years (Fig. 11), for instance, during the induction of conditioned reactions in response to a third stimulus after two preceding stimuli, perseveration of the word "don't," which was his reply to the inhibiting stimulus, was observed.

Disturbances of the verbal response as a result of inertia of the previously formed verbal connections were observed in all the oligophrenic children examined. During the formation of differentiation to duration, for instance, the children said that they pressed in response to the bright light and did not press in response to the dim one, which corresponded to the previously formed, verbalized differentiation by intensity and not to the differentiation by duration which was formed in this particular experiment.

In a comparative investigation of the after effect of the motor reaction in oligophrenic and normal children* (Ravich-Shcherbo, 1956), it was found that the reaction of the oligophrenics was

*The investigation was carried out on 20 oligophrenic children whose developmental histories are described in the present volume.

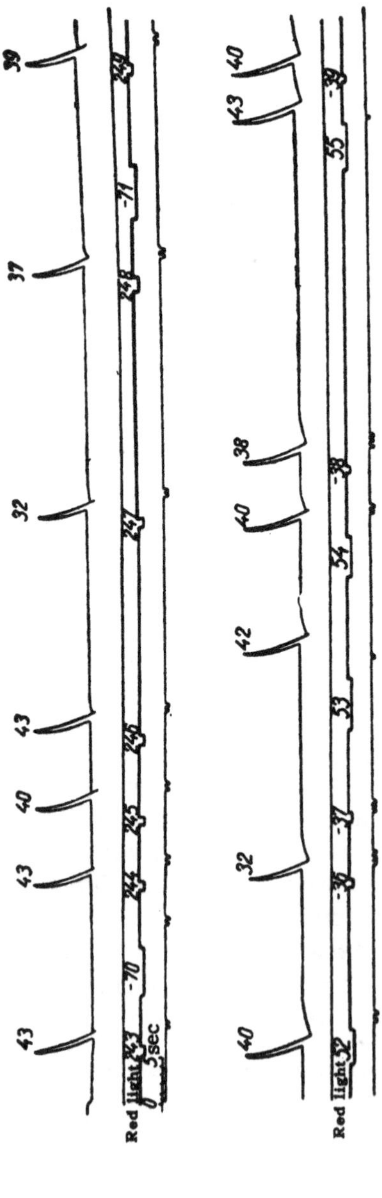

Fig. 10. Nina E., aged 13 years (oligophrenia). Difficulty of alteration of the conditioned meaning of the stimuli. Top line: motor reactions; third line from the top: marker of conditioned stimuli; bottom line: marker for verbal reinforcement.

characterized by general inertia and by many miss reactions but by few other errors. This investigator concludes from his findings that these phenomena may be explained by the inertia of the nervous processes in oligophrenic children. This view is strikingly confirmed when the experimental and clinical findings are compared in individual children. The children with the mildest degree of oligophrenia showed the smallest number of misses. In those children in whom the clinical findings indicated the most serious defect, the signs of inertia were much more marked.

Pathophysiological investigations indicate that among all the pathological changes in the higher nervous activity of oligophrenic children, a foremost place is occupied by the pathological inertia of the nervous processes. In several of the earlier experimental researches into the pattern of the higher nervous activity in oligophrenia, inertia of the fundamental nervous processes was clearly demonstrated. Il'inskii, for example, produced trace reactions experimentally in oligophrenics, and found that trace reflexes were formed slowly and were readily converted into available reflexes or disappeared completely. Il'inskii attributed the difficulty of formation of differentiation to the inertia of the fundamental nervous processes. Shnirman studied the interaction between reflexes in oligophrenics and also noted the marked inertia of the nervous processes. The difficulty in the formation of differentiation (the fixation or perseveration) of the last reflex to be reinforced is evidence, in Shnirman's opinion, of the lack of flexibility and mobility of the nervous processes. The degree of inertia of the nervous processes corresponds to the degree of retardation of the child.

The significance of pathological inertia as the most conspicuous of the various disturbances of the higher nervous activity in oligophrenia was shown even more convincingly by research carried out

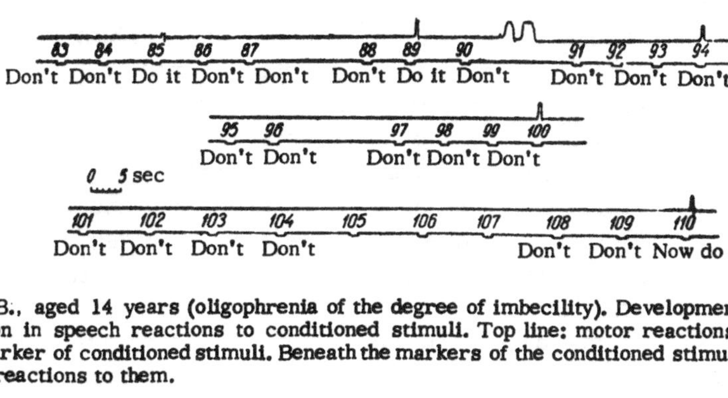

Fig. 11. Vova B., aged 14 years (oligophrenia of the degree of imbecility). Development of perseveration in speech reactions to conditioned stimuli. Top line: motor reactions; bottom line: marker of conditioned stimuli. Beneath the markers of the conditioned stimuli are the verbal reactions to them.

recently (Lubovskii, 1956; Ravich-Shcherbo; Martsinovskaya, 1955; etc.). The parameter of the phenomenon of mobility was first distinguished in an investigation of the peripheral nervous system in Vvedenskii's and Ukhtomskii's schools. The parameter of mobility in higher nervous activity was also studied in Academician I. P. Pavlov's school. Comparative-physiological research in Pavlov's school showed that the evolution of the nervous system proceeds along the lines of a progressive increase in the mobility or plasticity of its nervous processes. When studying the pathology of higher nervous activity, Pavlov attached great importance to disturbances of the plasticity of the nervous processes. Pavlov paid particular attention to perseveration in different mental diseases and interpreted it as a manifestation of the disturbance of mobility of the nervous processes, or pathological inertia.

The more important role of the parameter of mobility in the higher nervous activity is suggested by the results of a series of comparative-physiological investigations (Voronin, 1954; Biryukov; etc.). These investigations showed that the development of the general properties of the central nervous system in the course of its evolution proceeds mostly along the lines of an increase in plasticity of the nervous processes.

It was also shown in these investigations that the rate of formation of conditioned connections (one of the significant indices of the strength of the nervous processes) does not undergo much change in the course of evolution. Equilibrium of the nervous processes throughout the course of evolution is subject to individual variations and is a property related to the type of nervous system. Experimental research meanwhile shows that in the higher animals the conditioned reflexes are altered much more rapidly than in the lower. For example, in the course of repeated alterations in tortoises, the mobility of their nervous processes failed to show any response to training. In birds and rabbits each successive alteration of the signal meanings of the stimuli induced an appropriate response more rapidly than the one before. The mobility of the nervous processes is very amenable to training in dogs and baboons. The chimpanzee was especially outstanding in this respect. After three alterations, which were carried out extremely quickly, it was sufficient in subsequent experiments to use the stimulus once in its new signal meaning for the animal to react in suitable fashion to its next application.

The facts described show that the criterion of mobility may be used as an indicator of the qualitative differences in the higher nervous activity of the animals at different levels of evolutionary development. The experimental facts obtained by investigation of animals, the results of investigation of the higher nervous activity of oligophrenic children, and numerous clinical findings all point to the conclusion that a disturbance of the mobility of the fundamental nervous processes is the pathological change in the higher nervous activity which inhibits the possibility of the synthesis of complex functional systems and thus provides the basis for the most characteristic feature of oligophrenia.

It must be stressed, however, that inertia of the nervous processes is not the only pathophysiological peculiarity of oligophrenia, but merely the determining cause of the principal symptom. There is no doubt that during the comparison of the higher nervous activity of normal and oligophrenic children, the latter also show an appreciable decrease in the strength of the nervous processes, together with various disturbances of their equilibrium.

Our point of view is supported by a comparison of the clinical features of oligophrenia with the clinical features of related conditions which share some of its features (for instance, in cases of temporary retardation of development we do not observe any gross disturbance of perceptive activity in the clinical picture). During an investigation of the higher nervous activity of this type of child, Khomskaya discovered a weakness in their nervous processes and, in particular, a weakness of cortical inhibition, but in no case was a gross disturbance of the mobility of the nervous processes found. Even more convincing, we think, are the results obtained when we compare children with marked cerebral asthenia with oligophrenic children. In cases of marked cerebral asthenia the investigation of higher nervous activity showed a sharp decrease in the strength of fundamental nervous processes, especially weakness of active forms of inhibition, and also a disturbance of the relationship between excitation and inhibition. The investigation, however, showed no gross disturbance of the mobility of the nervous processes at the level of the second signal system. In the cerebral asthenias there was a decrease in working capacity, but no primary disturbance of perceptive activity was observed, i.e., the characteristic symptom of oligophrenia.

This comparison of the clinical picture with the pathophysiological findings in states similar to oligophrenia suggests that the inertia of the nervous processes, especially at the level of the second signal system, is responsible for the inertia of the connections once they are formed, and thereby prevents the formation of new connections in oligophrenia.

Does this mean that any degree of disturbance of the mobility of the nervous processes, arising at any stage of development of the personality, may give rise to that form of disturbance of the ability to abstract and generalize which is specifically present in oligophrenia? The answer to this question must be negative. The onset of inertia of the nervous processes in various diseases in adults, when complex forms of mental activity have already been established, cannot and will not lead to a defect with the same structure that is observed in oligophrenia.

Inertia, when it arises in the earliest stages of development of the child, leads to a disturbance of the creation of those complex functional systems which comprise the specific form of activity of the human cerebral hemispheres. This also leads to maldevelopment of all perceptive activity.

Whereas neurological investigation of oligophrenic children reveals a diffuse residual symptomatology of mainly cortical character, and electroencephalographic findings indicate a deep disturbance of the functional state of the cortical neurons, and whereas the study of the higher nervous activity shows the presence of pathological changes in the dynamics of the nervous processes, mainly in the form of a disturbance of their mobility, this cortical deficiency is manifested in the clinical picture as a maldevelopment of the most complex forms of mental activity, associated with a particular involvement of the second signal system. In the clinical study of oligophrenic children, the most prominent feature is a deficiency in their capacity for abstraction and generalization.

A faulty development in the abstract and generalizing functions of words was invariably observed in the course of our investigation of oligophrenic children. In the analysis of their perception of objects and their images, and of their perception of illustrative pictures, it was apparent that oligophrenics correctly perceive the discrete features of objects and individual objects themselves, but that the complex systems of connections which exist between objects and phenomena are not usually perceived by these children. That is why (as was shown by Solov'ev and his coworkers) the description by oligophrenics of objects perceived by them is always of a poorer, narrower, and more inert character. The perception of an illustrative picture and, even more so, of a successive series of pictures reflecting a given subject, is apparently a very difficult task for oligophrenic children. Oligophrenic children frequently list the separate details of pictures or repeat isolated firmly established thoughts, but they do not appear to be able to distinguish the significant features of images and to incorporate them in an evergrowing system of new connections. Similar difficulties are experienced by oligophrenic children in the understanding of passages of literature read to them. Where it is necessary to abstract the subject matter, and to forge a connection between the individual elements of the test in order to determine the underlying meaning, and sometimes to read between the lines, to identify the motives of the characters in the story and the moral of the passage as a whole, oligophrenics are usually limited to a mere statement of the obvious events directly described in the passage, or they may reproduce older and consolidated connections evoked in them under the influence of some part of the passage which was read to them. The perception of the passage by the oligophrenic child is therefore fragmentary and simplified in character and the more complicated operations of establishing a wide variety of connections and relationships between individual parts of the test are almost completely lacking. It is natural, therefore, that the understanding of metaphors, allegorical expressions, and proverbs is beyond the reach of oligophrenic children.

This maldevelopment of the abstractive and generalizing functions of speech, in fact, accounts for the character of the course of the various mental processes in oligophrenics. The work of Leont'ev (1931) and Zankov (1935) has shown that oligophrenics remember relatively easily obvious images of individual objects and individual words presented to them, but experience great difficulty when the operation of memorizing compels them to establish special auxiliary connections. Experience with logically reinforced memorizing, which in normal children leads to a wide extension of the range of memory, therefore does not improve, but may even impede the memorizing capabilities of oligophrenic children.

Defects of the abstractive and generalizing functions of speech are revealed with exceptional clarity in oligophrenic children by an investigation of the process of classification of visualized objects. This method of investigation is of the greatest diagnostic importance. As our results showed, the most severely retarded children, whenever a picture is presented to them, reproduce the firmly established visual connections formed by past experience, but they are in no condition to group together even small numbers of objects related to a single situation. Oligophrenics with a milder degree of intellectual deficiency easily classify in one group those objects which, in their experience, relate to a single concrete situation; for example they grouped objects together because they are found in a room, in the forest, on a table, etc., but were quite incapable of abstracting from objects presented to them (or from their images) any common feature through which objects usually found in different visual situations could be classified into a single category.

This process of generalization of objects on the basis of the preliminary identification of one feature, which, as was previously shown by Ushinskii, is a fundamental operation in any perceptive activity, is very difficult for oligophrenics to achieve, and this is specifically characteristic of these children. It is natural that this defect has an important bearing on the difficulties arising in oligophrenic children in the course of their education.

Considerable difficulties are also observed in these children during the initial stages of instruction in reading and writing. These difficulties are associated with the fact that the complex intermediate operations — the sound analysis of each letter and the fusion of the sound-letters into complexes — do not at once become an auxiliary method in these children for reading the word as a whole, and they often begin to acquire the character of an independent activity, in which the child does not perceive the meaning of the word that it has read. This defect later becomes one of the main obstacles to the understanding of reading matter. These difficulties of abstraction and generalization are also shown in obvious form when oligophrenic children are taught to count. The impossibility of forming a complex system of connections between a task expressed in words and the actual numbers and names lies at the basis of those difficulties which are experienced by oligophrenic children in the solution of arithmetical problems. It can thus be clearly seen that regardless of the method used to investigate oligophrenic children (clinical observation, experimental pathological investigation, investigation of the higher nervous activity), the predominant symptom of *maldevelopment of the power of abstraction and generalization* emerges as a conspicuous element.

This predominant symptom is characteristic of any oligophrenic mental deficiency, irrespective of the degree of severity and qualitative structure, thus permitting a group of conditions of differing etiology to be combined into a single clinical form. In some papers dealing with the study of oligophrenia, the entire symptomatology is described under various headings, most writers mentioning loss of memory, narrowness of perception, poverty of vocabulary, limitation of judgment, extreme weakness or absence of imagination and so on.

In contrast to the above, we distinguish a predominant and fundamental symptom, permitting the establishment of a regular correlation between the individual symptoms composing the picture of oligophrenic mental deficiency.

The importance of this delineation of the fundamental symptom during the analysis of different pathological conditions has been stressed by many writers. Goldstein (1924) based his researches on the correct assumption that in the analysis of a given pathological condition it is necessary to seek a fundamental disturbance which is responsible for a train of secondary symptoms. Luriya (1947) considers that an understanding of the changes observed in the aphasic in the form of a disturbance of speech, writing, and reading, and of inability to master grammatical forms and counting operations is only possible if a fundamental disturbance is assumed.

The demarcation of a fundamental symptom allows a deeper and more accurate understanding of the whole structure of the defect, i.e., an understanding of the interconnection between the individual symptoms and their mutual participation in the formation of the clinical picture as a whole. It is especially important to maintain this position during the analysis of anomalous development, when the investigator must treat the defect as a product of development and must attempt to find the fundamental symptom which led to the distortion of the subsequent mental development of the child. It is not by accident that for a hundred years different authors, using different methods of investigation, have discovered this fundamental symptom by some means or another.

Whereas the problem of the fundamental symptom is more or less clear, there remains the no less complicated question of the physiological basis of this fundamental symptom. Our numerous observations have shown that oligophrenic children are extricated with difficulty from their old stereotyped connections. This, in its turn, interferes with the formation of new connections in these children. We present herewith a few examples:

The teacher in the first class sets the children the following problem: "Three birds were sitting on a branch and two more flew to join them. How many birds were now sitting on the branch?" After the children had solved this problem (with the aid of the teacher), they were asked to think up other problems on their own. All the children repeated word for word the text of the problem which they had previously solved. The teacher suggested to the children that they alter its nature. The children who had been asked thereupon produced the following variation of the problem: "Three fishes were sitting on a branch and two more fishes flew to join them. How many fishes were now sitting on the branch?" It will be seen from the circumstances of this lesson why birds were replaced by fishes. This change was not accidental. Before turning to the solution of this particular problem, the pupils were at this period engaged in the analysis of the composition of the number 10, and this was illustrated by a table in which fishes were reproduced in color.

Many constantly recurring facts show that oligophrenic children give up their old stereotyped connections with difficulty. Oligophrenic children mastered arithmetical operations with two-figure numbers, but when some of them were asked to do a simple arithmetical example (add 6 to 12), most of the children gave the wrong answer (some children combined the two numbers to obtain 87, others 78, for the answer). The wrong answer was obtained because the children, in solving this problem, made use of the stereotype with which they had mastered the subject of addition of two-figure numbers: to the digit 1 representing "ten" in the first number to be added, the child adds the six "units" of the second number to be added, thereby obtaining seven "tens," and then to the two "units" of the first number to be added he adds the six "units" of the second number to be added, and thus obtains eight "units." The answer 78 is thus obtained. In the other case the child adds the two "units" to the six "units" and obtains eight "tens," and then adds the six "units" to the one "ten" and obtains seven "units" and the complete number 87. These children cannot change the mode of action to suit a change in the problem, but they set out to solve the new problem by the method to which they are accustomed.

If the children are set three or four problems of division with a remainder, they will solve all subsequent examples of division without remainder as problems in division with a remainder.

If the children, with the aid of the teacher, solve a problem formed of two questions, then after solving three or four problems of this kind, they will solve a problem consisting of one question by the method used in the solution of the previous problems. It is quite clear from the cases cited above that it is the old, inert connections which prevent the development of the process of perception. This phenomenon is demonstrated especially clearly in the incorrect solution of the arithmetical problem given above, in which the inertia of the pre-existing connections prevented the fulfilment of the task which was within the capability of these children.

We found inertia of pre-existing connections in oligophrenic children in the course of investigations by the method of classification of visualized objects. In the second year of education, in the Russian language program, ideas concerning animate and inanimate objects were developed. When naming a picture with the representation of a living object, the children asked the question "Who is that?" When naming a picture showing an inanimate object, they asked the question "What is that?" After a short time, in a special experiment on classification of the pictures, the same children were given the task of arranging the pictures into groups representing animate and inanimate objects. In this experimental investigation the questions "Who is that?" and "What is that?" were not envisaged as connected with the study of grammatical rules. Most children, however, when naming a particular picture, asked the question "Who is that?" or "What is that?" This experiment showed very clearly the inertia of the pre-existing connections in these children.

Experimental work by Vasilevskaya and Krasnyanskaya (1955) showed that a fundamental role in the dissociation between visual and word objects is played by the formation of inert verbal stereotypes. As the basis of maldevelopment of thinking, inertia of the mental processes was also observed during psychological investigations of mentally retarded children.

Kurt Lewin, for instance, in his dynamic theory of mental deficiency in children, deduces from the rigidity and inertia of the mental systems a direct and immediate tendency toward concrete thinking, which is a particular feature of the intellect of mentally deficient children. It must be agreed that inertia lies at the basis of the concrete thinking pattern of the mentally deficient child. In explaining this phenomenon, however, Lewin made certain mistakes. If inertia of thinking is, in fact, due to inertia in the emotional-volitional function, it is still completely unexplained what, in turn, causes inertia in the affective function. Inertia is observed in all forms of activity and in the behavior of oligophrenic children. This is clearly demonstrated by both clinical and pedagogic observations.

In a series of experimental researches into higher nervous

activity, attempts have been made to identify one of the parameters of higher nervous activity as being of greatest importance in oligophrenic mental deficiency. Kaz'min and Fedorov (1951) point out that strong negative induction in oligophrenics tends to impede the formation of the physical mechanisms in the second signal system lying at the basis of abstract thinking. These workers regard negative induction in the patients whom they studied as the principal physiological basis of mental deficiency. A similar attempt is to be found in the work of Gakkel' (1953). She considers that the fundamental characteristic of the higher nervous activity of oligophrenics is a weakness of the processes of excitation and inhibition.

A disturbance of the strength of the nervous processes undoubtedly plays an important role in oligophrenia. These pathophysiological features, however, cannot be regarded as the predominant characteristics of the fundamental symptom in oligophrenia, for gross disturbances of the strength of the main nervous processes are not invariably present in all degrees and varieties of this disability.

In this connection great attention must be paid to the fact that in the cerebral asthenias the strength of the fundamental nervous processes is profoundly disturbed, but no marked maldevelopment of the perceptive activity, i.e., the fundamental symptom of oligophrenia, is observed.

This applies to an even greater degree to the disturbance of the equilibrium between the fundamental nervous processes. Disturbances of equilibrium are not observed in all the clinical variants of oligophrenia (Lubovskii, 1956). As a result of a number of other diseases during childhood, of a traumatic or inflammatory character, the equilibrium of the fundamental nervous processes may be acutely disturbed (Khomskaya, 1956), but in these conditions no marked maldevelopment of perceptive activity is observed.

While disturbances of the neurodynamics of the fundamental nervous processes listed above are not invariably present, pathological inertia is observed in all variants of the defect, irrespective of the severity of the lesion. Hence it may be concluded that, against a background of maldevelopment of the whole higher nervous activity, a disturbance of the mobility of the nervous processes is of decisive importance to the development of the fundamental symptom of oligophrenia.

Maldevelopment of perceptive activity is also invariably reflected in the whole structure of the personality of oligophrenic children. In the earliest stages of education of oligophrenic children, they often do not understand the school environment, and they therefore do not know how to subordinate their behavior to the demands of the teacher. They have no attitude towards the teacher's estimation of their work, and are therefore unable to relate the work performed to the teacher's demands.

It is only in the course of organized education, bringing about the development of the child's personality, that these children gradually acquire the skill to subordinate their behavior to the teacher's demands, the skill to equate the teacher's estimation with the quality of the work done by the children themselves. Our observations show that such children develop elements of a critical attitude towards their work only at a particular stage of education, and only then are they able to assess a poor answer and to turn to the teacher with the request that they be allowed to answer again. Some oligophrenic children are able to respond critically to the higher estimation of the teacher. Such pupils subsequently develop along relatively favorable lines and adapt themselves well to the demands of an independent working life. The development of personality in oligophrenic children differs sharply from that of children with psychopathic conditions, in whom maldevelopment of the emotional-volitional function is the fundamental and predominant symptom. In children with psychopathic forms of behavior the understanding of a situation is not disturbed, but inability to control the behavior is observed. In contrast to this, oligophrenic children are characterized by another relationship. Their understanding of a situation is very limited. To the extent and degree to which oligophrenic children do begin to understand a situation, however, they are able to control their behavior. It may therefore be stated that in oligophrenic children the maldevelopment of the personality stands in close relationship to the level of development of their perceptive activity.

3. The Method of Investigation

The study of oligophrenia requires an adequate method of investigation. Such an adequate method may be a clinical method directed toward the study of the structure of the defect as a whole.

Until recently, in the United States, Great Britain, and other foreign countries, systems of tests have been widely used in the investigation of mentally retarded children. In a series of psychological investigations of mentally retarded children, especially in the work of Burt (1951–1955), different tests have been used, some of which were directed towards the investigation of the general attainment, others towards the investigation of special aptitudes.

Ultimately the I.Q. is determined, i.e., the ratio between the mental age and the actual age, and the level of normal development to which the child corresponds is estimated. The authorities responsible for these tests pay great attention to correlation between the tests. This type of study of the different forms of congenital mental deficiency is carried out in almost all clinical researches (Penrose, Tredgold, and others). The tests differ greatly. There are, for example, "projective tests," aimed at studying the emotional-volitional function, psychological tests, pedagogic tests, etc. Some authorities occasionally use the test method to study the parents of mentally retarded children.

Extensive testing is based essentially on the concept of the hereditary origin of mental retardation and of the purely quantitative retardation of normal development of the intellect in persons with congenital mental deficiency. Hardly any clinical studies have been made of oligophrenia. The true clinical study of these conditions has been replaced by testing, i.e., by the mechanical determination of the coefficient of mental development, and this, as we know, has led to gross theoretical and practical errors.

The neglect by many pathophysiologists of the clinical method of investigation has led to the fact that their experimental findings have not deepened our knowledge of the nature of oligophrenic mental deficiency. Pavlov found that observation of normal and sick animals and of human patients served as an inexhaustible source of material for scientific progress in the field of physiology. In his address to the Leningrad Society of Psychiatrists on the subject entitled "Psychiatry as an aid to the physiology of the cerebral hemispheres," Pavlov expounded with great clarity and precision on the role and importance of the clinical method of investigation.

A distinctive feature of the clinical method of investigation is the fact that it embraces not just an individual symptom, not any one aspect of anomalous development, not a single psychic function, but it studies the structure of the defect as a whole. A second and no less important feature of the clinical method of investigation is the principle of qualitative analysis of all the findings which are obtained both during observation on the child and in the course of experiments.

The structure of the defect as a whole may only be studied by a combination of careful analysis of each symptom separately, followed by their subsequent synthesis. The diagnostic value of each individual symptom depends on its manner of combination with other symptoms. The study of the combination of symptoms, their interconnection and their mutual dependence on each other is therefore of decisive importance to an understanding of the structure of the defect.

In the selection of a particular method, the most important factor is its adequacy for the task set by the researcher. In the study of the clinical picture of oligophrenia, it is therefore essential to use the clinical method. This is not meant to imply that the use of other methods of investigation is out of place in the study of mentally retarded children. For instance, experimental psychological methods directed at the study of the individual psychic functions, physiological experiments directed at the study of the dynamics of the fundamental nervous processes, etc., are of great value. Each method must be adequate for the purpose of the investigation. Any attempt to use the resulting experimental findings from a study of individual aspects or functions in order to solve the problem of the pattern of the structure as a whole must be profoundly misleading.

With the clinical method of investigation, when the diagnostic importance of each individual symptom is being assessed, it is necessary to compare it with other symptoms. For example, the child is instructed by means of a sign to carry out a series of movements of the articulatory system. If the child does not carry out these movements, this may lead to the erroneous conclusion that the child shows signs of oral apraxia. If this symptom is compared with other systems, however, its true nature is clearly revealed. The combination of the phenomenon of quasi-oral apraxia with integrity of the pronunciation aspect of speech, and the comparison with other features of the child, from which it is obvious that the child cannot perform elementary actions whether in response to a verbal command or to a sign, provide a basis for regarding the difficulties of movement of the articular apparatus in quite another manner.

When studying mentally retarded children, many research workers have used a wide variety of methods, starting from that of tests and ending with pneumoencephalography, but they have not made it their purpose to synthesize all their findings, and they have not therefore progressed towards the study of the structure of mental deficiency as a whole. The clinical investigation must be based on complexity, integration, concreteness, and continuity. By integration is meant the correlation of some findings with others concerning the child, and their study as mutually interconnected and interdependent phenomena.

Concerning the concreteness of the investigation (whether it be writing, reading, counting, the solution of arithmetical problems, the general behavior, the structure of experiences, etc.), it is essential to bear in mind the collection of concrete experimental results and observations in different conditions. The presence of concrete data and their analysis enables the understanding of what lies at the basis of a particular form of disturbance of behavior, activity or intellect.

The most significant feature of the clinical investigation is its continuity. By continuity is implied prolonged observations on the same child. The principle of continuity is most clearly demonstrated in the concept of the "zone of maximal development," put forward by Vygotskii. He showed that children, even with the same level of development of their perceptive activity, may solve the same problem in different ways when doing so independently. The divergence between the levels of solution of problems by a child with the help of adults and of solution of the same problems unaided defines the child's "zone of maximal development" or developmental capacity.

During clinical investigation the recognition of this factor is extremely important, for by means of this principle of investigation, we can not only measure what has already been attained in development but can also anticipate what is likely to emerge in the course of development. The study of the zone of maximal development may be utilized for differential diagnosis, for example in those exceptionally difficult cases when delay in development has to be distinguished from true oligophrenia.

The child of seven or eight years old has difficulty in forming ideas of arithmetical difference. If a child is given two groups of objects differing in number and is asked which group contains more objects, then even the mentally retarded child will give the correct answer without special difficulty. If the task is made more complicated, however, and he is asked how many more, it now becomes difficult for the child with temporarily retarded development and, in particular, for the oligophrenic child. After the first two or three demonstrations of difference, children with temporarily retarded development are then able to make the transfer to an analogous task. The oligophrenic child behaves quite differently. Repeated explanations to oligophrenics are not followed by the appearance of transference, i.e., they cannot do "tomorrow" by themselves what they can do "today" with the aid of an adult. The zone of maximal development is different in the oligophrenic.

In the study of different forms of anomalous development, the dynamic or continuous approach is especially important. The continuous study must be applied both to each individual symptom and to the interconnection and interdependence of the symptoms. In the study of each individual symptom it is important to understand its genesis and its role in relation to the age-period of development of the child.

It is well known that the same symptom may lead to different disturbances depending on the time of its appearance. For example, inertia of the mental processes, arising in the earliest stages of postnatal development, inevitably leads to maldevelopment of the generalizing function of the spoken word; the same inertia, but arising at later stages of development, cannot lead to these disturbances. The same thing is observed when the auditory function is tested. Deafness at an early age, before the function of speech has been established, leads to a severe maldevelopment of the whole function of speech, as has been shown by the work of Boskis (1953) and Vlasova (1954). The same degree of diminution of hearing in a child of school age does not lead to these disturbances. When I described the clinical picture of the chronic stage of epidemic encephalitis in children, I demonstrated the different role of identical disturbances, depending on the time of their appearance (Pevzner, 1941).

The essential feature of the clinical method is the complex nature of study, including as it does psychological experiments designed to investigate the perceptive activity of oligophrenic children. Only by the comprehensive study of oligophrenic children were we able to approach the problem of revealing the pathophysiological nature of oligophrenic mental deficiency.

In our investigations of the clinical aspects of oligophrenia we started from the indisputable position that behind the outwardly identical symptoms may be hidden different pathophysiological mechanisms, and we accordingly undertook the task of studying the higher nervous activity of these children. Experimental investigations of the neurodynamics of the fundamental nervous processes, like the investigation of the cortical rhythm by the method of electroencephalography, in conjunction with carefully studied clinical evidence, led to the discovery of the pathophysiological mechanisms responsible for the clinical findings and thereby deepened our understanding of the nature of oligophrenic mental deficiency.

The clinical study of oligophrenic children enabled the pattern of the anomalous development of these children to be analyzed. In the course of development of the anomalous child, specific features will inevitably manifest themselves, depending on the nature of the underlying defect.

4. Variants of the Defect in Oligophrenia

In spite of the fact that oligophrenic children share a common symptomatology, they possess certain features distinguishing them sharply from each other.

In accordance with the severity of the defect, oligophrenia may be divided into three groups: idiocy, imbecility, and feeble-mindedness (corresponding to the moron level in Western usage). In the case of idiocy we are concerned with a profound, diffuse lesion of the cerebral cortex and the subcortical formations. Involvement of the diencephalon is demonstrated in the clinical picture of disharmony, the presence of endocrine disturbances, and deformities in the structure of the skull and skeleton. In idiocy a gross disturbance of the cortical functions is observed. The formation of even the simplest conditioned reflexes is extremely difficult. In some idiots it was possible to produce natural motor reflexes, but conditioned reflexes in special laboratory conditions were induced in them only with great difficulty. The development of differentiation was impossible.

It is these characteristics of the higher nervous activity which are responsible for the gross psychic maldevelopment in idiocy. These children show severe disturbances in motor coordination, especially marked in relation to the fine movements of the hands. Many idiots show a disturbance of stance and gait, and stereotyped rhythmic movements are often observed in the form of swaying of the trunk, clapping of the hands, shaking of the head, or perseverative sucking of the fingers and toes. In idiocy speech development does not progress beyond the pronunciation of separate sounds. Idiots may sometimes awkwardly pronounce a limited number of words, representing the names of various objects, and certain cases of idiocy can be encountered where speech articulation is better preserved: these children may pronounce words and phrases whose meaning they do not understand. In idiots analysis and synthesis even within the limits of particular sensory or motor analyzers are very severely deranged. That is why they are incapable of mastering elementary school routines. These features are combined with the severest forms of maldevelopment of perceptive activity and with gross behavioral changes. Some idiots are almost completely incapable of reacting to the environment; others, on the contrary, show extreme motor restlessness: they run, jump, bite, and turn somersaults.

In imbecility there is every reason to believe that the lesion of the cerebral cortex is diffuse but relatively less marked than in idiocy, and that this also applies to the lesion of the subcortical structures, especially the diencephalon. It is for that reason that imbeciles show, to a less severe degree but nevertheless quite obviously, a disturbance of their physical development in the form of general dysplasia and structural anomalies of the skull (microcephalus, hydrocephalus).

Investigation of the nervous system of imbeciles confirms the hypothesis of the diffuse nature of the lesion. Besides the residual neurological signs indicating cortical damage, there are other symptoms showing a disturbance of the normal activity of the subcortical ganglia. The marked endocrine disturbances suggest that the process has also spread to the diencephalon. Faulty development of motor activity, although less pronounced than in idiots, is quite conspicuous in imbeciles. Motor function in these children is characterized by sluggishness and inhibition. Their movements show little differentiation, and often they cannot carry out an isolated movement.

Disturbances of the finer differentiated movements of the hands are quite obviously disturbed in imbeciles. The hands of imbeciles are limp, weak, and have little elasticity. That is why these children look after themselves so badly. The ability to dress and wash themselves or to make their beds requires certain definite skills which are not found in imbeciles. Imbeciles display marked distortions of personality development. For a long time these children do not realize that they are pupils and do not understand the teacher's requests. They walk about the classroom, stand beside their seats, eat during lessons, laugh for no reason, play with the visual aids, and pay no attention to the teacher's remarks. Certain imbeciles show imitative forms of behavior. The emotional characteristics of imbeciles have a definite influence on their behavior. Some of them are sluggish, apathetic, and listless; others, on the contrary, are active, good-natured, talkative, and at times their motor activity is restless and irritable. They usually show disturbances of speech development and in the understanding and pronunciation of the spoken word.

Perceptive activity is especially severely affected in imbeciles. The low level of development of analysis and synthesis within the limits of individual analyzers causes great difficulty when these children are taught elementary reading, writing, and counting. They remember the individual letters with great difficulty, for a long time they mistake letters which bear visual resemblance to each other or which denote similar sounds of speech. Still greater difficulties arise when sounds are merged into syllables and syllables into words. During instruction in elementary reading and writing a defect of the auditory analyzer and of synthesis may occasionally become apparent. After prolonged instruction, their reading continues to be purely mechanical in character: when they read they pronounce sounds and combinations of sounds without understanding the meaning of the words spoken.

Imbeciles find it especially hard to learn how to count. Even when they have mastered the technique of counting, they cannot correlate numbers and objects; the transition to abstract counting is beyond the grasp of many of them: they do not develop any understanding of number concepts and are only able to learn mechanically simple addition and subtraction and the multiplication table.

Faulty development of perceptive activity is revealed in imbecile children by their inability to understand the meaning of the easiest picture-story, and such pupils are usually limited to enumeration of the various objects represented.

Imbeciles and idiots differ not only in the severity of their defect, but also in their pattern of development.

Children at the feeble-minded or moron level differ appreciably from those at the two levels of mental deficiency described above. The principal pathogenic feature at this level of mental deficiency is a diffuse but relatively superficial lesion of the cerebral cortex. In certain cases there may be a combination of diffuse and focal lesions. In most feeble-minded children there is no involvement of the subcortical structures nor of the diencephalon.

Feeble-minded children show less severe abnormalities of physical development; in some cases of feeble-mindedness there is no abnormality of physical development. In certain forms of feeble-mindedness pronounced motor disturbances may be observed, but in most cases only the more complex movements are affected, and defects of motor function appear when the children have to carry out movements in response to a verbal command or in an imaginary situation.

Speech disturbances are less pronounced in the feeble-minded. So far as their behavior is concerned, they stand on a much higher level than the imbeciles. When given systematic instruction, these children learn to behave properly in school, master the special school curriculum, and can be trained for useful employment.

In spite of the fact that oligophrenic children have a common symptomatology, they also display features which clearly distinguish one group from another. These qualitative differences in children with a defect of the same general severity require a differentiation in educational approach. In the construction of a classification of oligophrenia it would be very tempting to proceed from a single principle, but the very complexity of the clinical picture of oligophrenia requires us to single out the several variants of defect, and to recognize a whole series of special features and their interrelations: the etiology, the time of onset of the lesion, and the qualitative peculiarities and extent of the disease process.

The study of the structure of oligophrenic mental deficiency and the differentiation of the special features of its pathogenesis, pathophysiology, and clinical pattern have provided us with a basis for the classification of oligophrenic states in childhood, in which four forms may be distinguished:

The first form of oligophrenia includes children in whom the maldevelopment of the most complex forms of perceptive activity is not accompanied by any gross lesion within the limits of any particular analyzer nor by any disturbances in the emotional-volitional function. The distinguishing mark of these oligophrenic children is their ability to undertake sustained purposeful activity. The special pathogenic feature of this form is a diffuse but relatively superficial and mainly cortical lesion, with no particular abnormality of the circulation of cerebrospinal fluid. In this form we are dealing mainly with a lesion of the higher layers of the cortex, the function of which is synthetic activity. The principal pathophysiological feature of this form is a disturbance of the mobility of the nervous processes, with absence of any gross disturbance of the equilibrium between excitation and inhibition.

The second oligophrenic group is characterized by the fact that a defect of perceptive function is associated with a gross disturbance of cortical neurodynamics. The gross disturbance of the cortical neurodynamics manifests itself both in behavioral changes and in a marked reduction of working capacity. No special disturbances of function of the individual analyzers are found in these children. The specific feature of the pathogenesis of these forms of oligophrenia is the association of a diffuse superficial lesion of the cerebral cortex with a disturbance of the circulation of cerebrospinal fluid, which leads to gross and characteristic changes in the cortical neurodynamics. This whole group of states may be divided into three subgroups in accordance with the nature of the disturbance of the cortical neurodynamics:

A. Oligophrenic children in whom the disturbance of the cortical neurodynamics is characterized by a predominance of excitation over inhibition.

B. Oligophrenic children in whom the disturbance of the cortical neurodynamics is characterized by a predominance of inhibition over excitation.

C. Oligophrenic children in whom the disturbance of the cortical neurodynamics is characterized by the weakness of both nervous processes.

A characteristic feature of the third group of oligophrenic children* is the maldevelopment of the higher forms of perceptive activity, combined with gross disturbances of the whole personality, distortions in the system of needs and motives, and disturbances in the emotional-volitional function. This fundamental defect is accompanied as a rule by specific defects in motor development.

The fundamental pathogenic basis for this form is the combination of a diffuse superficial lesion of the cerebral cortex with more severe disturbances of the anterior divisions of the cerebral cortex.

The higher nervous activity in this form is characterized not only by a general inertia of the nervous processes, but also by a particularly severe inertia in the region of the motor analyzer.

Finally, when the diffuse lesion of the cerebral cortex is complicated by a local lesion within the limits of a particular analyzer, we have the fourth form of oligophrenia. The higher nervous activity in this form is characterized by general changes in the dynamics of the nervous processes together with a very conspicuous disturbance of the cortical neurodynamics within the limits of the affected analyzer. In our clinical material the most frequently observed combination was a diffuse lesion of the brain associated with focal lesions in the region of the motor speech and auditory analyzers. In these cases, in addition to maldevelopment of complex forms of perceptive activity, specific disturbances of hearing and of the auditory speech system are observed.

*We have in mind oligophrenic children with a marked defect of the frontal areas of the cerebral cortex.

In contrast to the existing attempts to divide children with mental maldevelopment into harmonic and disharmonic, or into excitable and inhibited, we have distinguished four forms of oligophrenia on the basis of pathogenesis, pathophysiology, and clinical pattern.

The specific combination of basic pathogenic factors, pathophysiological, and clinical factors, together with individual additional factors determines the qualitative structure of the defect. This, in turn, determines the character of the corrective training procedures to be adopted.

Each of the forms which we distinguish may be divided into a series of subgroups. It is not within the scope of this book to describe that form of oligophrenia in which a diffuse, but relatively superficial lesion is combined with a local lesion.

CHAPTER 2

OLIGOPHRENIC CHILDREN—THE PRIMARY OR BASIC TYPE

The primary or basic type of oligophrenia includes those cases in which maldevelopment of the most complex forms of perception (which require a certain definite capacity for abstraction and generalization) is not associated with any gross lesion of any particular analyzer nor with any gross primary lesion of the subcortical regions.

It is characteristic of these children that they are able to work relatively well and to pursue consecutively and purposefully those activities which are within their grasp.

The subject matter of this chapter derives from a prolonged study of 43 oligophrenic children, of whom 20 were followed up for seven years and the rest for shorter periods (from one to three years). The results of the study are described below.

CASE 1

Vitya I., a boy of 15 years, a pupil in the imbecile class of a special school. No abnormal hereditary factors.

History. The boy's mother had four pregnancies. A daughter was born from the first pregnancy, now 18 years old, normal, and a good pupil. Our present case was the outcome of the second pregnancy. The child born from the third pregnancy died in the maternity home from some cause unknown to the mother. A normal girl, now six years old, was the product of the fourth pregnancy. In the sixth month of the pregnancy from which our subject was the issue the mother fell and sustained a blow on the abdomen. The course of labor was normal. From earliest infancy the boy was considerably retarded in his development. Vitya began to walk at the end of the second year of life, and to use single words at the age of three years. In early childhood he suffered from several children's infectious diseases, in the course of which he occasionally had febrile convulsions. Before reaching school age, Vitya was so retarded in his development that he was not accepted for the nursery nor the kindergarten.

When the boy was two years old, his mother took him to see a specialist, who already at that age made a diagnosis of oligophrenia. With the approach of school age, Vitya's retarded development became still more marked and obvious; he showed a severe retardation in speech and motor function, difficulties in spatial orientation and an inability to play with other children. At nine years of age he was accepted for the "imbecile" class in a special school for mental defectives.

Physical State. In his physical development the boy was considerably behind the normal for his age; there was also a microcephaly (head circumference 45 cm) and general dysplasia. Examination of the internal organs revealed a functional impairment of the cardiovascular system.

State of the Nervous System. Examination of the nervous system revealed bilateral residual neurological signs, more marked on the right: the right nasolabial fold was flattened, and the boy hopped poorly on the right leg. Motor activity was only very slightly differentiated, and it required a great effort for the boy to close one eye or to puff out one cheek. Changes of muscle tone reflecting faults of innervation were present. The tendon reflexes were brisk. The knee jerks were increased, tonic, and pendulum-like. All tendon reflexes were more marked on the right. The abdominal reflexes were sluggish and readily exhausted. The plantar reflexes were slightly exaggerated. Oppenheim's sign was slightly positive on the right side, and a crossed Babinski's sign appeared to a slight degree when Babinski's sign was elicited on the left side. No sensory dis-

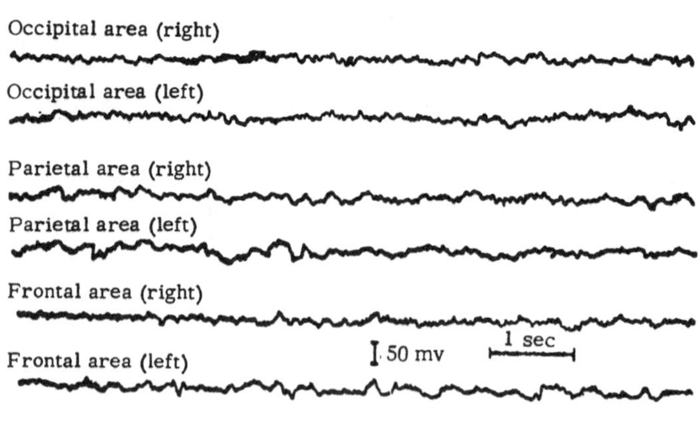

Fig. 12. Vitya I., aged 15 years, pupil in the imbecile class (oligophrenia, imbecile). The EEG shows an absence of α-rhythm, with β-rhythm predominant in all areas of the cortex.

turbances were present. Tests of tactile and proprioceptive discrimination, during sensory examination, revealed that inert motor speech stereotypes were readily formed.

Ophthalmological Examination. Visual acuity of the right eye 0.7, left eye 0.8. Optic fundus: the optic disc is pink and clearly demarcated, the veins large, the arteries of normal caliber and the periphery normal.

Otorhinolaryngological Examination. Hearing within normal limits.

X-ray Examination of the Skull. Microcephaly. Vascular markings indefinite and shadows slightly widened.

Electroencephalography. Investigation of the action potentials of the cerebral cortex showed diffuse pathological changes in the form of absence of α-rhythm, predominance of β-rhythms and the presence of slow waves of low amplitude in all areas of the cortex (Fig. 12).

The electroencephalogram showed an absence of delta-waves. No evidence was found of any well-defined pathological foci.

During investigation of the electrical activity of the brain by the method of rhythmic light stimulation, modification of the activity was recorded only in response to flashes of light with a frequency of 11, 12, or 13 per second (Fig. 13).

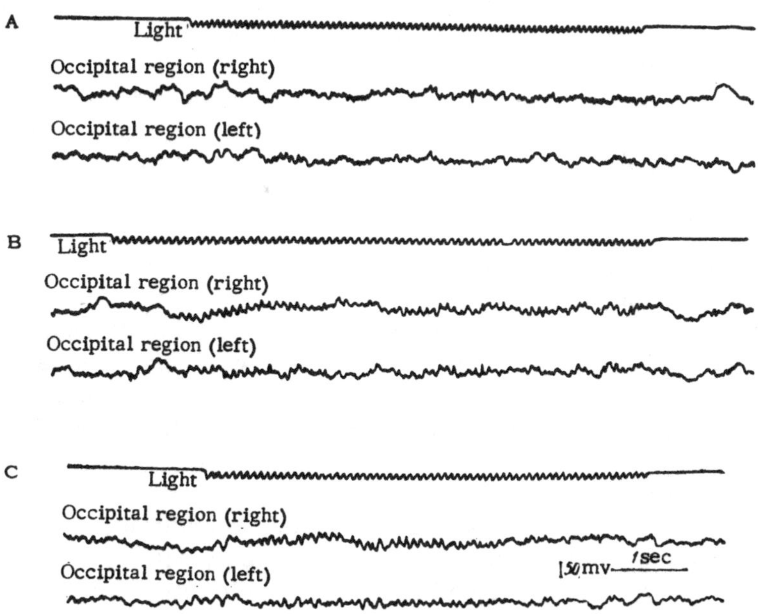

Fig. 13. EEG (of the same subject) during the application of a rhythmic light stimulus. A) Stimulation with rhythmic flashes of light (frequency 16 per second) causes no modification of the cortical rhythm. B) With flashes of light at a frequency of 12 per second, a relatively clear modification of the rhythm is recorded on the EEG. C) The same, when the frequency of the flashes of light is 13 per second.

With a higher flicker frequency (16 per second) no modification of the cortical rhythm took place. In this subject a relatively clear modification of the cortical rhythm was thus observed, though the range of frequencies capable of inducing such a modification was very narrow and did not exceed the frequency of the α-rhythm.

Investigation of the Higher Nervous Activity. Simple positive connections and simple differentiation of color were readily established and were stable. Other unrelated stimuli had no significant influence on the established systems of connections. Differentiation was not disinhibited by an increase in the frequency of application of the stimuli. The connections were also well maintained after removal of the stimuli. The boy correctly gave expression to the established simple connections with verbal statements.

The formation of more complex connections, i.e., the differentiation of light signals by their intensity and especially by their duration, created great difficulties. The production of such connections was made easier by means of a stereotype of alternated signals. During the formation of the more complex connections a correct response was obtained, with some delay involving the formation of a system of adequate motor reactions. During the formation of differentiation of signals based on their duration, for a long time the pattern of the formation of the preceding simple connections was repeated in stereotyped fashion. The older inert stereotypes were repeated for an especially long time because of the formation of a conditioned reaction based on the principle of alternation (every other signal).

Mental State

Visual Analyzer. Pictures shown to Vitya were correctly named by him, though his replies were somewhat slow. Continuous- and broken-line drawings were recognized with difficulty, and he did not always recognize pictures of objects shown to him upside down.

Spatial Orientation. Vitya was able to orientate himself in space. He had developed the idea of right and left. He copied elementary figures made of sticks or matches rapidly and correctly, but more complicated tasks confused him.

Motor and Motor-Speech Analyzers. In tasks concerned with postural movements, Vitya could cope satisfactorily with simple tests, but complicated tests caused him considerable difficulty or were even impossible. Dynamic movements presented very great difficulty. He could construct an elementary sentence properly.

Phonemic Hearing. Vitya could understand speech addressed to him.

He could repeat correlated phonemes satisfactorily, and was not embarrassed by an extension of the scope of the problem.

When performing simple tasks, Vitya showed no evidence of gross focal cortical disturbances. With complicated tasks, difficulties became apparent within the limits of some particular analyzer, a situation which could be regarded as a disturbance of analytico-synthetic activity.

Cognitive Function and Behavior. Vitya was a diligent, attentive, and orderly pupil. During his class work he would listen carefully to the questions asked by the teacher and after only momentary preliminary reflection would answer.

Vitya's behavior was completely under control. He conformed to all the school rules, and was especially well-behaved and disciplined when a stranger entered the classroom. At such a time he was able to keep the other children in order.

Emotionally, Vitya was composed. Within the limits of his understanding he was upset by poor marks and pleased with good marks. He was to some extent able to consider a task set for him and thus showed the rudiments of a critical attitude. Vitya behaved in a manner appropriate to the situation: he was confused when he was placed in an unaccustomed situation; at recess and in the company of other children he was at ease, and with older people he was restrained, polite, and attentive.

Vitya always willingly went to the doctor for examination, displaying neither diffidence nor negativism on these occasions. The relatively composed emotional make-up of the boy was also revealed in the course of clinical conversation with him alone: for example, tears came to his eyes whenever his father, who lived apart from his family, was mentioned.

Vitya did not have an unduly high opinion of himself. When he compared himself with the two best pupils in the class, for example, he thought that he was more stupid than they, and offered the explanation: "Because I am a poor student."

The principal symptom determining the structure of the disability in this case was a gross maldevelopment of perceptive activity, so that the child was deficient in his ability to abstract and generalize. This principal symptom manifested itself regardless of the task put to the boy. During the investigation of postural movements, for example, Vitya could cope with simple problems, but if they were made slightly more complicated they were apparently beyond his capacity.

The same pattern was revealed when the boy was asked to name the objects shown in pictures. When they were presented to him the right way up, and slowly, he could recognize all the pictures, but if the picture were presented to him upside down, he could no longer recognize the object which it showed.

This disturbance of recognition was also clearly demonstrated during clinical conversation with the boy. Elementary orientation toward the environment was possible for Vitya. He could give his correct address, could discuss with whom he lived at home, knew where his mother worked, but he was unable to appreciate and understand the situation as a whole. He could say with confidence what work was done by an engine-driver, a doctor, or a teacher. Vitya did not understand a question put to him unless it was formulated in a sufficiently concrete manner. If he was asked to name the days of the week, he would usually reply, "I don't know." In response to the easier question, "What day is it today? " he would reply, "It's night now." The boy's reply was nothing more than a verbal stereotype. If the doctor himself mentioned the name of any day of the week, however, Vitya would then name all the other days of the week, in both the proper and reverse orders. If Vitya was then asked to give the names of the months, he would name the days of the week, i.e., he would reproduce the verbal sterotype of the previous task. If the examiner himself named one of the months, Vitya would then give the names of the months in the proper order, both forward and backward. If he was then asked what seasons he knew, he would recite the names of the months. If this question was accompanied by the direct instruction, "Vitya, look through the window. What time of year do you think it is now?" the boy would then give the right answer.

The maldevelopment of the cognitive function was demonstrated especially clearly in an experiment on classification of pictures. Vitya failed to understand the instructions he had been given, simplified his problem, and, guided by the word "arrange," placed all the pictures in a row irrespective of their content.

After further explanation and considerable simplification of the instruction, in this experiment Vitya found conceptual categories in relation to concrete situations. For example, he grouped together the pictures illustrating a tomato, radish, beet, and cucumber, motivated by the fact that all these grow in a kitchen garden. He grouped together the pictures illustrating a goat and a cabbage, because "goats like cabbage." He was unable to group the picture of a deer with any other, because no suitable picture was available.

Even when Vitya grouped the pictures presented to him and

representing different objects in accordance with some indication of their common category, his spoken remarks showed that the boy did not have in mind in such cases any essential features of the objects. For example, he grouped together pictures of a knife, a fork, and a frying pan, but this was motivated as follows: "We cut bread with a knife, and we eat from a frying pan with a fork."

When the experimenter suggested that the group be added to, Vitya added pictures representing vegetables to pictures of cooking utensils, giving the following explanation: "Vegetables grow in the kitchen garden, then they are cooked in pans, cut up and eaten at table."

A year later, when the school syllabus introduced generic concepts, Vitya was able to choose correctly, at the request of the experimenter, pictures illustrating vegetables, cooking utensils, furniture, and clothing, but in the subsequent course of the experiment, during the extension of the group, he added pictures of fruits and vegetables to those of animals. He gave the correct names to each separate category, but this did not prevent him from grouping them together, motivated by the fact that animals may eat both fruit and vegetables. When the experimenter remarked that animals, fruits, and vegetables cannot be grouped together, Vitya quickly took away the apple, the reason for this being that the fox may eat it. Thus the same motive impelled Vitya in one case to group these pictures together, and in the other to separate them.

This example shows that the categories present here are only formal and mechanically learned, not reflecting a true level of development of the child's thought. The task of establishing the points of similarity and difference between a cat and a dog also revealed paired concrete forms of thought in the child: he could not distinguish a single essential sign, but compared the pictures of the cat and dog in terms of irrelevant signs: "The cat is grey with white spots, the dog is white with a brown spot;" "The cat has whiskers but the dog has none;" "The dog has a crooked tail but the cat's tail hangs down." Comparison was achieved by means of dedesignation: "The dog has legs and the cat has legs;" "The nose is similar and the eyes are similar."

Maldevelopment of the cognitive function was shown even more clearly in Vitya's understanding of passages from stories. The following excerpt was read to the boy from the story "Little Sasha." "Little Sasha woke up in the morning feeling very bad. His mother gave Sasha some medicine, took her umbrella and basket and went away." After the second reading of the story, Vitya could almost repeat the passage word for word. In reply to the question, "Why did Sasha feel bad when he woke?" Vitya at first replied: "Because he was little," and the second time: "Because his mother went away." In reply to the question, "What was the weather like?" he replied "The weather was bad because it was autumn." In reply to the third question "Where did mother go?" Vitya replied "Mother went to work."

Thus it can be seen that Vitya did not analyze the passage, but replied to each question separately, without considering it in relation to the passage as a whole. Nor did he understand that the answer to the question could be found in the passage.

Although Vitya remembered the subject of the story well, he was unable to establish any rational connection between the separate parts of the story. The next story which was read to him was "A Place for Everything." "As soon as Serezha wakes, he begins to look for his things. One stocking is on the chair, the other under the table, one boot is under the bed, and the other is not in the room at all. Serezha wastes his time every morning and he is late for school."

In this story the child has to understand that, in order not to be late for school in this concrete case, everything must be in its proper place. In his reply Vitya recited the usual sequence of actions necessary for going to school. "You must get up, dress, wash, eat, and then go to school." In reply to the investigator's question "What do we call Serezha when he is always late for school?" he gave an answer to the question as it was formulated without any relation to the passage from the story—"Serezha was big."

These investigations thus demonstrated the maldevelopment of the generalizing function of the spoken word in this boy, the predominance of the visual system of connections over the verbal, and the severe inertia of the verbal stereotypes which develop. In Head's experiment the predominance of the first signal system over the second was shown particularly clearly. In the course of this experiment the subject, who sits opposite the experimenter, is instructed to perform the same movements as the experimenter himself. The fundamental condition of Head's experiment is that it opposes a verbal instruction to a visual signal, thereby creating a state of conflict in the subject. It is therefore a suitable experiment for studying the predominance of the first or second signal system.

At the beginning of this experiment, in spite of the fact that crossed reactions were required by the verbal instruction, Vitya persistently gave mirror images of the experimenter's actions, obeying the direct visual signal. The experimenter then asked Vitya if he was doing the test correctly. After this question the boy began to compare the position of his hands with those of the experimenter, and replied that he had done the test correctly.

Subsequently the principle of the correct solution of the problem was completely hidden by the experimenter, who set it in the final form as follows. "If I raise this hand, you must raise the other hand." After this instruction Vitya was still unable to suppress the mirror reaction.

This means that the final form of the instruction did not become an effective link in the organization of his motor reaction, and the latter remained just as direct as it was before. The experiment again convinced us that in this case the visual system of connections clearly predominated over the verbal system, as shown by the impossibility of shifting from the direct reaction to a reaction based on the indirect stimulus of speech.

As a result of systematic instruction, Vitya acquired a number of skills. He read fluently and, in reply to questions, could give the content of an easy story, adhering accurately to the text. He could write a simple text from dictation, although mistakes were found in his writing because of his ignorance and lack of understanding of the rules of grammar. We found no mistakes with Vitya indicating a lowered capacity for work, in the form of omission of letters, syllables, words, or of gaps and transpositions.

Complicating factors did not interfere with the process of writing. For example, if Vitya was asked to write with his tongue gripped between his teeth, this did not lead to an increase in the number of mistakes.

In the course of a long period of training, Vitya learned to count. He could count up to twenty and back again, and could also count in tens, both up and down the scale. Vitya replied slowly, deliberately, and correctly. He could count by twos (2,4,6,...), but this was not a form of group counting, for he worked each item out one at a time. Vitya also managed to retain the details of a problem while he carried out a particular action. He also studied the multiplication table. Despite all these achievements, the boy could not comprehend the meaning of the most elementary arithmetical procedure. Vitya had no true understanding of number concepts, even up to ten. He solved his arithmetical problems of addition and subtraction up to ten only by the aid of his fingers. If he was given a problem in which he could not use his fingers, then he was unable to solve it. For example, when he was asked how many he must add to 8 in order to make 10, he looked helplessly at his fingers for a long time before replying that he did not know.

The boy had no clear idea of tens and units. For example, his wrong answer to the problem 20 + 10 was 12. He understood 10 as ten, and 20 as two units. [The Russian word for twenty begins with the word two.] He could easily retain in his memory and solve a problem of three components, adding them one at a time by the aid of his fingers. When solving the problems: 6 + 2 - 3 = 5; 6 + 4 - 2 = 8, and 4 + 3 - 5 = 2, he remembered the details of the problem very well, thought for a long time, and did not make a single guess. The operations were carried out on his fingers. When solving the problem: 14 + 2 = 16, he counted: 14 + 1 = 15; 15 + 1 = 16.

Vitya experienced particular difficulty in the solution of arithmetical problems. If he were asked to do the following problem: "One boy had 6 apples and another had 3 apples more than that; how many apples had the two boys?" he would retain in his memory the details of the problem and be able to repeat them. He could not, however, establish the necessary connections of reasoning, and he could do no more than perform isolated arithmetical operations. His first attempt was to add 3 to 6, i.e., to replace the solving of the problem by a simple arithmetical operation. When he was told that this answer was wrong he began to subtract 3 from 6, and obtained 3, after which he multiplied 6 by 3 and replied that the second boy had 18 apples and the first had 6. In this way he applied all the arithmetical operations he knew to the solution of the problem.

The maldevelopment of the cognitive function, and the boy's inadequate power of generalization and abstraction thus showed themselves very clearly in all these cases. With this maldevelopment as background, no gross defects were found in Vitya within the confines of any particular analyzer.

Vitya readily understood when people spoke to him and could correctly repeat a phrase that was difficult to pronounce. He could distinguish an individual sound from a complete word, or choose a word beginning with a particular sound. For example, when selecting words beginning with the letter "k" he easily chose kotenok, kartoshka, kamen', kastryulya, and kartochki. Vitya was able to read and write, although with great difficulty. It may be concluded from these findings that no gross disturbances of speech were present. We may remember that during the investigation of the individual analyzers, we also found no gross defects. A distinctive characteristic of Vitya was the fact that his capacity for work was relatively intact. He was attentive, diligent, and industrious, and did any job within his power both carefully and well. Vitya was one of the most successful pupils in his work.

Principal Stages of the Child's Development. Three stages in the development of this boy can be distinguished. The first stage covers the period before the beginning of systematic education. We shall be right in saying that in the first stage we are dealing with a very gross maldevelopment of the whole of the analytical-synthetic activity, so that a serious degree of mental deficiency could be diagnosed in the earliest stages of the child's development.

The second stage began with the time when the boy's corrective training began, which was planned to meet the requirements of his particular defect. Even at the end of the first year of education, a perceptible shift in his development had occurred. Different parts of his mental equipment were found to have developed at different rates. Vitya showed the greatest improvement in the development of his emotional-volitional functioning. In the second year of his education he was a disciplined pupil and usually behaved correctly in a situation which he understood. He developed the ability to critically evaluate the things his teacher brought to him. He showed himself affectionate toward his family, other children, and the teacher.

The capacity for abstraction and generalization developed much more slowly in the boy. The development of individual skills was much more rapid than that of his power to reason, so that the level of his reading ability was higher than the level of understanding of what he had read. With organized education, however, the boy made good progress in his general development.

The third stage in development began when Vitya started work in the school workshop, and was characterized by further compensation of his condition. This compensation was more obvious in relation to the development of his emotional-volitional functions. The boy's behavior became even more orderly. Not only did he now show a well-developed attitude toward a situation, but elements of a critical outlook appeared toward himself and his future.

At this stage a considerable development of the level of analysis and synthesis took place within the limits of individual analyzers. The boy also made good progress toward mastering reading, writing, and counting, and also acquiring skill at work. At this stage, however, the maldevelopment of his power of abstraction and generalization became very obvious, showing itself in the difficulty which Vitya experienced in the solution of the most elementary arithmetical problems, in the understanding of the rules of grammar, and in recognizing the subject of a story or of a picture.

Clinical Analysis of the Case

The fundamental etiological factor in this case was an intrauterine lesion of traumatic origin. While still in the maternity home, the doctors had drawn attention to the considerable disturbance of the child's development. The series of childhood infections, which were accompanied in our patient by occasional convulsions, must be regarded as the reaction of a defective brain to the particular physical disease.

The maldevelopment of complex forms of mental activity arising in consequence of the early intrauterine damage to the central nervous system gives grounds for making a diagnosis of oligophrenia in this case. So far as the degree of his deficiency is concerned, the boy may be regarded as an imbecile. An attempt may be made to analyze the qualitative nature of the defect and the factors responsible for it. The qualitative aspects of the clinical picture are determined not so much by the etiology of the disease as by its pathogenesis. By pathogenesis we understand the nature and the distribution of the pathological process itself.

With regard to the nature of the disease process in our case, this consisted of hemorrhage into the brain as a result of the abdominal injury sustained by his mother at the end of the sixth month of pregnancy. With regard to the distribution of this traumatic lesion of the brain, there is every reason to suppose that it was mainly localized in the cortex. The predominantly diffuse lesion of the cerebral hemispheres was confirmed by the EEG findings.

The neurological findings also demonstrate the cortical character of the lesion for the child showed paresis of the facial nerve only, and disturbances of tone due to faulty innervation. Although the lesion was diffuse and bilateral, the predominantly right-sided symptoms were clearly evident, showing that the left cerebral hemisphere had suffered the greatest damage.

The characteristic pattern of this case was further determined by the fact that with a diffuse and early lesion of the cerebral cortex, no localized symptoms were observed.

The absence of gross localized symptoms was revealed by the psychopathological state of the patient (no defect of individual cortical functions). The EEG findings also indicated absence of foci of pathological activity. It may therefore be assumed that the hemorrhage, which took place in the intrauterine period, spread mainly over the convex surface of the cerebral hemispheres.

The next distinctive feature of this case is the fact that whereas Vitya's cognitive functions showed considerable maldevelopment, his emotional-volitional function was relatively intact. He was diligent, attentive, and a disciplined pupil, capable of responding to a situation. He showed appropriate emotional responses, was attached to his parents, affected by failure at school, was able to appreciate the value of the things he was taught, and was even critical in an elementary way of work which he had done. All in all, these features indicate the relative integrity of his emotional-volitional functions and are of considerable importance in determining the whole clinical picture. By starting from the pathogenic aspects of this case, and, in particular, from the distribution of the lesion, it is possible to understand the structural peculiarities of the defect, in which relative integrity of the emotional-volitional function is associated with gross maldevelopment of the cognitive functions.

As pointed out above, the investigations which have been described suggest that in this case the lesion was mainly cortical in character. A further special feature of the structure of the defect in this case is the fact that Vitya retained the ability to work: he was steady, did not tire easily, finished a job which he started, and worked carefully and accurately. His ability to overcome difficulties in the performance of individual tasks enabled him to acquire the elementary attainments of reading, writing, and counting. This remarkable fact is due to the absence of disturbances of the cerebrospinal fluid dynamics or of the cerebro-vascular system in the residual stage of the disease.

The distinctive structure of the defect in this particular case was thus determined qualitatively by a combination of gross maldevelopment of cognitive functions (the ability to abstract and generalize) with a relatively intact emotional-volitional function and good capacity for work, and by the absence of any severe focal defect involving a particular analyzer.

Of particular interest in this case is the comparison of the clinical and pathophysiological findings. Investigation of the boy's higher nervous activity showed that simple connections and simple differentiations were formed rapidly and easily and became quite stable. More complex systems of connections were formed slowly and were less stable. During the formation of still more complex connections, for example, differentiation of signals based on their duration, discrepancies emerged between the direct reactions and those dependent on verbal systems, for having previously formed the correct system of reactions, in his response he reproduced the old, inert verbal connection.

Investigation of the higher nervous activity as a whole showed that, while this was generally disturbed, the mobility of the fundamental nervous processes was particularly affected, and this was shown to its greatest degree in the verbal system of connections. It is this pathophysiological feature, namely the disturbance of the mobility of the fundamental nervous processes, which plays the most significant role in the production of the basic symptom of this condition, the maldevelopment of the cognitive functions.

CASE 2

Vera Z., a girl of 14 years, a pupil in the fourth class at a special school. No abnormal hereditary factors could be discovered.

History. The mother of our subject had had five pregnancies. The eldest son had died in the war at the age of 22 years. Three children had died in early childhood from various infectious diseases. Our case was the product of the fifth pregnancy.

During pregnancy the mother's health was poor as a result of difficult living conditions. The child was born at full term, but as a result of a transverse fetal position, the girl suffered severe asphyxia at birth. Her early development was considerably retarded: she cut her first teeth at the age of two years, began to walk at three, and spoke her first words at the age of four years. At $1^1/_2$ years the child suffered from a disease of unknown etiology which was accompanied by a solitary fit with transient loss of consciousness, after which she gradually recovered her strength. After this illness the general retardation of the child's development was even more marked. It was only when she reached kindergarten age that she began to babble a few words, but subsequently the tempo of speech development increased considerably.

The girl showed no interest in toys. She hardly listened to stories and did not understand what they were about. Only at the age of seven or eight years did she begin to play with younger children.

Before going to school her behavior caused no difficulty. Vera was taught to keep herself clean and tidy comparatively easily. She learned to obey adults and do as she was told. At eight years of age Vera began to attend regular public school. In her mother's words, the girl went to school willingly and was diligent, attentive, and obedient. Because of difficulties which the girl began to experience during instruction in elementary reading and writing, she began to develop feelings of frustration. After one year of instruction in regular school she was transferred to the second class of a special school; in spite of her diligence, attentiveness, and industry, the girl still experienced considerable difficulty in learning. She remained behind for a second year in the third and fourth classes.

Physical State. In physical development the girl was considerably below the normal height and weight for her age. The structure of her skeleton showed general dysplasia and her skull was deformed. The head circumference was 53 cm. The facies was pinched and long, and the chest constricted. The skin and mucous membranes were pale and the palate high. On examination of the internal organs, pulmonary breath sounds were weak, heart sounds muffled with rhythm regular, pulse rate 72 per minute but of poor volume. Digestive organs were normal.

State of the Nervous System. The pupils reacted well. When the eyes were closed, twitching of the orbicularis oris muscle was observed. The tongue deviated to the right, and the right nasolabial fold was flattened. Her voice was thick, with a slightly nasal quality. Some weakness of the distal muscle groups of the right upper limb was noted. Disturbances of tone, ascribable to denervation, were noted in the lower limbs, more marked on the right. The knee jerks were equal. The ankle jerk was increased on the right. Mayer's sign was increased on both left and right. The palm-chin, labial, nodding, and sucking reflexes were elicited. The Babinski reflex was positive on both sides.

Ophthalmological Examination. Visual acuity of the right eye was 0.1, left 1.0. Vision was corrected by glasses. Eye grounds were normal.

Otorhinolaryngological Examination. A slight degree of deafness was found.

X-ray Examination of the Skull. The skull was spherical in type. The pattern of the inner table of bone was obliterated. Base of the skull increased in density. The sella turcica was very small, the sutures obliterated, and the vascular markings increased.

Electroencephalography. A clearly defined α-rhythm of 11-12 per second was recorded in all cortical regions. A somewhat less marked α-rhythm was noted in the anterior regions of the cortex.

In the occipital and parietal regions the α-rhythm was combined with small slow waves of 4-6 per second and with occasional epileptoid bursts. The slow waves were more prominent in the parietal regions (Fig. 14).

Modification to a frequency of 17 per second appeared over small areas (Fig. 15, A). At a frequency of 10 per second, modifi-

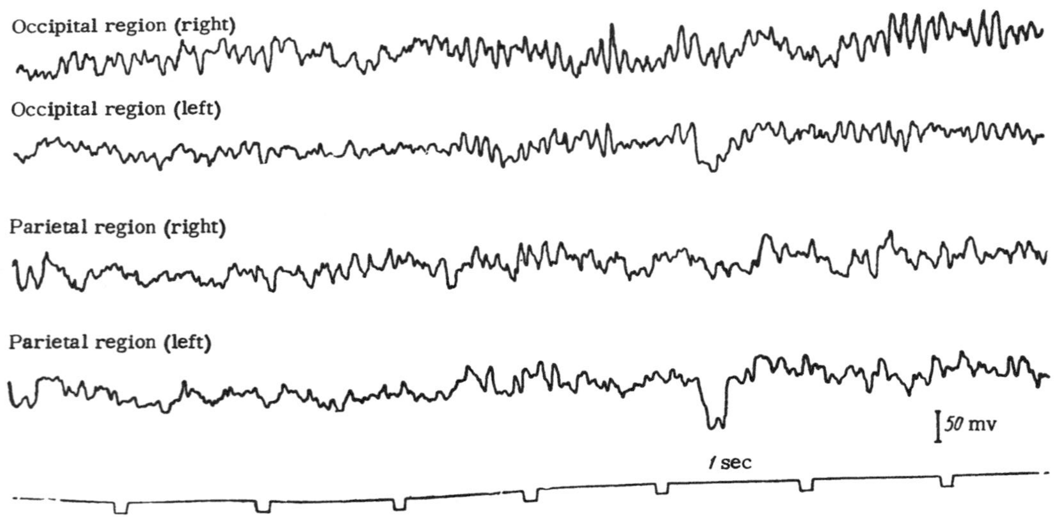

Fig. 14. Vera Z., 14 years old, pupil at a special school (oligophrenia, at feeble-minded or moron level). It is clear from the EEG that in the occipital regions of the cortex the α-rhythm occurred in combination with slow waves of 4–6 per second. In the parietal regions the slow waves were more marked.

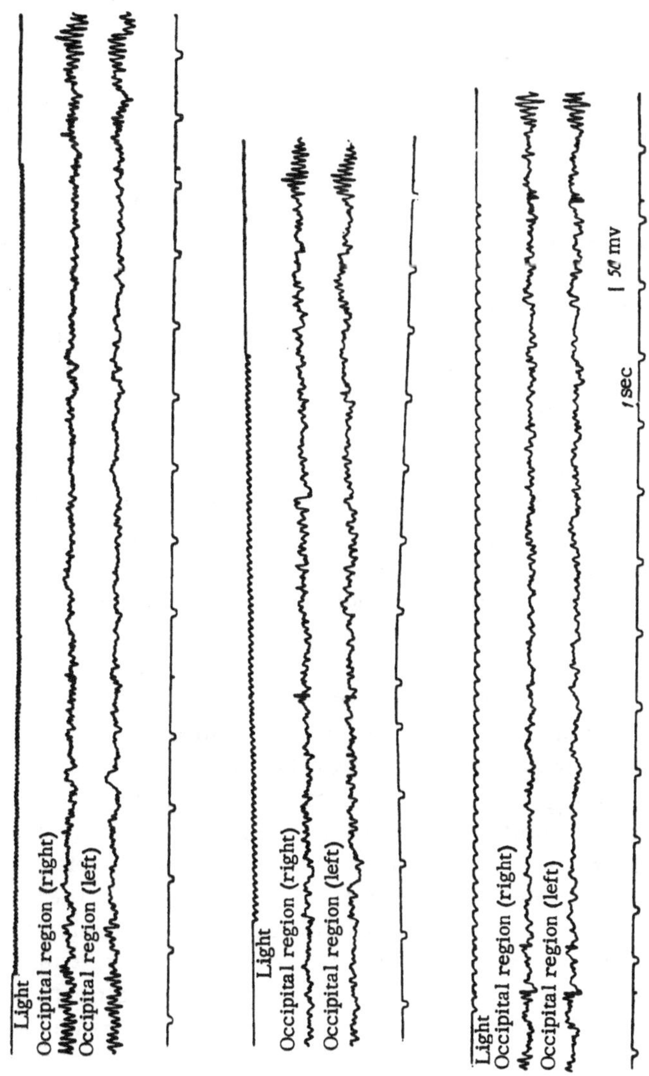

Fig. 15. EEG (of the same subject) during the application of a flicker stimulus. A) Stimulation with rhythmic flicker of 17 per second caused ill-defined modification of the cortical rhythm B) With flicker of 10 per second a relatively clear modification of the rhythm was recorded. C) At a flicker frequency of 5 per second, no modification was noted.

cation was relatively clear (Fig. 15, B). At a lower frequency (5.5 per second) no modification was demonstrable (Fig. 15, C).

The electroencephalogram, taken in a state of relative rest, gave no indications of gross abnormalities of the electrical activity of the brain.

Only isolated epileptoid waves and ill-defined slow waves were present in the central regions of the cortex. The application of a functional load (rhythmic flashes of light) caused a reduction of cortical functional mobility, as shown by the ill-defined and irregular modification of rhythm in response to high-frequency flicker. However, the moderate degree of modification of the cortical rhythm in response to light flashes of average frequency, the absence of modification at low frequencies and the absence of reactions of the parabiotic type provided no evidence of gross neurodynamic disturbances.

Investigation of the Higher Nervous Activity. Simple positive conditioned connections and simple differentiation of light signals according to their color were achieved rapidly. Alteration of simple systems of connections took place readily, and no clear indication of imbalance of the fundamental nervous processes (the predominance of one of them) was noted on these occasions. The verbal report associated with the formation of simple systems of connections and their alteration was adequate and sufficiently complete. The simple systems of connections possessed considerable stability and were well maintained until the next experiment. During the formation of a finer degree of differentiation after alteration of the system of connections setting this differentiation in motion, a tendency was observed for the restoration of the old system of connections (i.e., that existing before the alteration).

More complicated forms of differentiation were produced very slowly; for instance, differentiation by duration was formed only after 18 combinations of the differential signal with negative reinforcement. During the production of complex forms of differentiation, the verbal statement retained for a long time a pre-existing inert verbal stereotype, which itself was the verbal reflection of a previous and simpler differentiation. Alteration of the complex systems of connections not receiving adequate verbalization was slowed, suggesting an inertia of these connections. Old positive connections returned after cessation of reinforcement following alteration of the complex systems of connections, indicating the presence of a marked degree of inertia of the nervous processes.

Mental State

Visual Analyzer. When she was shown pictures representing separate objects, she named them correctly. She gave her replies slowly but deliberately. She recognized pictures presented to her upside down only after a prolonged scrutiny. The girl also recognized outline drawings correctly, but also rather slowly.

Spatial Orientation. She was well orientated in space. She understood the meaning of "right" and "left." She copied figures made from sticks correctly, difficulty arising only when the task was made considerably more complicated.

Motor and Motor-Speech Analyzers. Tests of postural movements presented no difficulty. Dynamic movements were difficult. Oral movements were not disturbed. The child had no particular difficulty in repeating phrases even when difficult to pronounce.

Phonemic Hearing. Vera understood what was said to her, repeated correlated phonemes correctly, and was not embarrassed by extension of the scope of the problem.

Investigation showed the absence of localized cortical disturbances during the performance of a task involving any particular analyzer. Difficulties in the performance of tasks arose only when these were made more complicated.

Cognitive Function and Behavior. During her entire school attendance Vera was one of the most diligent pupils. She attended her classes punctually, listened carefully to the teacher's explanations, kept her textbooks and exercise books clean and neat, ran errands for the teacher with the greatest willingness, and carried out her routine duties well. She introduced order into the class, and she took care to see that the plants in the room were always watered in time. Vera looked after her classmates and, when any of them were ill she gave their parents the assignments the child missed.

During her second year at school the girl developed appropriate attitudes towards the teacher's opinion of her. A bad opinion greatly upset her, but on account of her intellectual inadequacy, she could not relate the teacher's opinion to the quality of her own work in carrying out a task.

Some conspicuous and characteristic difficulties were noted in her behavior. Being by nature very diligent, hard-working, and industrious, at the same time she frequently hindered the work of the class. This state of affairs, paradoxical at first glance, becomes clear when the structural pattern of her disability is analyzed. The girl's increased activity, her persistence, and her strong tendency to complete a task which she had been set, combined with the very low level of development of her cognitive functions led to some peculiar difficulties in her behavior. Vera asked the teacher innumerable questions and would not keep quiet until she had grasped her explanations. She would not allow even one word which she did not understand to pass. During dictation, for example, she encountered the phrase "The group (kollektiv) of girls sowed the vacant land (pustyr')." In this sentence she did not understand the words "kollektiv" and "pustyr'," and actively sought to have them explained. She was angry and irritable if she did not understand the teacher's explanations and persistently asked for further explanation.

The first sentence was followed by a second and a third in which she also met words that she did not understand. Vera therefore continually asked questions, which hindered the work of the class. In this way the child's positive qualities, combined with her general intellectual inadequacy, led to characteristic difficulties in her behavior.

Proof of this statement is provided by Vera's high sense of discipline and her ability to work hard when carrying out some task which was within her capacity. She was capable of working very productively. She carried out many domestic duties satisfactorily: cleaning the rooms, washing the clothes, making simple purchases. When working in the bookbinding workshops throughout the year she got excellent grades and her punctuality in this work was an example to all the other pupils. All these aspects of the girl's behavior stand out against the background of her general intellectual deficiency.

Maldevelopment of the capacity for abstraction and generalization was very marked in Vera. This was demonstrated especially clearly when her cognitive functions were tested. For instance, in an experiment in which she had to reject one unsuitable picture from four that were presented to her, she exhibited forms of reasoning based on dual situations. For example, she was shown pictures illustrating a table, a hen, a cock, and a duck. She rejected as unsuitable the picture of the cock, her argument being that the cock was colored black and yellow. On making a second attempt to solve this problem, she rejected as unsuitable the picture of the table, giving the explanation, "The table does not fit because it stands in a room." When given pictures representing a duck, a carrot, a cabbage, and an onion, the girl rejected as unsuitable the picture of the duck, justifying her choice by the fact that the duck swims in the water but all the others are green.

The girl was thus unable to select an unsuitable picture on the basis of the generic concept, and she made her choice by irrelevant signs (i.e., color) or on a basis of dual concrete connections (the duck swims in the water).

After a detailed explanation, she was asked to classify pictures. In spite of the explanations which she had received, she arranged the pictures into groups, working on the quantitative principle, i.e., with four pictures in each group. This was nothing more than a stereotype, established during the performance of the previous task. This stereotyped connection was extinguished by means of prolonged explanation, and the girl then began to arrange the pictures singly, which may be regarded as the restoration of another old connection (before the experiment on classification of pictures the girl was shown pictures representing separate objects). Attempts followed to classify pictures on the basis of color, so that she grouped the picture of a fox with that of a carrot. The selection of individual objects in terms of color was also converted into stereotyped activity, which was very stable. The experimenter's attempt to put all the vegetables together met with a sharp protest from the girl, who declared that this was impossible because the cabbage is green and the carrot yellow.

When the task presented to the girl was simplified and she was asked to choose pictures representing animals, kitchen utensils, or clothes (i.e., in this experiment the examiner relied on categories learned by the girl), she did this correctly.

When the experiment was repeated eight days later, considerable difficulty again arose, connected with the presence of indirect verbal stereotypes. At the beginning of the experiment, for instance, Vera used the categories which she had learned, and grouped together pictures representing animals, vegetables, and kitchen utensils, but she only put four pictures in each group, i.e., the performance of the task was hindered by the inert stereotyped connection from the previous experiment, in which she had to reject the fourth superfluous picture. Later on she again began to classify pictures by color, and thus she grouped together pictures representing a cow, a pencil box, and a table. This classification by color, however, was interwoven and supplemented with concrete objects grouped in pairs. For example, the pencil box, calendar, jug, and overcoat were grouped together by the girl because all these objects are found in a room.

It is clear that in the course of the experiment concerned with classification of pictures, Vera displayed a very obvious maldevelopment of her capacity to abstract and generalize, together with inertia of connections once established in her verbal system.

The maldevelopment of Vera's cognitive functions was also revealed in her understanding of passages from books. She could remember an easy story that was read to her, and could tell what it was about almost word for word, but she was quite unable to understand the meaning of the story and to reach the appropriate conclusion. We presented her with a passage from the story "What Did Serezha Think?"

"Serezha lived in a big house with his mother. The others who lived in the house were Tanya, Vera, and Misha, with their mother and father, and an old woman called Irina Petrovna. The old woman often told stories to the children. The children enjoyed listening to her very much. One morning the old woman said to the other people living in the house, 'I felt ill this morning and I have only just got up. My room is not tidied, my dishes are not washed and I must go to the doctor.' The old woman went off to see the doctor, and Serezha ran to the other children and said, 'Tanya, Misha, Vera, come quickly, I have thought of something. There is something that we must all do.' Question: 'What did Serezha think?"

Vera listened attentively to the story and correctly described what it was about but she was unable to establish the necessary bond of meaning between the old woman's words and the decision made by Serezha. She confused elements of her own experience with individual fragments of the story and replied that Serezha decided to tidy the room because the room needed tidying, and she tidied the room at home every day.

The story "Medicine" was next read to Vera. "Tanya's mother fell ill. The doctor prescribed some nasty medicine for her. The little girl saw that her mother had trouble drinking it, and said to her, 'Give it to me, mother, and I will drink the medicine for you.'"

In reply to the question whether Tanya did right, Vera confused elements of her own experience with individual fragments of the story read to her, and said, "The medicine should have been drunk by the old woman, because she was old."

Vera grasped the meaning of story-pictures with great difficulty and could not arrange them in any related order. In a simple series she was able to establish the necessary connection between the pictures, but before this connection had been established, she went through a ritual of enumeration of individual objects. If the task was made slightly more complicated she was unable to cope with it. She regarded each picture as a finished episode. She correctly described what was represented on each separate picture, but was quite incapable of establishing the necessary connection between pictures joined together by the development of a common story line.

Despite this low level of development of cognitive functions, Vera learned to read and write and to do elementary counting. She read correctly but without adequate expression, because she had a poor understanding of the meaning of what she read. She read Oseeva's story "The Sons," but could not understand its meaning. The girl read purely mechanically, without following the sense at all: for example, when she read a page ending with the first syllable of a word, she did not proceed to the next page but declared that she had finished the story.

She learned to write with great difficulty and very slowly. The girl experienced no particular difficulty in the analysis of sounds and letters, but the most difficult part of writing for her was to understand the rules of grammar and to be able to apply them, although by virtue of her ability to take great pains, she ultimately mastered this difficulty too.

In the course of her education, Vera experienced special difficulty in learning to count. Nevertheless she successfully solved complicated arithmetical problems by herself, memorized her multiplication table well, and could do mental sums. She performed each task presented to her with great attentiveness and concentration. Division with remainder was a difficult challenge for Vera. She had to have additional tutoring to explain this work. She worked each problem many times before she got the correct answer. In the course of this work Vera often sought the teacher's help. She had the same sort of difficulty when dividing two-digit numbers by two-digit numbers. This was taught by the tedious method of splitting the operation up into component elements. Whereas many of the other pupils in the class, as they became proficient in a particular part of the syllabus, changed from long to shorter methods of solution of the problems, Vera continued to employ mainly the long and laborious methods of solution.

For example, when she was asked to divide 75 by 15, she divided the number of tens of the dividend by the number of tens of the divisor ($70 \div 10 = 7$). She multiplied the result by 15. She carried out multiplication in the same way: $7 \times 10 = 70$; $7 \times 5 = 35$; $35 + 70 = 105$. She compared the number which she had obtained for a long time with the dividend, and only after considerable reflection was she convinced that the quotient was incorrect. She then took another quotient (6) and again solved the problem with the same long method. The number 90 which she obtained was compared with the dividend, and again she was convinced that the wrong quotient had been taken. After these two tests she took the number 5 and again repeated the whole cumbersome operation to solve the problem, to be convinced after trial that she had again chosen the wrong number.

This form of solution, which she used each time with unusual thoroughness and punctiliousness, enabled the child to master this part of the syllabus.

In the course of her education, Vera was asked to count "in her head." This is usually done badly by the group of oligophrenic children who have a poor capacity for work. Vera performed this task without a single mistake. For example, she subtracted from 50 by three's mentally, and after each operation she repeated aloud the number remaining. After carrying out this problem, she was given one rather more complicated: to subtract mentally from 100 by eighteens. She performed this task too without a single mistake.

On each occasion she would mentally repeat the same roundabout operations, which caused her to take a considerable time for the solution of the problem. For example, she subtracted 18 from 46 as follows: 46 - 6 = 40; 40 - 10 = 30; 30 - 2 = 28. She used this type of solution every time. Before replying, Vera checked herself. All these examples reveal her relatively high level of diligence in regard to her work, which was a conspicuous characteristic of this girl.

Vera experienced great difficulty in the solution of arithmetical problems. She could not correlate the method of formulation of the problem with the numerical data or the nomenclature.

When she was a pupil in the fourth class of the special school, she could solve by herself the simplest problem by the method of easy stages. For example, she was asked the following problem. "Three girls each found 5 flowers. How many flowers did they find altogether?" She gave the correct answer, "All the girls found 15 flowers."

She reached a solution in the following way. "The first girl found 5 flowers, the second girl found 5 flowers, and the third girl found 5 flowers: 5 + 5 + 5 = 15." When she was asked if this problem could be solved in another way, of her own accord she changed the arithmetical operation and solved it by multiplying 5 by 3.

More complicated problems were beyond her capacity. When, for example, she was asked to formulate a problem to incorporate the following: "Two boys each caught two fishes and two girls each caught four fishes," she was unable to do so. When the experimenter formulated the problem asking Vera for the total number of fishes caught, she solved it as follows: 2 × 2 = 4; 4 × 4 = 16. The girl substituted two arithmetical operations for the solution of the problem, the second being a stereotype of the first.

The same problem was presented to her a second time, but in a very concrete form. But even posing the problem in its most concrete terms did not enable Vera to solve the problem, and she again repeated exactly the same method of solution that she had previously used. It may thus be seen that methods of counting which she had studied and learned by heart enabled her to solve arithmetical problems correctly, but in every case in which the girl had to incorporate additional methods, in which a bond of reasoning had to be established between the separate elements of the problem, she was unable to master the problem.

Principal Stages of the Child's Development. Three stages can be distinguished in the girl's development. The first stage covers the period before her organized education began. From an analysis of this stage of the girl's development it follows that emotional-volitional disturbances were absent. Vera was attentive, quiet, diligent, and orderly in her behavior. At the same time she showed gross maldevelopment of her cognitive functions.

The second stage in her development began with the time she first went to the regular school. At this period, because of difficulties in her lessons at school, the girl developed a number of secondary symptoms in the form of irritability, an increased tendency to fatigue, and headaches. Education in the ordinary school was found to be beyond her capacity. In view of her attentiveness and diligence, however, while still at the ordinary school Vera mastered the rudiments of reading and writing, and she was accepted for the second class at the special school.

The third stage began with the girl's admission to the special school. She had to be left back for a repeat year in the second, third, and fourth classes, because she could not learn to count, could not understand what she had read, and could not cope with the solution of arithmetical problems. Over the whole period of her education, however, a considerable shift took place in her development. The most obvious development involved her emotional-volitional function. She developed a good attitude towards the work she had to do and an interest in doing it. She learned to overcome her difficulties and to take a responsible attitude towards work. Progress in her analytico-synthetic activity within the limits of individual analyzers took place at a slower rate than the development of her emotional-volitional function. The child's capacity for abstraction and generalization developed especially slowly.

Clinical Analysis of the Case

There are grounds in this case for assuming that the disturbance of early development is associated with trauma at birth, resulting from the transverse position of the fetus. The laterally compressed skull and the prominent frontal tuberosities are a sign that the head was compressed during labor, which may have been followed by multiple hemorrhages on the convex surface of the cerebral cortex.

The fit with the transient loss of consciousness from which the girl suffered at the age of $1^1/_2$ years appeared to be the reaction of a defective brain to a physical disease of unknown etiology.

The fundamental etiological factor was thus a natural lesion of the central nervous system, and the fundamental pathogenic factor was multiple hemorrhages on the convex surface of both cerebral hemispheres. The clinical picture is mainly determined by the pathogenesis. We may attempt to show how the pathogenic factors which we have mentioned above may be revealed in the clinical picture.

The neurological findings confirm the correctness of our hypothesis regarding the mainly cortical character of the lesion in this case. This is demonstrated by the complete integrity of the movements of the tongue, unaccompanied by associated movements, whereas movements of the upper facial muscles also provoked movements of the lower facial muscles. The presence of reflexes of oral automatism (sucking, labial, palm-chin reflexes) also indicate a lesion of both hemispheres. The very circumscribed residual paresis (weakness of the right upper limb distally), the innervation disturbances of tone and the bilateral Mayer's sign in turn suggest that the lesion was cortical in character.

In this particular case, against the background of a diffuse lesion, clear evidence was present of a right-sided symptomatology: the tongue deviated to the right, the right nasolabial fold was ill-defined, weakness of the distal part of the right upper limb was present, the innervation disturbances of tone were more severe on the right, the left hemisphere was more severely affected. We consider this fact to be highly significant, for in diffuse lesions of the cerebral cortex in oligophrenia the left hemisphere is found to be more often more severely involved.

The electroencephalogram, taken in a state of relative rest, also demonstrated a diffuse lesion of the brain.

Let us try to understand the structural pattern of the defect in our patient in terms of the pathogenic factors. The fundamental, predominant and definitive feature of the structure of the defect in this case was the inadequacy of her cognitive function, as shown by maldevelopment of her capacity for abstraction and generalization. The early but not gross, diffuse lesion of the cortex of both hemispheres inevitably led to a disturbance of the whole of the girl's higher nervous activity, and especially of the mobility of her fundamental nervous processes, which was clearly revealed during the experimental investigation of her higher nervous activity. In the clinical picture we also detected inertia of connections once formed, especially in the verbal system.

The disturbance of the mobility of the nervous processes, developing from earliest childhood, played a particularly important role in the maldevelopment of the second signal system, and led to the maldevelopment of the generalizing function of words and, subsequently, to maldevelopment of the whole cognitive function. The structure of Vera's defect was distinguished, however, by the fact that a low level of development of the cognitive function was combined with relatively intact emotional-volitional function. From her earliest childhood Vera showed no difficulties in behavior. She was quiet, attentive and did as she was told by her elders. When at school the girl took an interest in her lessons. She was able to surmount obstacles, was diligent and painstaking and tried to complete tasks given to her. She had an appropriate attitude towards the teacher's opinion of her.

The absence of disturbances in the subcortical formations and the relative integrity of the subcortical-cortical connections account for the relatively adequate level of development of emotional-volitional functions in this case. The qualitative aspects of the structure of the defect were also determined by the fact that Vera had no gross disturbances within the limits of a particular analyzer, as a result of which, in spite of the severe maldevelopment of her cognitive function, she was able to acquire the skill to read, write, and count relatively easily and confidently. The relatively intact motor function was to a large extent responsible for the girl's subsequent productivity when at work.

The pattern of the structure of the defect, like the integrity in the emotional-volitional function, was also connected with the pathogenic features of this case. The presence of a diffuse but superficial cortical lesion leads to the fact that the clinical picture of the oligophrenia is determined purely by the leading manifestation, i.e., by maldevelopment of the capacity for abstraction and generalization.

An essential factor which determined the nature of the structure of the defect in this particular case was the fact that the girl retained the will to work. Vera hardly ever showed signs of fatigue in the course of her activities at school. She always had an air of efficiency, and for that reason her writing never contained mistakes as a result of inattentiveness (missing letters, syllables, or words). She learned by heart the rules of grammar, retained them in her memory and knew how to use them. The girl's capacity for work played a most important part in her education.

The physiological basis for the ability to work satisfactorily is the adequate strength of the fundamental nervous processes and the relatively normal balance between excitation and inhibition, as has been experimentally confirmed. In order to understand the relative integrity of working capacity in this case, the results of the electroencephalographic studies are of particular interest. The application of a functional load (rhythmic light stimuli) revealed a lowered level of functional mobility of the cortex, as shown by the ill-defined modification of the rhythm in response to high-frequency flashes of light. However, the satisfactory degree of modification of the cortical rhythm with average flicker frequencies, the absence of modification at low frequencies and the normal duration of the reactions give reason to believe that in this case no gross disturbances of the cortical neurodynamics were present.

The early lesion of the cerebral cortex, leading to maldevelopment of the cognitive function, forms a basis for the diagnosis of oligophrenia. The qualitative features of the structure of the defect were determined by the association of a gross maldevelopment of the cognitive function with a relatively less severe disturbance in the emotional-volitional function, combined with a high capacity for work, in the absence of any gross focal disturbances of the individual analyzers.

In this case of oligophrenia we are therefore dealing with a diffuse lesion of the cerebral cortex with no gross focal manifestations. An important pathogenic consideration is the presence of normal cerebrospinal fluid dynamics and normal cerebrovascular system in the late residual stage.

The structure of the defect was determined qualitatively by the fundamental leading manifestation of oligophrenia: maldevelopment of the capacity for abstraction and generalization with preservation of relatively intact emotional-volitional function, in the absence of focal gross defects within the limits of individual analyzers. In view of the foregoing details, this case may be classified with our primary or basic type of oligophrenia.

CASE 3

Tanya A., aged 14 years. This girl is a pupil at a special school. There were no abnormal hereditary factors.

History. The mother of this girl had six pregnancies. Three children are healthy. Two children died at an early age from various infectious diseases. The subject of this report was the product of the sixth pregnancy during the difficult conditions prevailing in 1941. Delivery took place at term. From an early age the child showed severe dystrophy and considerable retardation of development. Because of the dystrophy, Tanya was sent to a special sanatorium, where she spent two years and from which she returned in good physical health, but with grossly retarded mental development. She could not walk or talk before the age of $3^1/_2$ years, and was very lethargic and apathetic, hardly reacting at all to the environment. From three to five years of age, Tanya remained in the special sanatorium for dystrophic children. After her discharge from the sanatorium, i.e., at the age of five years, a considerable change was seen in her development. During the period from five to seven years she learned to speak well, to play eagerly with other children, and to develop an interest in toys. Tanya was easily taught to keep herself tidy and she did as she was told by her elders. At eight years of age, Tanya attended regular school. She attended classes eagerly, and was attentive, neat, and diligent. From the beginning Tanya had a great deal of difficulty with her school lessons. She remained behind for a second year in the first class. After two years of education in the ordinary school, Tanya was transferred to the second class at a special school.

Physical State. The girl's physical development was normal for her age. The head circumference was 52 cm. There was no abnormality of the internal organs.

State of the Nervous System. The pupils reacted briskly. A slight deviation of the tongue to the right was observed and the left upper limb was very slightly weaker than the right. The toes of the left foot moved less freely. She could not hop. Muscle tone was normal. During physical effort she complained of pain, and the big toe of both feet adopted a position of extension. The tendon reflexes were brisk but with no pathological features. The abdominal and plantar reflexes were brisk and equal.

Ophthalmological Examination. Acuity of vision of both eyes 1.0. Optic fundus normal.

Otorhinolaryngological Examination. Hearing within normal limits.

X-ray Examination of the Skull. Shape of the skull rather oxycephalic. Pattern of the inner table of the skull obliterated. Ill-defined decalcification along the course of the coronary and lambdoid sutures. Vascular shadows slightly intensified.

Electroencephalography. A clearly defined but irregular α-rhythm was recorded in the posterior regions of the cortex (especially in the occipital regions). Slow waves (4-6 per second) were recorded in all areas of the cortex, and were especially pronounced in the parietal regions (Fig. 16).

The application of a rhythmic light stimulus caused no modification of the cortical rhythm in this girl. The addition of tactile stimulation of the same frequency to the light stimulus, however, led to the appearance of a fairly clear modification (Fig. 17).

Investigation of the Higher Nervous Activity. The motor reactions in response to a direct, spoken order were well stabilized. Superfluous movements of a perseverative character were observed. Simple positive conditioned connections were quickly established. Primary generalization extended only to the stimuli closest to the positive signal. Simple differentiation was also quickly established. The connections when established were stable; extrastimuli had only an insignificant influence on them (and mainly at the beginning of the investigation of the child).

The conditioned meaning of the positive and inhibitory stimuli was readily and quickly reversed; under these circumstances no sign of the preponderance of one nervous process over the other was observed.

The girl gave full and developed verbal accounts of the establishment and modification of simple connections, and reacted adequately to the verbal equivalents of direct stimuli. More complex forms of differentiation were produced much more quickly in Tanya than in other oligophrenic children, although in the course of formation of newer and newer complex conditioned connections, the process was slowed, adequate verbal accounts appeared after a delay, and were finally supplanted by the repetition of the inert verbal stereotypes established in the child during the previous experiments in which simpler connections were formed.

Inertia of the verbal connections appeared especially prominently if the establishment of the new complex system of connections began after considerable consolidation of the preceding system of conditioned reaction and differentiation. Disturbances of delayed inhibition were observed. During preliminary instruction, all connections were formed easily.

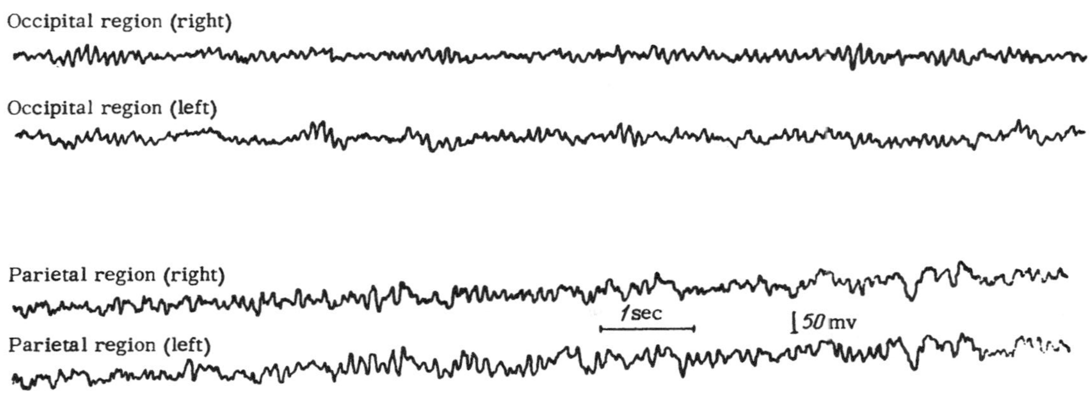

Fig. 16. Tanya A., aged 14 years, pupil at a special school (oligophrenia, feeble-minded degree). The EEG shows that a relatively well marked α-rhythm is recorded in the occipital regions of the cortex. In the parietal regions the α-rhythm is combined with slow waves of low amplitude.

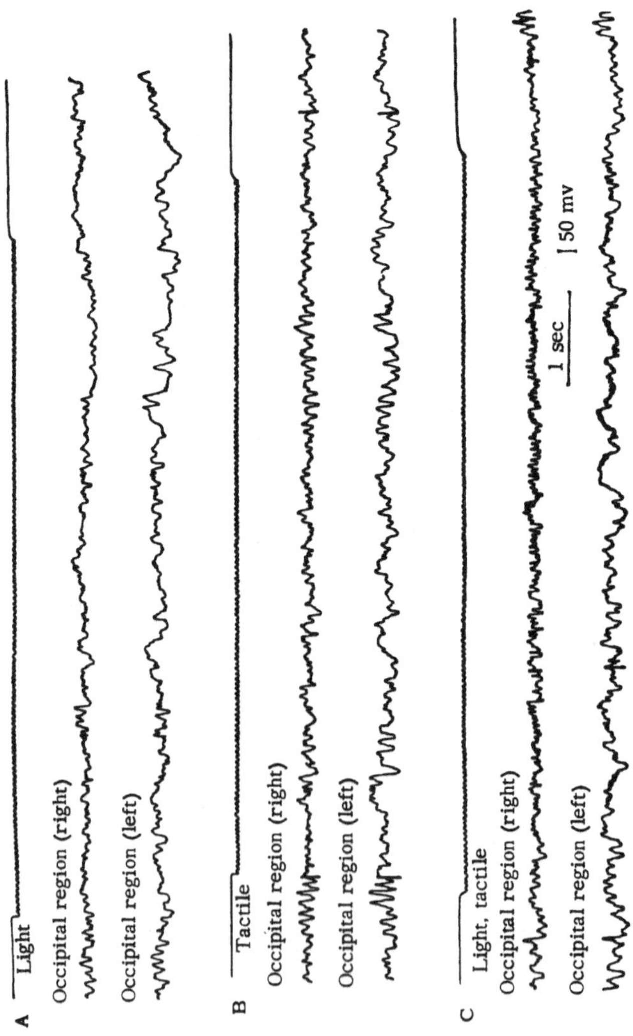

Fig. 17. EEG (of the same subject) during the application of a rhythmic light stimulus. A) Stimulation with flashes of light with a frequency of 18 per second causes no modification of the cortical rhythm. B) A tactile stimulus of the same frequency also causes no modification. C) Synchronous light and tactile stimuli induce definite modification. Frequency of stimulation as before.

All these findings thus indicate that in the presence of pathological inertia, manifested to the greatest extent in the verbal system, and with some degree of weakening of active inhibition (which was shown only during the formation of complex differentiation), the girl's higher nervous activity was characterized by a relatively high concentration of the nervous processes and by the absence of any pathological preponderance of one of them.

Mental State

Visual Analyzer. We examined the girl twice. At the end of the second year of instruction, Tanya correctly recognized pictures shown to her representing individual objects. She gave her answers with a minimum of delay, and she never gave impulsive, hasty or rash replies. On re-examination (in the fourth year of education) she showed no difficulty in recognizing pictures presented upside down, outline drawings, or crossed-out figures.

Spatial Orientation. Tanya was well oriented in space. She had the notion of right and left. She copied figures made with sticks correctly at her initial examination, but if the task was made more complicated, considerable difficulties ensued. At the next investigation Tanya could also manage to do the more complicated problems.

Motor and Motor-Speech Analyzers. No difficulty was discovered during investigation of postural movements. Isolated tests of dynamic movements were accomplished with difficulty. Oral praxis was not affected. Her sentences were complete and grammatically correct. The girl showed some indistinctness in the pronunciation of sibilants (only at the first investigation), but when she was investigated in the fourth year of her education her pronunciation was correct.

Phonemic Hearing. The girl's understanding of speech was not disturbed. Tanya repeated correlated phonemes well, even when the range of the task was considerably extended. The fact that Tanya mastered her initial elementary reading and writing comparatively easily in the regular school showed that her speech function was preserved.

Investigation showed the absence of localized cortical disturbances in the performance of tasks requiring the participation of any particular analyzer.

Cognitive Function and Behavior. From the first days of her study at the school Tanya was well disciplined, diligent, and eagerly carried out the duties given to her by the teacher. In the second year at school the girl showed an obviously appreciative attitude towards the high regard paid by the teacher for her successes, and even elements of a critical attitude towards the work which she did.

Tanya's emotional function was intact. She was very attached to her mother, paid heed to her opinions, and helped her. Tanya was upset if she overheard the teacher remark to her mother on some of her failings. Tanya showed considerable discrimination in her attitude towards other children. With some she was friendly, some she helped, and others she was sorry for. She often gave her school books to children who had none, and went to the boy next door to use his books to prepare her lessons.

Among Tanya's good qualities was her ability to help the more backward pupils under the guidance of the teacher. For example, she looked after the little girl K., and helped her to prepare her lessons. She did this systematically, patiently and without being reminded.

During her education and training, Tanya learned to behave in a cultured manner: she greeted her elders, was always ready to oblige them, and her conduct was always most orderly. When strangers visited the class, Tanya was not only the best behaved girl but an example for the rest of the children to follow. Of her own initiative she found the teacher's telephone number and called him when he was ill to find out how he was, and then excused herself for having troubled him. After her third year of education at the special school, Tanya showed herself very adaptable in practical matters and possessed of a great deal of independence. She made quite long trips about Moscow on complicated errands (for example, buying provisions in shops). However, although essentially a well-disciplined, quiet, and attentive girl, she sometimes behaved improperly. Tanya was persistent and active, and in all circumstances tried meticulously to carry out the job she had been given. According to the school rules no child is allowed in the classroom during recess. If any child came into the classroom when Tanya was on duty, then without turning to the teacher for help, she would herself reprimand the offender. Though the teacher reminded her that this course of action was wrong, this usually had no effect on Tanya's behavior.

From time to time the teacher asked Tanya to take certain articles back to the apparatus room. The girl eagerly took the articles as requested back to the room where they belonged. Soon she came back and explained to the teacher that only the technician was there, and so she had brought the articles back. It did not occur to her to leave the articles and to look for the person in charge of the apparatus room. A very detailed analysis of all her behavior was necessary before Tanya could carry out this particular errand.

It will be seen from the examples given that the girl's inability to grasp a situation and to change her behavior to meet changing circumstances led to behavioral disturbances. It is clear from the observation that the girl found it very difficult to extricate herself from a complicated situation. Occasionally it was Tanya's turn to be on duty, but she did not carry out all her obligations. The teacher decided to test how far Tanya would understand an indirect approach. On Tanya's duty day, and in Tanya's presence, therefore, the teacher suggested to the class that they choose another girl, hoping that Tanya would realize why her chores were relinquished to another. However, Tanya could not see any connection between the fact that the teacher had chosen another girl to tidy the classroom and the fact that she had failed to carry out her duties on the previous day. Only when the teacher pointed out her mistake directly did Tanya react in an appropriate manner.

Thus in every case when the girl understood the situation she behaved properly, but when the situation became more complicated mistakes appeared in her conduct, as a result of the maldevelopment of her cognitive functions and the inertia of her mental processes. She could not change her mode of reaction to meet a changing situation.

The maldevelopment of her capacity for abstraction and generalization showed itself clearly in the girl's cognitive function. For instance, in the experiment on the classification of pictures, Tanya used the categories she had learned by heart. She could correctly arrange the pictures in separate groups (furniture, clothes, animals), but if she was asked to extend the groups, then concrete situational forms of reasoning became dominant. She grouped the picture representing a table with pictures of a candy, a ball, a pair of scissors, or an inkstand, only because all these objects could lie on a table. Or else she grouped together pictures representing wild animals with pictures of trees and flowers, because animals live in the woods where trees and flowers grow.

Characteristic difficulties appeared in her understanding of passages from stories. When a story was read to her she remembered it, could say what it was about, and could even draw suitable conclusions. If the task was made rather more difficult, however, Tanya was unable to cope with it.

This was demonstrated when the following story was read to her. "Tanya's mother was ill. The doctor prescribed a nasty medicine for the patient. The girl saw that the mother had difficulty drinking it, and said, "Mother, let me drink the medicine for you."

In reply to the question whether the girl did the right thing, she replied that the girl was wrong, because only her mother should drink the medicine and the girl might become ill if she drank medicine that was not for her.

Tanya understood picture-stories and, if they were easy, could arrange them in proper order. If the task was made more difficult, she could say correctly what each picture showed separately, but she found it difficult to establish a connection between pictures having a common theme.

Tanya did not experience any undue difficulty in mastering elementary reading and writing. When she entered the second class of the special school she had some skill in reading, writing, and counting. During her period of education at the special school Tanya was quite capable of coping with the syllabus. The girl made mistakes in writing because of her inability to make use of the rules of grammar, but gradually she mastered the various items in the curriculum. When writing by dictation or by copying Tanya made no mistakes, omissions, or transpositions; the girl was able to check the work she had done and to note and correct any errors. She read fluently and expressively, although she did not always understand the meaning of what she had read. She learned poetry by heart comparatively easily and remembered it for a long time.

The girl experienced considerable difficulty in mastering various arithmetical operations. Nevertheless, her thoroughness in carrying out particular tasks and the plan of solving arithmetical problems by easy stages, with her knowledge of the multiplication table—all these factors taken together enabled Tanya to master arithmetical operations up to the standard of the syllabus. She found the solution of arithmetical problems particularly difficult. She had a poor grasp of the conditions of the problem and was unable to establish a rational connection between the verbal formulation of the task, the numbers and the names.

For example, she was given the following problem. "In the morning a pioneer fetches 25 pails of water, and in the evening even 18 pails more. How many pails of water does the pioneer fetch altogether?" This problem was discussed and solved in class. Tanya formulated the first part correctly, and chose the arithmetical operation to suit the formulation, i.e., to 25 pails she added 18 and obtained 43. The second part she formulated properly, but instead of adding 25 to 43 she subtracted it. This indicates that the girl had memorized the formulation of the problem, but did not understand the way in which the problem must be solved. In her answer she wrote that altogether the pioneer fetched 18 pails of water. The fact that the number 18 was the same as that given in the original problem did not mean anything to her at all, and she did not realize her mistake.

Principal Stages of the Child's Development. Four stages in the development of the child may be distinguished. The first stage covered the period before she went to school, and was characterized by severe retardation of development.

The second stage began shortly before school age, when she stayed for a long time in a sanatorium for dystrophic children and made considerable progress in her development. It was at this period that the comparatively rapid development of her motor and speech functions was observed. The girl began to show an interest in her surroundings: she played eagerly with other children. At eight years of age she began to attend the regular school.

The third stage in her development was during the period of her attendance at regular school. The most intensive development here took place in her analytical-synthetic activity, making it possible for her to master elementary reading and writing, and arithmetic. The pattern of her emotional-volitional functions also underwent considerable development. Side by side with the development of these good qualities, however, difficulties in the girl's education emerged.

The fourth stage in Tanya's development covered the period of her education at the special school. It was at this stage that her emotional-volitional functioning underwent special development. Tanya was well disciplined, efficient, attentive, painstaking, and critical of both herself and her surroundings. The level of general development of the child was very considerably raised.

Clinical Analysis of the Case

The fundamental etiological factor in this case was the severe, prolonged, and early dystrophy. The mild and mainly cortical neurological symptomatology, the changes in the electroencephalogram and the marked severity of the principal manifestation in the form of maldevelopment of the capacity for abstraction and generalization give grounds for regarding this as a case of oligophrenia.

The qualitative nature of the structure of the defect in this case also was determined by the association of maldevelopment of the cognitive functions with a relatively intact emotional development, combined with a high capacity for work and an absence of any gross disturbance in the function of individual analyzers.

The clinical analysis of this case reveals with great clarity the connection between the pathogenesis and the clinical picture. All the investigations that were made point to the mild and mainly diffuse nature of the cortical lesion. The mild residual neurological manifestations, mainly cortical in character, the absence of gross changes when the action potentials of the brain were recorded in a state of relative rest, and the absence of modification of the cortical rhythms by high-frequency flashes of light indicate a low level of functional mobility of the cortical neurones.

Investigation of the higher nervous activity showed a disturbance of the mobility of the nervous processes with relative integrity of both the strength of the fundamental nervous processes and the balance between excitation and inhibition. The clinical picture, which was characterized by the presence of the principal symptom only, i.e., oligophrenic mental deficiency, corresponded to these pathogenetic features.

Analysis of the principal stages of this girl's development also confirmed that the understanding of the pathogenic features of the first variant of disability in oligophrenia was correct. The absence of primary disturbances in the subcortical formations ensured an adequate level of development in the girl's emotional-volitional function as a result of proper corrective training. The absence of any gross defects in individual cortical functions enabled the girl to develop various skills and to be capable of elementary reading and writing even at the ordinary school level of instruction. The most persistent feature of the case, however, was the maldevelopment of the cognitive function.

Taken as a whole, the clinical analysis given above gives grounds for regarding this case as a first variant of oligophrenia.

In addition to pupils at special schools, we also examined a group of oligophrenic individuals who had finished their training at special schools. Among these cases we found clear evidence of the fundamental form of oligophrenia.

CASE 4

Yura F., aged 24 years (male). After the successful completion of his training at the special school he worked in a furrier's workshop. His mother mentioned several of his good qualities. He was well disciplined, a good worker, and helped his mother look after the house.

History. This man's mother was twice pregnant. One child died at an early age from scarlet fever. The case under discussion was the child born of the second pregnancy. The course of the pregnancy was normal, but the child was born in severe and prolonged asphyxia. His early development was characterized by absence of any severe retardation. The boy's intellectual backwardness came to light during the year when he attended the ordinary school. There he was a disciplined pupil; however, from the first days of his attendance he had great difficulty with his lessons. After a year of unsuccessful education at the ordinary school, Yura was transferred to a special school.

Physical State. His physical development was normal for his age. No abnormality of the internal organs was found.

State of the Nervous System. Slight residual symptomatology. Right-sided hemisyndrome.

Ophthalmological Examination. Visual acuity of both eyes 1.0. Optic fundus normal.

Otorhinolaryngological Examination. Hearing within normal limits.

Electroencephalography. The α-rhythm was recorded only in the posterior regions of the cortex. In all regions of the cortex pathological slow waves were recorded. In the temporal regions of the cortex rapid variations of potential were predominant.

The EEG was suggestive of an ill-defined, diffuse lesion of the brain.

X-ray Examination of the Skull. Microcephaly. Base of the skull flattened. Bones of the vault thinner than normal. Cranial sutures ill defined. Pattern of the inner table of the skull obliterated. Shadows of the transverse and sagittal sinuses slightly intensified. Shadows of the Pacchionian bodies moderately intensified.

Investigation of the Higher Nervous Activity. Investigation of the higher nervous activity revealed: adequate strength of the fundamental nervous processes, which were well balanced and inert, especially so at the level of the second signal system.

Mental State

Visual Analyzer. Yura correctly recognized pictures shown to him, whether upside down or not, as well as crossed-out and outline figures.

Spatial Orientation. Yura was well orientated in space. He correctly copied figures made from sticks, and had no difficulty in this when the problems were made more complicated.

Motor and Motor-Speech Analyzers. No difficulties were discovered during the investigation of postural movements nor during the solution of a series of problems involving dynamic movements. Oral praxis was not disturbed. No disturbances were found in speech pronunciation.

Phonemic Hearing. His understanding of speech was complete. Yura repeated correlated phonemes correctly even when the scope of the problem was considerably extended.

This investigation demonstrated the absence of localized cortical disturbances during the performance of tasks involving the participation of any analyzer.

Cognitive Function and Behavior. Yura was subdued, confused, and constricted in a new situation. He had a well-developed attitude towards praise and reproach, and also to some extent towards his own failures. He reacted feebly to the difficulties arising in the course of the experimental investigations, which in turn lowered the quality of his replies. When performing isolated tasks he was efficient. Investigation of his cognitive functions showed considerable maldevelopment of his capacity for generalization and abstraction. During the classification of pictures he showed concrete-situational forms of reasoning. He grouped together pictures representing a briefcase and a table, his explanation being that the briefcase has to lie on a table. "Where else can it lie?" he added at this juncture.

When extending the groups, he arranged together pictures of a chair, a table, and an inkstand, explaining this action as follows. "These must all go together so that you can write. You cannot write with your finger or hand, and in order to write you have to sit on a chair and not on the floor. One table can be taken from another group, because only one table is necessary. The scissors must be placed on the table in order to cut the paper, and the key should be put here because you cannot cut paper with it."

He placed the goose, turkey, sucking-pig, and goat in the group of domestic animals. "The goat gives milk. The pig, if it is cut up, gives pork. But I don't know about the turkey, for I haven't seen many of them."

During an experiment on generalization based on verbal instruction, he was asked to arrange the pictures: 1) the dog helps the man, and 2) the dog looks after the puppies. The subject was asked not only to arrange the pictures into groups, but also to explain why he placed a particular picture in a particular group. This experiment showed that Yura was able to regulate his activity by verbal instruction and to analyze visual material correctly. When, however, he was presented with a task requiring a higher level of abstraction and generalization, verbal instruction did not serve to regulate his activity, but he turned to visual material, and was guided entirely by concrete-situational connections. These connections were of prime importance to him for both generalization and differentiation; for example, when adding the third picture (a hunter with his dog) to the fourth (a first-aid dog), he gave the explanation, "Close to the forest something may attack the hunter, for example a wolf, and the dog may save him because it is a first-aid dog. If the hunter is not badly wounded, the dog may bring a bandage and iodine."

In the experiment the subject has to remember words by means of pictures. In order to remember a word by a picture he must establish a rational connection between the word and the picture. In fact, he could cope with this task only in the simplest cases, and if it was made more complicated he could not solve the problem. For example, when the subject had to form a rational connection between the word "dinner" and the picture "fork," he was quite incapable of doing so ("You eat with a fork and not with your hands.").

During the determination of similarity and difference, the concrete nature and the inertia of the connections, once formed, were revealed. He read the story "The Four Wishes" (from "Our Mother Tongue" for Class 1) but completely failed to understand it in spite of the fact that he read certain passages over again and discussed them with the teacher. He understood metaphors literally. He said that you could say "golden head," but it was better to say "clever head," because no man could have a head of gold.

He understood proverbs equally literally. For example, he understood the proverb "Don't spit in the well, for it is drinking water" to mean "If you spit there, the water will be fouled. It is better to spit near the well, or even further away."

His defective capacity for generalization and abstraction was clearly apparent when he tackled arithmetical problems. It was not easy to show or help him. After being shown many times how to do a simple problem, he would usually solve it only with the aid of the experimenter.

Clinical Analysis of the Case

All the data which we have presented, namely the abnormal development, severe disturbances of cognitive functions, slight residual right-sided neurological symptoms, EEG findings indicating an ill-defined, diffuse lesion of the brain represented by slow waves over the entire cortex, — all these provide justification for the diagnosis of oligophrenia in this case. The structure of the defect is determined qualitatively by the general diffuse cortical pathology, without any gross focal disturbance of any particular analyzer. The investigation of the conditioned reflex activity revealed no gross changes in balance between the fundamental nervous processes.

Yura's behavior was not particularly abnormal: he was well disciplined, orderly, hard working within the limits of his capabilities, and critical of himself and of his environment.

The dominant and decisive manifestation of the defect in this case was maldevelopment of the capacity for abstraction and generalization. The experimental investigations of the cognitive processes described above, and the analysis of the basic elements of his scholastic activity (reading, writing, problems) show that the difficulties in his mastering of school tasks resulted from the inadequate development of his cognitive functions.

Qualitative differences in the structure of the defect in this subject were revealed at the various stages of development. In the earlier stages of his education the principal difficulty was that Yura had an insufficient grasp of the subjects on account of the general mental retardation. At later stages of his education, when Yura was reasonably efficient and rational and normal in his behavior, the same difficulties still appeared in abstraction and generalization.

Investigation of Yura at this stage, during organized work, still showed with great clarity that our decision to regard him as belonging to the primary type of oligophrenia was correct. Because of his ability and desire to do useful work and the absence of any gross disturbance of behavior and character it is perfectly possible for him to be placed in productive employment.

ANALYSIS OF ALL THE RESULTS OBTAINED

Special Features of Early Development. A characteristic feature of any form of oligophrenia is the disturbance of mental development at the very earliest stages of life of the child. A specific feature of the children of this particular group is the relatively late manifestation of their defective development. At the nursery age, for instance, those in contact with the child did not notice his defect. In the nursery behavior was normal. There were no complaints from the kindergarten regarding the behavior of these children, although the supervisors observed that their general mental development was defective. Most of the children of this group, in whom the defect was not of a gross degree, before being admitted to the special school had spent from one to four years in the ordinary school, where again there were no complaints about their behavior. They were orderly in their conduct, persistent and purposeful in the performance of their various duties. The chief difficulty in their education was due to the poor grasp that these children had of problems presented to them.

X-ray Examination of the Skull. Qualitative analysis of the findings described on previous pages shows that a specific feature of the pathogenesis of this particular variant of oligophrenia is a diffuse, and mainly superficial lesion of the cerebral cortex, without involvement of the subcortical formations and without any disorder of the cerebrospinal fluid system in the chronic or residual stage of the disease. This unique feature of the pathogenesis has been confirmed by a series of investigations. The results of X-ray examination of the skull in children of this group clearly indicate a series of changes brought about by the persisting early lesions of the central nervous system. These features are as follows: changes in the dimensions of the skull, obliteration of the pattern, and flattening of the base of the skull. In a number of cases the cranial sutures can hardly be distinguished, but condensation or even calcification of the sutures is seen, especially in the coronary suture.

On X-ray examination of the skull of children with this variant of the defect, certain other distinctive features are seen. In these cases we do not observe the digital impressions so characteristic of the type of case where cerebrospinal fluid disturbances are much in evidence. The absence of disturbances of the cerebrospinal fluid dynamics was demonstrated during the investigation of two pupils from a special school who were admitted to the Institute of Neurosurgery because of naso-orbital herniation. These children were given a comprehensive investigation. So far as the qualitative structural pattern of their defect was concerned, these children belonged to the primary group or type. They were successful pupils in their special school, whose maldevelopment of cognitive function was associated with a preservation of good working capacities and good emotional-volitional functioning in the absence of any gross focal disturbance of any particular analyzer.

Pneumoencephalography in these children showed no disturbance of cerebrospinal fluid dynamics. Comparison of X-ray and pneumoencephalographic findings with the clinical picture suggests that the absence of any disturbance of cerebrospinal fluid circulation has an important bearing on the peculiar mode of development of the higher nervous activity, and subsequently plays an important role in the clinical picture as a whole.

Neurological Investigation. The mainly diffuse nature of the cortical damage is also confirmed by the results of investigation of the nervous system. Neurological examination showed a mild, disseminated cortical symptomatology in the form of differential pareses and central type changes of muscle tone. In contrast to children with other types of mental defect, neurological examination of these children did not reveal any inconstancy of the individual neurological signs.

Investigation of the Electrical Activity of the Brain. The absence of gross changes in the cortical neurodynamics in this particular form of oligophrenia is also confirmed by the results of electroencephalographic investigations. Recordings of the electrical activity of the brain in a state of rest are characterized, in contrast to other variants of oligophrenic defect, by the relatively milder abnormalities of the electroencephalogram. By way of example we show a typical EEG (Fig. 18).

The electroencephalogram shows a clearly defined α-rhythm, periodically alternating with slow waves of low amplitude (delta-waves, indicating a more serious abnormality in the functional state of the brain, are absent in the EEG).

The unique qualitative features of this variant of mental defect are demonstrated especially clearly during recording of the electroencephalogram when a functional load was applied (rhythmic light stimuli). In contrast to the other group of oligophrenic children in whom EEG frequency changes were either not induced, or induced only in response to very low frequencies, in these subjects a relatively well-marked modification was recorded in response to frequencies of from 7 to 13 flashes of light per second, i.e., to frequencies not exceeding the frequency of the α-rhythm (Fig. 19).

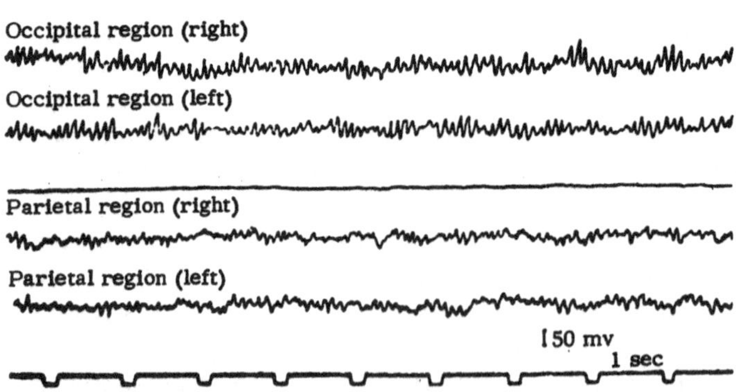

Fig. 18. Nina L., aged 14 years, a pupil at a special school. The EEG shows a well-marked α-rhythm; slow waves of low amplitude in the central areas of the cortex. Delta-waves absent.

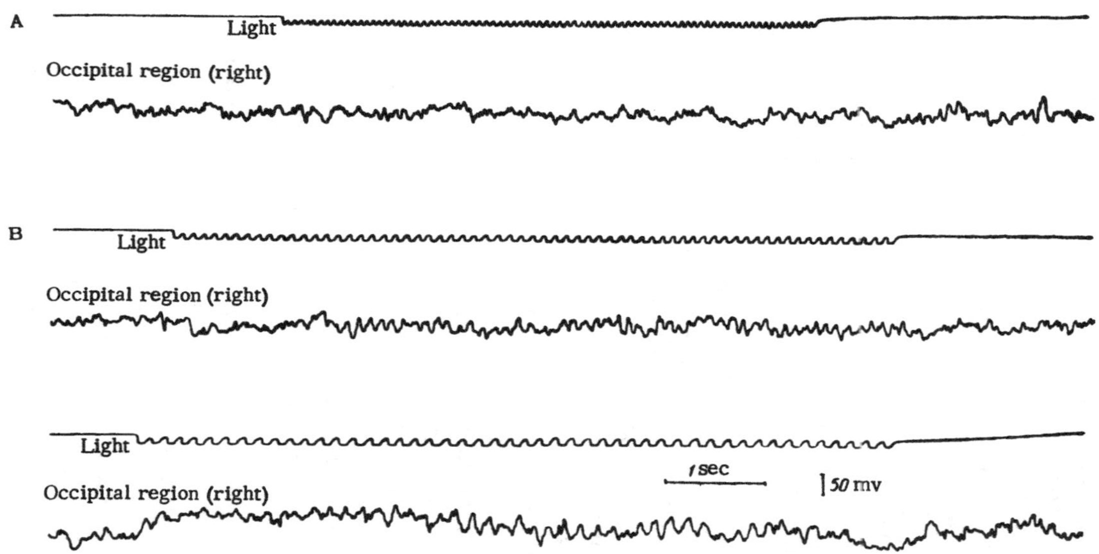

Fig. 19. EEG (of the same subject) during the application of a rhythmic light stimulus. A) Frequency of rhythmic stimulus 17 per second, no modification of the cortical rhythm is induced. B) Reduction in the frequency of stimulation to 8 per second leads to the appearance of a modified rhythm. A flicker frequency of 7 per second causes a relatively marked modification of the rhythm.

In all these cases the induced change of EEG frequency is fairly well defined and lasts for 6-7 seconds, i.e., it attains the normal duration. The induced frequency change and its normal duration together indicate that gross neurodynamic disturbances are absent in this form of oligophrenia.

An understanding of the special features of the higher nervous activity may thus be derived from the special pathogenetic features, i.e., the absence of gross changes in the cerebrospinal fluid and vascular systems.

Special Features of the Higher Nervous Activity. The investigation of the simple motor reaction to a direct verbal command shows certain special features in this group of children, distinguishing their reactions from those normally observed: primarily, superfluous movements of a perseverative character, appearing after the frequent repetition of the command, and also a retarded stabilization of the conditioned reactions.

It must be pointed out, however, that in contrast to oligophrenic children belonging to the other clinical variants, in the oligophrenics of this group the stabilization of the conditioned reactions is incomparably more marked and takes place relatively rapidly. The tonicity of the first motor reactions to a command is less well marked.

The formation of simple positive conditioned connections takes place readily in these children, mainly after one or two combinations. Simple differentiation is also produced rapidly. Generalization of new stimuli extends in most of these children only to stimuli addressed to that analyzer which receives the conditioned signal (in the mildest cases, only to those very similar in quality), and only in certain oligophrenics of this group is a wide generalization of stimuli observed beyond the limits of the analyzer to which the positive stimulus is addressed.

Simple positive and differential connections are very stable in these children, and are well maintained after removal of reinforcement, can be reproduced after considerable intervals of time, and are influenced only slightly by extrastimuli (external inhibition and disinhibition).

The children give an adequate verbal projection of these connections. The modification of the conditioned meaning of the stimuli takes place quickly and easily, and there are no signs of the preponderance of one or the other nervous modality.

More complicated forms of differentiation (by duration, by the alternation principle) are developed slowly, as in all oligophrenic children, which indicates some degree of weakening of active inhibition and, in particular, the inadequate participation of the verbal system in the formation of these connections. The latter factor is also confirmed by the gross disturbances of the verbal projection which are observed during the formation of these connections. The verbal projection in these cases consists merely of the reproduction of the inert verbal stereotypes formed in previous experiments. During the modification of complex connections, manifestations of inertia are also observed.

Systems of simple conditioned connections are readily formed in oligophrenics of this group by the method of preliminary instruction. When these have been formed they have the same qualitative characteristics as the connections formed in response to speech reinforcement. The manifestations of inertia were perhaps slightly more marked during modification of the connections induced through instruction. Relatively greater disturbances were observed during the formation of "conflict" connections by means of preliminary instruction, which indicated a weakness of the regulating function of the second signal system.

The results of the investigation of the higher nervous activity of the oligophrenic children of this group, taken as a whole, demonstrate that although pathological inertia and considerable disturbances of the interaction between the signal systems are present, there are no gross pathological changes in the relative strength of excitatory or inhibitory nervous processes of the kind which would lead to severe disturbances of equilibrium, and the concentration of the nervous processes is relatively well maintained.

Investigation of Individual Cortical Functions. The distinctive feature of the pathogenesis of this variant of the defect is shown clinically by the absence of gross focal cortical signs. The absence of a localized symptomatology is also confirmed by the results of electroencephalographic investigation. In no child belonging to this variant of the defect were foci of pathological activity discovered.

Investigation of the cortical functions reveals no gross deterioration in the children of this group. Their visual analysis and synthesis are preserved. They recognize actual objects presented to them, and also pictures of various objects shown to them even when shown upside down. They also recognize geometrical figures and crossed-out pictures. Difficulty in the recognition of pictures representing various objects when shown upside down, or broken-line drawings of objects was noted in the children of this group during the initial stages of their education or when a more severe degree of oligophrenia was present.

During the investigation of spatial orientation in these children, no gross abnormalities were noted. They have a proper understanding of "right" and "left" and they correctly copy figures made from sticks. They are well able to carry out such tasks as the arrangement of tiles into patterns. During the performance of all these tasks, the children are quite orderly and purposeful in their behavior, without being hasty or impulsive.

As a rule children with this variant of the defect have no gross localized lesions affecting the motor analyzer. During the investigation of postural movements these children do not experience any special difficulty. Some difficulties in the performance of isolated tasks relating to dynamic movements are due to inertia, resulting in awkwardness in switching from one movement to another. In the children of this group no focal disturbances are found in either the auditory or the motor-speech analyzers. They understand what people say to them, and they can construct elementary grammatically correct sentences. Only in the initial stages of education do these children appear to be speech-inhibited, a disability which is overcome in the process of education and training. The children can discriminate well between correlated sounds, and the widening of the scope of the problem does not detract from their performance, which distinguishes them sharply from the group of oligophrenic children who have severe disturbances of the cerebrospinal fluid and vascular systems (with widening of the scope of the problem these children usually slip into motor-speech stereotypes). Even when the defect is of a considerable degree of severity, as in our first case (Vitya I.), we found no dysfunction of the auditory analyzer. Without much difficulty the boy could discriminate between an individual sound and a whole word, or could select words beginning with a particular sound.

It was this preservation of elementary cortical analysis and synthesis that enabled the children in this group to master elementary reading and writing even when they received their education in regular classes.

Peculiarities of Cognitive Activities. The distinctive pathogenetic features of this condition lead in the course of development to characteristic pathophysiological changes and, as pointed out above, the parameter most affected is that of the mobility of the nervous processes. Inertia of the nervous processes, arising in the very earliest stages of development of the child, leads to disturbances in the formation of the complex functional systems which are specific for the activity of the cerebral hemispheres. This difficulty in the formation of complex functional systems subsequently leads to developmental disturbances in the abstracting and generalizing functions of speech.

The clinical picture of the defect in this first or primary group of oligophrenics in our classification is determined by one fundamental deficiency, which betrays itself when the child is presented with any task demanding a certain level of development of the generalizing and abstracting functions of speech. The severity of this developmental deficiency, as is clear from the clinical observations described above, may vary from case to case.

The more marked the defect the more clearly does this fundamental symptom emerge and with it the underlying distinctive pathophysiological features. Oligophrenic children do not grasp the significance of a task presented to them, and instead of solving it, they carry out some other form of activity, oversimplifying complex tasks by reducing them to some partial individual elements.

Oligophrenic children find difficulty in grasping the element of reasoning in any problem, and the fundamental symptom of oligophrenia is therefore demonstrated in these children no matter what investigation is carried out. While grasping the meaning of a picture-story, they find it difficult to establish a complex system of connections between the separate elements. They are unable to understand a passage from a story, especially in cases when they must independently reach a conclusion from what has been read to them, or when a story has a hidden meaning or a missing link. The inadequate level of development of generalization and abstraction is shown with special clarity when various forms of classification are attempted. Children belonging to this oligophrenic group seldom abandon their habit of thinking in terms of visual situations, and under these circumstances show a tendency to stereotypy.

The fundamental symptom in oligophrenia is based upon a distinctive disturbance in the interaction between the two signal systems. In the normal child not only are all forms of activity mediated through the joint activity of the two signal systems, but the verbal system, which plays a direct part in the creation, reinforcement and alteration of each connection, achieves the leading role in this process.

Through the operation of this verbal system, the creation and reinforcement of the connections take place quickly and do not require prolonged "learning by heart" and constant external reinforcement. As a result of this abstracting and generalizing function of speech, the connections that are formed become relatively independent of the direct afferent signal channels, and may even sometimes be formed in opposition to such signals.

Finally, the connections that are formed acquire exceptional mobility.

The facts obtained in the course of investigation show that the interaction between the two signal systems in children with this variant of the defect is characterized by certain quite distinctive features. As experimental research and clinical observation have shown, in this particular group of children simple forms of analytical-synthetic activity are performed with effective interaction between the two signal systems, and at this level of activity speech takes a fairly active part in the formation, reinforcement, and alteration of simple forms of differentiation. As the task is made increasingly complicated, however, a dissociation of the activity of the two signal systems occurs, and a firmly consolidated verbal stereotype can then be repeated for a long time through the secondary system of connections. At the level of complex analytical-synthetic activity, the verbal system of such a child loses its organizing function.

Experimental investigation of the interaction between the signal systems in oligophrenic children of this type thus showed with complete clarity the fundamental and leading manifestation of oligophrenia, namely maldevelopment of the capacity for abstraction and generalization.

Characteristics of the Emotional-Volitional Function. An essential feature of children showing this particular variant of the disability is the relative integrity of their emotional-volitional function. In no case did we find any indication of marked disturbances of behavior, of restlessness, irritability, or of lack of discipline.

In their observations, the supervisors of the kindergarten encountered no training difficulties and no improper behavior among these children. They were most attentive children. Stereotyped behavior patterns were created in them with particular ease. Their histories also demonstrated that their emotions were adequately developed (attachment to their families, kindness, affection). As regards their volitional characteristics, it must be mentioned that they were attentive, diligent, and painstaking. During their period of education in regular schools it was noticed that these children were attentive and that they behaved properly when they were in a situation which they understood. While attending special schools these children were also very orderly in their conduct. Analysis of the developmental trend in this group of children reveals considerable development in their emotional-volitional function. For instance, in the course of their education, not only do they develop an understanding of their situation and an appreciation of the teacher's opinion of them, as well as a certain critical attitude towards their own work and their prospects, but they also acquire a responsible attitude towards their obligations. Nevertheless, in spite of the integrity of their emotional-volitional function, the maldevelopment of their cognitive function leads to certain peculiarities in the behavior of the children of this group.

Although hardworking, active and diligent, they become difficult in any situation which appears conflicting and incomprehensible to them. They interpret all the teacher's instructions literally and carry them out equally literally. When the situation becomes complicated and they are compelled to abrogate or modify a decision which they have made, characteristic difficulties arise because of their failure to understand the situation. Often during lessons in class these children behave badly; being active and purposeful, they may keep up an endless chatter of questions during the lesson, and will not stop until they grasp the teacher's explanation. It is difficult and sometimes impossible to explain to such a child that he is disturbing everybody and behaving badly. If, for example, the teacher said to such a child, "If ever you don't understand something, don't hesitate to ask," this statement would be catastrophic for the child. It is for this reason that these hardworking, orderly, and purposeful children can under certain circumstances become difficult in their behavior. This feature is also explained by the inadequate mobility of their nervous processes, as a result of which they cannot alter their behavior to meet changing conditions.

Such a child, when on duty in the class, seeks to obtain absolute observance of all the rules from his classmates, and should any pupil run into the classroom during recess, the pupil on duty will try to put him out of the classroom without any regard for his strength, and may even start a fight with the offender. This does not happen because of the increased excitability and irritability of these children, but purely because the oligophrenic strives by every means in his power to observe the school rules. Thus in the absence of primary disturbances in the emotional-volitional function, as a result of the maldevelopment of their cognitive function, maldevelopment of all the more complex forms of behavior may arise secondarily in these children.

Characteristics of Motor Activity. Investigation of the motor activity of these children revealed no apparent deficiencies of the motor analyzer. The deficiencies of cognitive function, however, induced secondary effects in the organization of complex motor acts. The children showed no appreciable signs of general motor awkwardness nor of disturbances approximating apraxia: they easily and quickly learn to look after themselves, and they can quite skillfully perform an assortment of tasks requiring some degree of manual dexterity.

During the gymnastics and handicrafts periods they can follow instructions and work in an orderly and purposeful manner. Their movements are well under control and they can carry out a task consisting of three to eight elements in the correct order. Difficulties arise only when they are required to carry out movements in response to verbal commands without any accompanying demonstration.

These children experience special difficulty when required to perform complex groups of movements in a situation in which visual and verbal components stand in conflict with each other. During the period for rhythmic exercises, for example, the children are arranged opposite each other in pairs, and each member of the pair must perform movements of an opposite character. In every case which we investigated, such children could not follow verbal instructions but could only follow the movements of the control group.

Thus in spite of the preservation of their motor function, some maldevelopment of the generalizing function of speech is apparent in the organization of their movements. Any normal child given a similar task would first create the verbal connection "I must do the opposite." This verbal connection regulates his movements so that he carries them out properly. In oligophrenic children these tasks are performed on the basis of visual, direct connections, so that these children are incapable of coping with the problem.

Some Special Characteristics of Children of this Group Emerging in the Educational Situation. Maldevelopment of cognitive functions is definitely responsible for the difficulties which the children in this oligophrenic group experience in the course of their education. When they are learning elementary reading and writing, they have considerable difficulty in the analysis of the sound value of each letter and in the fusion of sound-letters in complexes. Nevertheless the absence of gross speech defects, their capacity for hard work, and their application to the tasks given to them enable them to master the technique of reading in many cases even while attending an ordinary school.

It must be pointed out that the transfer from the reading of a word to the comprehension of the meaning of what has been read is very greatly hampered in these children. They can read fluently but completely fail to understand the meaning not only of the story as a whole but also of the separate words. Later, this gap between the technique of reading and the understanding of what has been read is widened and acts as the main obstacle to the understanding of a passage read by the child.

The extended time spent on an introduction to letters in the special schools, the special methods of education, the careful distinction made between the sounds of speech and the greater precision of their pronunciation, and in particular the special attention given by the teacher to the analysis of the sound composition of speech—all these approaches have allowed even children with a rather severe degree of intellectual deficiency to master the reading skills.

In learning to write this group of children showed no difficulties in visual organization; nor were any difficulties observed in these children during writing instruction attributable to deficiency in phonemic hearing. They were quite able to follow correct sequences in writing both words and sentences. No missing letters, transpositions, blanks, or displacement of separate elements were observed. Their difficulties in learning to write were mainly associated with their inadequate understanding of the rules of grammar. It was especially difficult to teach the children to count. In the initial stages of their education the children readily learned the sequence of numbers, but they had difficulty carrying out arithmetical operations. Gradually in the course of their special education, these difficulties were usually overcome, and these children learned to do arithmetical operations. Their education in the various divisions of the syllabus took place at a very slow tempo, by breaking each operation down into component elements, in an extended form of solution.

Investigations by Nepomnyashchei (1956) on this group of oligophrenic children demonstrated that the considerable defects in the abstracting and generalizing functions of their speech led to extreme difficulty in the consummation of even the simplest mental performance by these children. They always had to break the action down into individual component parts.

Children with this variant of defect manifest productivity in all kinds of activity that lie within their capacity. Such children, when carrying out various school tasks such as writing, reading, or solving problems, are always purposeful, active and productive so far as their capabilities allow.

The qualitative analysis of the structure of the disability in children with the first variant of oligophrenia thus showed that the clinical picture is dependent on the pathogenesis and on the resulting distinctive features of the higher nervous activity. The fundamental pathogenetic factor is a diffuse lesion mainly affecting the cerebral cortex, with relative integrity of the subcortical formations and absence of disturbance of the circulation of cerebrospinal fluid.

These pathogenetic features lead to specific changes in the higher nervous activity, which are characterized by disturbances in the mobility of the nervous processes, with the strength of the fundamental nervous processes relatively well maintained, and with the balance between excitation and inhibition preserved.

The specific features of the higher nervous activity are, in turn, responsible for the specific features of the clinical picture, which is characterized by the presence of the fundamental sign; maldevelopment of the cognitive functions is, in turn, responsible for the secondary maldevelopment of all aspects of the personality. This qualitative pattern of the structure of the defect which we have described may be detected in lesions of varying severity, i.e., in both imbecility and feeble-mindedness. We observed this form more commonly in oligophrenic children at the feeble-minded or moronic level of retardation.

Differentiation Between Children with the First Variant of Oligophrenia and Children with Temporary Retardation of Development. In the case of children with this variant of oligophrenia, the diagnosis, like the differential diagnosis, presents certain difficulties. The differentiation between children with oligophrenia and children with a temporary retardation of development [academic backwardness or pseudo-retardation] may be a particularly complicated task.

In temporary retardation of development the child is arrested at some early level of development. For instance, having reached school age, he continues to retain preschool interests (play). He cannot be included in school activities nor appreciate school tasks and carry them out.

The absence of skills and interests where school work is concerned leads to confusion between this group of children and oligophrenics. In spite of an apparently marked similarity, however, they differ in many ways from oligophrenic children. In the latter group the disturbance of complex mental functions appears through the whole course of development, and assumes characteristic forms at each age period. In children with a temporary delay of development, the maldevelopment of the complex functions bears a temporary character and is gradually and completely overcome. In children with a temporary retardation of development there are no specific motor disturbances, such as we observe in oligophrenic children. They may perform a given motor act in response to verbal instruction, and give an appropriate motor response for an imaginary situation. There is one particularly clear difference between children with the first variant of oligophrenia and children with a temporary delay in development, which is revealed by investigation of their cognitive function. As we have already pointed out, in oligophrenic children the maldevelopment of their cognitive functions is manifested by inability to grasp a picture-story and to understand the meaning of an easy story. Children with temporary retardation of development, even though they may be unsuccessful pupils at school and acquire hardly any academic skill at the end of the school year, may understand the meaning of a story which has been read to them, and may arrange in the proper order a series of pictures and understand the theme of a picture-story.

The difference between children with a temporary retardation of development and children with this first variant of oligophrenia is as follows: 1) in children with a temporary retardation of development difficulties in learning elementary reading, writing, and arithmetic are combined with a fairly high level of development of the cognitive functions. Such a combination is not characteristic of oligophrenic children; 2) children with a temporary retardation of development are capable of utilizing help which is offered to them. By solving a given problem with assistance, they use this assistance in the solution of similar problems. This demonstrates that these children possess far superior potentialities for future development.

Oligophrenic children cannot utilize to a sufficient extent any assistance that is offered to them. Prolonged observations which I made on 25 children with temporary retardation of development showed that it is this ability to take advantage of proferred aid and the ability to make rational use of what has been learned in their subsequent education, that makes it possible for these children to subsequently become successful pupils in the ordinary school. The pattern of development of these children thus differs from that of oligophrenic children.

Ways of Compensation. The dynamic investigation of oligophrenic children of this group showed that the clinical picture is determined by the fundamental sign: maldevelopment of the most complex forms of mental activity. The qualitative structure of the disability also determines the character of the corrective training required by these children. In working with these children it is necessary above all to use teaching methods which are aimed at the development of cognitive activity.

In the course of this work, especially in the early stages, it is important to develop analytical-synthetic activity within the bounds of each analyzer, and to teach these children to carry out a given task in response to the teacher's verbal command. In the process of performing individual tasks these children must abstract from the old inert connections, stimulate the formation of new connections, and learn to make use of new impressions.

The prolonged introductory period of study of the letters of the alphabet in the special schools, the analysis of the sound values of each letter, and the fusion of sound-letters into complexes usually make it possible for these children to learn the technique of reading, but they often do not grasp the meaning of what they have read. With such children it is therefore necessary to explain constantly the meaning of words in the course of their instruction, so that in the future they will be able to grasp the meaning of passages which they read.

When these children are learning arithmetic it is very easy to note their tendency to keep repeating a series of numbers in a stereotyped way, It is therefore necessary to break down an arithmetical operation into separate elements, to first construct it as a chain of objective operations, to designate each individual operation verbally, and then gradually transfer it into a vocal plan.

The organization of the behavior of a child with the first variant of oligophrenia presents no special difficulties, although here again it is necessary to take account of specific features. It must be remembered that these children behave adequately only in a situation which they understand, and situations must therefore be explained to them. Such children must learn to modify their actions and their conduct in accordance with changing situations. Methods of teaching such as these will help children with this kind of disability to develop in the right direction. This progress in their development has been observed most clearly in the emotional-volitional function. After keeping such children under observation for five years, we found that not only were they able to behave in class and to obey the teacher, but also that their behavior had acquired certain cultivated attributes, and that they had a conscious attitude towards learning and a critical attitude towards the work they did.

It was also easy to observe the development of analysis and synthesis within the individual analyzers in these children. As a result of their education, they no longer have difficulty carrying out individual tasks addressed to any analyzer. Through education the cognitive functions of children with this variant of oligophrenia also developed to a significant, though moderate, degree.

Of the 43 children with this form of oligophrenia, seven completed their education at the special school and are working in industry. Reports were obtained on all these children showing that they were coping satisfactorily with their duties. The remaining 36 children are still attending the special school.

The good compensation for their disability in the children with this form of oligophrenia is due to the fact that the corrective training which they receive at the special school promotes their development.

CHAPTER 3

PATHOGENESIS OF THE SYNDROME OF OLIGOPHRENIA WITH GROSS DISTURBANCE OF THE CORTICAL NEURODYNAMICS

It is a characteristic feature of all oligophrenic children with gross disturbance of the cortical neurodynamics (Chapters 3, 4, 5, and 6) that maldevelopment of the complex forms of cognitive function takes place in these children against a background of considerable disturbances of the equilibrium of the fundamental nervous processes. This supplementary pathophysiological mechanism also forms the basis for the characteristic clinical picture of this form of oligophrenia.

Besides the maldevelopment of the cognitive function, i.e., of the fundamental sign of oligophrenia, the clinical picture also shows several additional features. These include typical behavioral changes and a marked reduction in the capacity for work. In our cases the psychopathological manifestations were extremely unstable and shifting, and were sometimes paroxysmal in character, from which it was assumed that they were due to disturbances in the flow of cerebrospinal fluid. A clinical investigation carried out on this group of children revealed that these manifestations were indeed connected with the presence of a disturbance of the flow of cerebrospinal fluid in the residual stage of the hydrocephalic disorder.

In order to clarify the problem of the connection between a disturbance of the cortical neurodynamics in oligophrenia on the one hand and hydrocephalus on the other we examined some aspects of the etiology, pathogenesis and clinical features of hydrocephalus. There are indications of the role and significance of hydrocephalus in oligophrenia in a paper by Golant (1935). He points out that when oligophrenics were investigated by the method of pneumoencephalography, a moderate degree of internal and external hydrocephalus was observed, together with secondary hydrocephalus due to atrophy of the brain substance. The presence of a diffuse dilatation of the subarachnoid spaces was established as evidence of cortical atrophy. Hydrocephalus is not an independent nosological form, but a syndrome arising in connection with some abnormality of the cerebrospinal fluid system

The principal site of accumulation of the cerebrospinal fluid is in the subarachnoid spaces. Another place in which the cerebrospinal fluid collects is the cisterna magna, situated between the cerebellar tonsils, the medulla oblongata and the margin of the occipital foramen. This is the area where we find the foramen of Magendie, through which the cavity of the fourth ventricle communicates with the cisterna magna. The lateral recesses of the fourth ventricle terminate in Luschka's foramen, which connects the cavity of the ventricles with the subarachnoid space of the basal cisterns, and primarily with the lateral and median cisterns of the brain.

Besides these places where the cerebrospinal fluid may accumulate peripherally, there are also central internal receptacles, namely the ventricular cavities. By means of the foramina of Monro, each lateral ventricle communicates with the third ventricle, and the latter communicates with the fourth ventricle by means of the aqueduct of Sylvius. The fourth ventricle forms a direct path of communication by means of the foramina of Magendie and Luschka between the central receptacle of cerebrospinal fluid and the subarachnoid fluid spaces. The exact physiology of the cerebrospinal fluid is not understood. Most researchers at present consider that the vascular plexuses play a part in the formation of the cerebrospinal fluid. It is not yet known with certainty whether the vascular plexus is the only organ to produce cerebrospinal fluid or whether other tissues, especially the ependyma of the ventricles, the meninges and the nervous parenchyma also produce cerebrospinal fluid. A group of Soviet workers conclude from their experiments that the cerebrospinal fluid is produced by the vascular plexuses and is absorbed through the subarachnoid spaces of the brain and passes into the venous blood stream. Other authorities consider that absorption of the cerebrospinal fluid takes place along the perineural and lymphatic channels of the brain and spinal cord, and that the formation of the cerebrospinal fluid takes place in the brain tissue itself.

There is no agreement on the etiology and pathogenesis of hydrocephalus. Foreign investigators (Virchow, Strumpel, Oppenheim, Hoffmann, Leyden, Schultz) have related hydrocephalus to hydromyelia and syringomyelia. The attempt to relate these processes is based on the incorrect assumption of these workers that hydrocephalus, like syringomyelia, is a congenital manifestation. The problem of the etiology of hydrocephalus has been tackled much more productively in the Russian literature. Muratov (1899) postulated a fundamental exogenic factor in the etiology of hydrocephalus. Troshin (1902), in his paper "The pathological anatomy of internal hydrocephalus," expresses doubt about the possibility that idiopathic forms of hydrocephalus may exist, and offers weighty evidence in favor of its inflammatory origin. Klossovskii and Nikitin (1936), in a series of experimental researches, showed convincingly that hydrocephalus is the result of inflammatory processes. The inflammation is most frequently localized to the meninges, the ependyma and the vascular plexuses. The foramen of Magendie or Luschka may be closed by adhesions, thereby causing closed hydrocephalus. All the subsequent work by Soviet investigators has convincingly shown that the fundamental etiological factors in hydrocephalus are inflammatory, traumatic and neoplastic diseases of the central nervous system. Arendt (1948), for instance, in his monograph "Hydrocephalus and its surgical treatment," points out that the fundamental etiological factor in the production of hydrocephalus is infection of the central nervous system. Of the 84 cases of hydrocephalus which he cites, developing in the postnatal period of life, in 75 cases the condition appeared immediately after an attack of some infectious disease. First place among infectious diseases is occupied by cerebrospinal meningitis. The importance of cerebrospinal meningitis in the etiology of hydrocephalus has been discussed by many Russian or Soviet authorities: Filatov (1912); Popov (1925); Margulis (1926); Leonov (1930); Langova (1938); Skvortsov (1938); Astvatsaturov and Glauberman (1938). The pathological–anatomical investigations of Skvortsov (1938) and Smirnov (1935) also showed clearly that in cerebrospinal meningitis changes take place in the meninges, the ependyma of the ventricles, and the subependymal glia. These changes interfere with the drainage and resorption of the cerebrospinal fluid, thus leading to its retention in the ventricles of the brain and the cisterns. In the initial stages of cerebrospinal meningitis these workers found cerebral edema. Various other infectious diseases in children may also be responsible for the subsequent development of hydrocephalus. Parainfectious meningoencephalitis, secondary meningitis after pneumonia, or acute intestinal infections may also be complicated by hydrocephalus. Arendt describes the connection between malaria in the mother during pregnancy and the subsequent development of hydrocephalus in the child. Serous meningitis may also play some part in the etiology of hydrocephalus. Depending on the time of onset, hydrocephalus may be described as congenital or acquired, or in relation to its course—acute and chronic, and according to its localization—internal and external. In accordance with the character of the disturbance of the cerebrospinal fluid system we can distinguish: hydrocephalus with a disturbance of communication of the cerebrospinal fluid – closed occlusive, and a type due to failure of resorption – aresorptive. The etiology and pathogenesis of hydrocephalus and the physiology of the circulation of the cerebrospinal fluid are adequately discussed in the literature, but the question of the structure of mental deficiency in hydrocephalus has received very little attention in the literature, although there are reports that hydrocephalus is accompanied by various degrees of mental deficiency in nearly every paper on hydrocephalus. Muratov (1899), in his clinical lectures, in describing the mental state of patients with hydrocephalus, mentioned a diminution in their mental capacities varying from complete idiocy to the milder degrees of mental deficiency. In his description of the mental features of these patients, Muratov pointed out that they are unaware of their pathological state and had no critical attitude towards themselves and their environment. For example, in contrast to normal children who usually react in a pained manner to an offensive nickname, not only did a hydrocephalic child not object to the name "big head," but also used it himself. The inventory of ideas of such a patient was extremely limited. He would reply from time to time with stereotyped sentences that he had learned by heart, without realizing the meaning of what he said. Voznesenskii (1928) considered that the typical features of mental deficiency associated with hydrocephalus were: a depression of all mental functions, general inertia, and memory difficulties. Pakhorskii pointed out their lability of affect and tendency to euphoria. Foreign writers (Bonhoeffer, Blomberry, etc.) confine themselves to general remarks on the mental changes in hydrocephalus, and point out that in association with a background of feeblemindedness, these patients may have a good mechanical memory and even an ability to learn foreign languages and music. Turetskii and Model' (1936), in their description of hydrocephalus, point out that most children remain severely mentally retarded. Simson (1925) observed that children suffering from hydrocephalus had a good memory for sound forms. They memorized nonsensical sounds far better than those which made sense; sentences which included abstract ideas were memorized particularly badly. In some cases of hydrocephalic children,

Simson observed an ability to do mechanical calculation even in a setting of general mental deficiency.

In order to determine the pattern of the structure and dynamics of mental deficiency in patients with organic lesions of the brain complicated by hydrocephalus, we examined 20 patients with chronic early open forms of hydrocephalus. Before turning to a description of the structure of the mental deficiency as a whole, let us consider certain clinical cases.

CASE 1

Anya F., aged 10 years. This girl had been originally admitted to the Institute of Neurosurgery at the age of one year with a chief complaint of blindness.

History. The early development of the patient until the age of $7\frac{1}{2}$ months was normal. At the age of $7\frac{1}{2}$ months she had an attack of cerebrospinal meningitis, after which her head increased considerably in size and she became unable to see, crawl, and stand. During her first hospital stay it was found that this patient had an open hydrocephalus following the meningoencephalitis, with considerable impairment of cortical processes from the distended ventricles. Burdenko's operation of omental drainage was performed on this patient, after which she improved. She began to see and to move about, though with difficulty, and she subsequently developed speech and a mechanical memory. In 1938, at the age of ten years, the girl was readmitted to the Institute of Neurosurgery.

Physical State. The skull was hydrocephalic, the circumference of the head being 61.5 cm. On percussion of the skull a box-like sound was obtained. No abnormality of the internal organs was found.

State of the Nervous System. There was a divergent strabismus; the visual acuity of both eyes was 1.0. Investigation of the optic fundus showed some dilatation of the veins. The patient walked with her feet wide apart, holding on to surrounding objects, and leaning forward. If she stood with her feet together she had a tendency to fall forward. An intention tremor was present in the right hand. The tendon reflexes of the upper limbs were increased, slightly more so on the right. The knee and ankle jerks were increased equally. The clonus of both ankles rapidly disappeared. Bilateral positive Babinski's sign. Plantar reflex diminished. The finger-nose test showed awkwardness of the left upper limb, with slight shaking movements.

Mental State. Anya's presenting problem was primarily her increased excitability, which made contact with her extremely difficult. She chattered incessantly, speaking to adults, to children, to anybody at all, or even to herself. She knew many stories, proverbs, and songs, readily memorized what she heard, confused much of it, forgot some of it, and joined it to something else to create a chaotic and at times nonsensical hodge-podge. In this setting of hyperexcitability her capacity for work was markedly reduced. The girl could not perform the simplest task by herself, even one well within her capabilities, simply because she could not concentrate on it. The marked restriction of work capacity also became apparent when individual analyzers were tested. Though capable of correctly naming objects illustrated in pictures, the girl often gave incorrect answers on impulse. Often her replies disclosed fragmentary cognition; the girl recognized only part of an object shown to her. When she was shown a picture illustrating a certain object, she developed side associations which she could not inhibit. At the same time, with a little outside help in composing her behavior, she had no difficulty in recognizing pictures illustrating various objects when presented to her upside down.

In visual perception she thus showed lack of clarity, fragmentation, and also signs of pseudo-optic agnosia. All these disturbances, however, were transient in character, were combined with a proper recognition of objects and depended a great deal on how much the girl was concentrating. No gross chronic disturbances of spatial synthesis were found in Anya. If she concentrated, she correctly recognized her own right and left hand and those of another child, and could copy a simple pattern of matches as demonstrated. The girl could finish these tasks only with the teacher's assistance; otherwise she would be distracted and would not complete it. She showed no disturbance of the speech function: she readily repeated a sentence that was hard to pronounce, correctly understood what people told her, and had enough of a vocabulary to be able to construct sentences correctly. No motor disturbances were found in this girl; she could correctly reproduce any position of the hand indicated to her and experienced no particular difficulty in performing various exercises in dynamic movement. These features contrasted with the underlying severe maldevelopment of cognitive functions. When describing a story-picture, the girl produced a haphazard list of the various objects which met her eye. She made no attempt to grasp the meaning of what was represented and did not distinguish the more important elements of the picture, in fact sometimes omitted them. The maldevelopment of the generalizing function of speech was shown with special clarity in the experiment in which a fourth superfluous picture has to be discarded. Of the four pictures offered to her, she would reject one picture for a quite unimportant reason. In the picture classification experiment she could group together only pictures that were identical.

The maldevelopment of the cognitive function and the sharp diminution of her capacity to work were demonstrated still more clearly during her experimental education. The girl remembered letters with difficulty, but her most characteristic feature was her extremely poor fixation of what she learned by heart. Letters which she had learned by heart one day would be regarded by her as quite unfamiliar next day. After she learned a certain number of letters by heart, the girl often gave wrong answers, naming letters which she was shown incorrectly. She could not advance to reading by syllables, for she could not fix her attention on her work. Even greater difficulties appeared when she was learning to count. She succeeded in learning numbers up to ten by heart. Attempts to instruct her in elementary number concepts were unsuccessful, for in reply to all the questions she was asked, she would repeat in stereotyped fashion the series of numbers which she had learned by heart.

Clinical Analysis of the Case

After an attack of meningoencephalitis at the age of $7\frac{1}{2}$ months, our patient developed an open hydrocephalus. At one year of age the child already showed marked retardation of development and deterioration of vision. At the same age Burdenko's operation of omental drainage was performed. The operation greatly improved the drainage of cerebrospinal fluid, which had a beneficial effect on our patient's development. Her vision was restored, her behavior improved and speech developed. The presence of mental deficiency was definitely established, however, nine years after the operation. The structure of the disability here is determined qualitatively by the fact that a gross disturbance of cortical neurodynamics stands out against a background of severe maldevelopment of the cognitive functions.

CASE 2

Kolya P., boy aged 10 years. Admitted to the Institute of Neurosurgery because of recurrent headaches.

History. The course of pregnancy and labor in the mother was normal. At the age of three months the patient suffered from an illness accompanied by high temperature, vomiting, and convulsions. Soon afterwards some increase in the size of the head was noted. Up to the age of four the boy was described as listless, he played little with other children, but loved songs and stories and remembered them easily.

During the war the patient was evacuated, and suffered from severe malnutrition and edema. In 1944, on his return to Moscow, he began to attend kindergarten, where he was soon found to be undisciplined, talkative, and idle. At the age of eight years he began regular school, but in class he would not pay attention to the teacher nor react to correction, and often laughed or cried inappropriately. After an unproductive six months in regular school, he was transferred to a special school.

Physical State. The skull was hydrocephalic, with a head circumference of 58 cm. In his physical development the child was slightly backward for his age. No abnormality of the internal organs was found.

State of the Nervous System. The eyes were deep-set, with anisocoria, sluggish reaction to light, no convergence, poor fixation of gaze, with divergence of the eyes observed at times. Other cranial nerves intact. Movements adequate in range, but choreiform hyperkinesis seen in the digits; movements rapid, fidgety, clumsy, and imprecise; tone low. Stable in Romberg's position, rapid gait. All tendon reflexes increased. Knee and ankle jerks increased on the left more than the right. Oppenheim's test positive on both sides, and a hint of a positive Babinski on the left. No meningeal signs present.

Pneumoencephalography. Air entered the anterior and posterior horn of the left lateral ventricle. The ventricle was wide and approximately spherical in shape. The right lateral ventricle was not filled with air, presumably on account of closure of the foramen of Monro. A large accumulation of air was observed in the cisterna chiasmatica. No essential change was note in the pattern of the subarachnoid spaces. The third ventricle was dilated. The results of pneumoencephalography indicated a large internal open hydrocephalus of the left lateral ventricle. The incomplete filling of the right lateral ventricle with air was due to sequelae of an inflammatory process. Lumbar puncture: CSF pressure 200 mm water, protein 0.099 percent, cells $^{2}/_{3}$, all other tests negative.

Mental State. The boy was extremely active, fidgety and restless. When in the doctor's consulting room he was constantly moving from one place to another, grasping every object in front of him, grimacing and laughing for no reason. When taken to the pets' corner he showed no interest in the animals but asked tiresome, stereotyped questions, without waiting for an answer: 'And who are you?; "And what are you doing here?"; And what's your name?"; etc. He repeated the same stereotyped questions with nearly every adult he met; without waiting for an answer to one question he would ask another.

Against this background of general hyperexcitability, he showed a marked incapacity for work. While a pupil in the third grade of a special school, he was sometimes unable to carry out the most elementary activity: he could not construct a simple pyramid, could not pay attention until a bit of instruction was completed, quickly picked a pyramid to pieces, and then just as quickly and haphazardly dropped the rings on the rod.

During investigation of individual analyzers, no gross localized defects were discovered: he recognized all pictures representing various objects that were shown to him whether they were right or wrong side up, and easily recognized outline drawings of objects. Along with some correct answers, however, the boy often gave incorrect and impulsive answers. The boy's spatial concepts were also preserved. He recognized the directions: "to the right," "to the left," "forward," "backward," etc. He could arrange matches in the form of a given figure. These correct answers could only be obtained from him if he was concentrating and had some incentive to complete the given task, otherwise his answers were absurd and impulsive.

So far as the motor analyzer was concerned, no gross disturbances were found here either: the boy, with some organization of his attention, could easily reproduce a position of the hands demonstrated to him, and he had no special difficulty carrying out very simple dynamic movements.

The boy showed no gross disturbance of speech function: he had an adequate vocabulary, knew many sayings, often repeated clichés, and easily learned to read and write.

No gross disturbances of the individual cortical functions were thus found. At the same time, analysis and synthesis within the bounds of the various analyzers showed specific changes in their activity. Kolya could not retain an instruction that was given to him, but often responded piece-meal fashion, drifting away from the problem and losing touch with its individual elements. Not only did the boy fail to retain an instruction given to him from outside, but he could not maintain an intent arising within himself. For example, when he was sitting in the garden he saw a horse passing by, whereupon he brightened up and expressed the desire to go horseback riding. He got up and tried to run to the horse. On the way he met a boy who spoke to him about something, so that he forgot his original intention, and quietly returned to his place. All these features appeared in a setting of maldevelopment of cognitive activity. Any task which called for a certain level of abstraction and generalization was carried out by the patient with great difficulty. For instance, in the picture classification experiment he grouped them together in accordance with signs of no consequence. He was unable to grasp the significance of a story with a hidden meaning. When describing a picture-story he could not identify the more important subject matter. The maldevelopment of his cognitive functions, like the diminished capacity for work, was clearly revealed in the course of his education: the boy memorized individual letters comparatively easily, but progressed to reading of syllables only with great difficulty because of his poor capacity for fixing his attention. When he had mastered the technique of reading, the boy still read carelessly and hurriedly, often by guessing, and from time to time lost his place.

The boy was prone to make certain mistakes in writing: repetition of individual letters, syllables and words, omission of letters and words, and transpositions.

In calculation, he showed a tendency to replace the solution of elementary arithmetic problems with a series of numbers reproduced in stereotyped fashion.

When his attention was sufficiently organized, the boy could give the correct names of a number of objects arranged on a table, but at the same time he could not count them. Kolya was very confused by the solution of even simple tasks. His difficulties arose not only because of his inability to form connections of meaning between verbal expressions, numerical data, and names, but also because of his inability to concentrate on the problem. He could not remember the conditions of the problem and lost sight of its component elements.

Clinical Analysis of the Case

In this particular case we are concerned with a residual stage of meningoencephalitis, from which the boy suffered at the age of three months.

The hydrocephalic skull (circumference of the head 58 cm)

and the results of pneumoencephalography clearly confirmed the presence of a gross degree of open hydrocephalus. With regard to the qualitative aspects of the structure of the disability there was a combination of marked maldevelopment of the cognitive functions with the specific signs of this particular clinical picture. Among these specific signs we included general disinhibition, increased tendency to distractability, impulsiveness, a tendency to drift away from an assigned task, and an inability to retain instructions.

The maldevelopment of the cognitive functions in this case was permanent in character, for even if the boy could be organized and assisted to complete a set task he could nevertheless solve it only at the level of his capacity. The behavioral changes as well as the marked reduction in work capacity were more unstable in character and were basically due to disturbances of the circulation of the cerebrospinal fluid.

* * *

The treatment of hydrocephalus is directed mainly towards improving the flow of cerebrospinal fluid. We shall therefore attempt to examine what changes take place in the structure of the mental deficiency associated with chronic hydrocephalus when therapeutic measures are applied. We made a careful investigation of patients before puncture and appropriate treatment with hypertonic solutions, and after puncture. In several cases we observed that the state of these patients was slightly improved after puncture and suitable treatment. They were better able to concentrate and could perform elementary tasks which had been impossible for them before treatment. After treatment these children could master the elements of reading, do elementary sums, and recognize pictures which were shown to them, and they took part more readily in organized games and activities. We obtained particularly convincing results in relation to the changes in the structure of the disability in hydrocephalus when we observed a group of patients in the children's department of the Burdenko Institute of Neurosurgery before and after operative treatment. The operation was designed to improve the drainage of the cerebrospinal fluid. We shall describe some of these cases:

CASE 1

Igor' K., boy aged 10 years. He was admitted to the children's department of the Institute of Neurosurgery complaining of marked enlargement of the head and difficulty in walking.

History. The patient was born from a second pregnancy. Labor was prolonged, but until the age of $2\frac{1}{2}$ months the child developed normally. At the age of $2\frac{1}{2}$ months, for no apparent reason the child's head began to enlarge considerably. He walked badly, and from the age of two years spent all his time in bed. From three to eight years the patient suffered from time to time from attacks of headache and vertigo, which were accompanied by psychosensory disturbances. During these attacks the boy felt that objects were falling on him and that the houses were leaning in a peculiar way, he sometimes had double vision and objects appeared to be very close to him or, conversely, very far away. During this period the patient's temperature was raised for a brief interval of time for no apparent cause. His mother thought that the boy's mental development was adequate: he chattered a lot, easily memorized separate words and expressions used by adults, and was reasonably attentive.

Physical State Before Operation. His chest was barrel-shaped and his neck short. There was an excessive deposition of fat on the chest, abdomen, and thighs. No abnormality of the internal organs was found. The skull was hydrocephalic in shape, with well-developed frontal and parietal tuberosities. The circumference of the skull was 62 cm, the transverse diameter 17.5 cm and the longitudinal diameter 22 cm. Percussion of the skull produced a cracked-pot sound. Percussion was painless. The fontanelles were closed.

State of the Nervous System Before Operation. The pupils were equal and reacted promptly to light and adequately to convergence. A slight pallor of the optic disks was noted, more marked on the left than the right. No signs of congestion. Visual acuity: right eye 0.6, left eye 0.4. Perimetry with the hand showed a small concentric constriction of the visual field to white, red, and green light. No hemianopsia present. Paresis of fixation of gaze on upward gaze. The tongue deviated very slightly to the right. Active movements of the upper limbs were full in range, adequate in strength and unchanged in tone. Active movements of the lower limbs were slow, the power of the muscles of the leg was reduced and their tone increased, and the limbs were adducted. Adiadokokinesis was present in both hands. The patient carried out the finger-nose test awkwardly with tremor of the hands; when standing the lower limbs were semiflexed at the knees and the thighs were pressed tightly together. While walking the boy lifted his feet off the ground with difficulty. There was no impairment of sensation. The tendon reflexes were brisk, and there was a bilateral ankle clonus. Babinski's, Oppenheim's, and Gordon's signs were present on both sides.

Otoneurological examination revealed a disturbance of the mechanism of experimental nystagmus in the form of dissociation to the left and slight tonicity.

X-ray Examination. Gross changes in the skull and sella. Digital impressions hardly visible in relief. The picture suggested open hydrocephalus.

Mental State of the Patient Before Operation. Consciousness lucid. Orientation towards the environment preserved in an elementary manner. The patient was usually in a slightly excited euphoric state, spoke a great deal, and repeated everything that he heard about him. The patient's statements convinced us that he did not understand the meaning of the words which he uttered. There was a gross disturbance of the cortical neurodynamics in this patient. He could not perform the most elementary task because of his indifference to it. It was discovered with difficulty that the patient knew his letters. This did not prevent him, however, from identifying the letter "A" correctly and then immediately calling it something else. When engaged in an exercise he often wrote what was not given in the example. He was able to carry out arithmetical operations involving numbers up to 10, but besides giving correct answers he would also give wrong ones. For example, if he could concentrate his attention and organize it, he could state correctly that 2+3=5. If the question was repeated, however, he might give a wrong answer: 6, 7, or 8. During the experiments and lessons, the patient was very easily distracted and readily intruded into his conversation anything that happened to engage his attention. The patient's speech superficially seemed to be well developed, but in fact consisted of the repetition of remarks of those around him word for word. All these features of behavior and activity emerged in a setting of maldevelopment of the capacity for abstraction and generalization, in the absence of gross defects within the bounds of individual analyzers.

The clinical picture before operation thus consisted of the following signs: a hydrocephalic skull; spastic paraparesis of the lower limbs, with an increase in tone mainly affecting the adductor muscles of the thighs; considerable changes in the skull and sella turcica; pallor of the optic disks, without signs of stasis; and a mental deficiency of characteristic structure, which was determined by the maldevelopment of the mental functions and a severe disturbance of the cortical neurodynamics. It could be concluded from these findings that this was a case of open hydrocephalus, possibly resulting from an attack of meningoencephalitis in early childhood. The absence of headache and papilledema, and tests of the cerebrospinal fluid dynamics confirmed the presence of open hydrocephalus in this case.

On February 2, 1948, the operation of omental drainage by Burdenko's method was performed on this patient. A bed was made beneath the long muscles of the spine through which an omental drain was taken down to the site of a laminectomy. The peritoneal cavity was closed in layers. The dura and arachnoid were opened for a distance of 2 cm. The cerebrospinal fluid flowed freely under increased pressure. The omental drain was fixed by a suture to the dura mater. The muscles, aponeurosis, and skin were closed in layers.

During the first two days after operation the patient was apathetic, showed no spontaneous activity, spoke little, and occasionally complained of headache and vertigo. Subsequently his condition gradually improved. His postoperative course was smooth. A further investigation of the patient was made 12 days later.

Condition of the Patient After Operation. No abnormality of the cranial nerves was found. Active movements were full in range but slightly decreased in strength; the muscle tone in the lower limbs was slightly increased, but much less than before the operation. Special remedial exercises which were undertaken with the patient after operation had good results. With a little assistance he began to move about the ward independently. After the operation a considerable change occurred in the patient's mental state. Against the background of his existing intellectual deficiency, which remained stable, the boy's capacity for work improved greatly. He became quieter and better able to concentrate, and he managed to perform elementary tasks comparatively easily; he no longer confused the names of letters and easily learned the technique of reading. For a period of $1\frac{1}{2}$ months after the operation the boy received individual tuition every day, in the course of which he learned the elements of reading, writing, and arithmetic.

CASE 2

Kira K., an eight-year-old girl. She was admitted to the children's department of the Institute of Neurosurgery because of mental retardation associated with hydrocephalus.

History. Pregnancy followed a normal course, but before the child was one month old her mother noticed that the head was considerably enlarged. At this time the child had several infectious diseases (chicken-pox, whooping cough, pneumonia), following which her condition deteriorated still further: she developed attacks of dyspnea with cyanosis of the face and distal parts of the limbs but without convulsions, lasting 1-2 minutes and followed by sleep. Initially these attacks were repeated several times a day, but later they became less frequent, taking place once or twice a month, and at the age of $3^1/_2$ years they ceased completely. Since she was six years old her parents had noticed that the girl was greatly retarded in her mental development.

Physical State Before Operation. The skull was hydrocephalic, circumference of the head 65 cm, longitudinal diameter 24 cm, transverse diameter 20.5 cm. No abnormality of the internal organs.

State of the Nervous System. Pupils regular in shape. Reaction to light satisfactory, to convergence weak. No signs of congestion of the optic fundus observed, optic disks pale. Visual acuity of the right eye 0.3, left cyc 0.4. Eyc movements unrestricted, no hemianopsia. The range of active movements of the upper limbs was full and the muscle power good but uniformly diminished. The range of movements in the hip joints was diminished and that of the knee and ankle joints was full. Muscle power diminished. All movements were greatly retarded, and the muscle tone was increased in the upper and lower limbs. Forced movements of choreoathetoid type were observed in the upper limbs, against a background of dysmetria and ataxia. During the performance of coordination tests signs of dysmetria appeared. For instance, during the performance of the finger-nose test, in addition to missing the target, a coarse tremor of the hands was observed. The tendon reflexes in both upper and lower limbs were equally increased. Bilateral ankle clonus was present. Babinski's sign was inconstant on both sides, and Oppenheim's sign was present on the left. The abdominal reflexes were equal.

Grossly abnormal hydrocephalic skull. Lumbar puncture: CSF pressure 240 mm water, proteins 26.0 mg percent, Pandy +, Nonne-Apelt +, cells 42/3. Ventricular puncture: CSF pressure 120 mm water, proteins 7.7 mg percent, Pandy +, cells 3/3.

Encephalography. No air in the ventricles. Traces of air were found in the cisterns in the region of the sella turcica and in the neighboring fissures. Tests of the cerebrospinal fluid dynamics demonstrated open hydrocephalus.

Mental State of the Patient Before Operation. The girl's consciousness was lucid. Elementary orientation towards her surroundings was preserved. Speech articulation was sufficiently well developed. Her speech mimicked the speech of adults, with repetition of whole sentences but without any grasp of their meaning. The child's capacity for orderly thinking was severely defective. She could not apply herself to even the simplest practical activity. She did not understand the meaning of the simplest picture and could only recite a list of the various items in the picture, with no grasp of action and with absolutely no understanding of a situation. The patient's active memory was poor. She learned a few words by rote with difficulty, and in the course of this learning her memorization curve at first rose rapidly and then fell sharply. The girl remembered all the songs she listened to on the radio and could repeat them without making a mistake. Although her grasp of pictures representing objects was reasonably good, at times she made stupid mistakes, associated with the disturbance of her deliberate activity. She was unusually easily distracted and introduced accidentally heard words or visual images into her activities or conversation. The patient was euphoric and lacking in judgment. Burdenko's omental drainage operation was performed on this patient. The postoperative course was uneventful and at the present time the patient's condition is satisfactory.

Condition of the Patient After Operation. Examination of the patient after operation showed an improvement in both the neurological and mental states. The hyperkinesis and ataxia of the upper limbs had decreased. She began to stand, holding on to a chair, and moved about with difficulty. Her spastic paresis was less obvious. The patient's mental state had considerably improved. She developed an elementary attitude towards her surroundings. She was able to listen to instructions and to carry them out, which had been quite beyond her power before the operation. She was able to undertake an easy task. She began to have daily individual tuition, as a result of which she mastered the rudiments of reading and writing.

The increase in the size of the head, the spastic quadriparesis, the hyperkinesis in the upper and lower limbs of choreoathetoid type, the marked dysmetria of the limbs, the slight exaggeration of the reflexes, the nystagmus during experimental testing, the tinnitus and vertigo, the low albumin concentration in the ventricular CSF, and the normal composition of the lumbar CSF, and also the characteristic picture of mental deficiency with the disturbance of cortical neurodynamics typical of hydrocephalus — all these were evidence that in this particular case we were dealing with hydrocephalus. In this patient too, as in the preceding case, there was an obvious improvement after operation.

Postoperative clinical observations showed an improvement in the physical state of these patients: their headaches ceased, their appetite improved, they became more cheerful, more active, and livelier. The signs of stasis observed in the optic fundus in some cases usually disappeared in the course of a few months postoperatively. In the few cases in which epileptic fits were observed before the operation, after operation they became much less frequent or disappeared altogether. We observed marked improvement in the mental state of our patients. This improvement did not take place because of any change in the permanent signs associated with the process of atrophy of the cerebral cortex. The improvement manifested itself clinically mainly because the children became more attentive, more purposeful, and more capable of working. Before the operation for instance, the patient usually did not grasp the meaning of an object which was shown to him (a picture, a letter, or a number), and even when the object was correctly recognized its image was apparently quickly erased. But after operation it could be demonstrated in a series of experiments that an object was comprehended much better. Whereas before operation the children were extremely inattentive and intruded into their speech everything they heard around them, were quickly distracted, did not retain instructions and were thus incapable of education, after the operation they became more attentive, could retain elementary instructions and carry out tasks, and made definite progress under individual tuition.

Changes thus took place in the structure of the disability as a result of the operation. The operative procedure improved the drainage of cerebrospinal fluid and thereby lowered its pressure. The decrease in the pressure of the cerebrospinal fluid increased the cortical activity, which lead to an improvement in the capacity of these patients for work. It may be regarded as proved that the diminished work capacity and the characteristic behavioral changes of these patients were due to a disturbance of the flow of cerebrospinal fluid in the central nervous system.

Clinical Analysis of the Cases

A characteristic sign of the physical state of these patients is their general dysplasia, with a tendency in some cases to excess fat deposition. The disturbance of the metabolic functions is explained by the presence of prolonged intraventricular hypertension. In lesions of the brain complicated by hydrocephalus, the disturbance of the central nervous system expresses itself in various forms of paralysis, in hyperkineses, and by disturbances of coordination of movement and posture. Hypertonia and hypotonia of muscles and various pathological reflexes are observed.

The craniographic findings indicate changes in the configuration of the skull, thinning of the bones and increased digital markings. Pneumography makes it possible to judge the presence of an internal and of an accompanying external hydrocephalus. In chronic hydrocephalus with a prolonged course the cerebrospinal fluid will be diluted and will approximate distilled water in its composition. In organic lesions of the brain complicated by hydrocephalus, we find characteristic features in the structure of the disability, the analysis of which will help us to better understand the structure of the disability in those cases of oligophrenia where there is a gross disturbance of the cortical neurodynamics.

The results of clinical investigation have shown that two series of symptoms may be distinguished in the structure of the disability in hydrocephalus. One series manifests itself as a maldevelopment of cognitive functions. These children have difficulty in forming complicated types of mental activity in all tasks which require a certain level of development of the capacity for abstraction and generalization. In these children too, the maldevelopment of the cognitive functions bears a permanent character and is due to changes in the brain substance itself. The other series of symptoms in an organic lesion of the brain complicated by hydrocephalus is characterized by a disturbance of the cortical neurodynamics. These symptoms take the form of a severe reduction of the capacity for work and of disturbances of purposeful activity. They are of a general cerebral character and appear when any problem is presented to the child, but also induce peculiarities of behavior. These children are very easily distracted and fatigued and their behavior is aimless. They cannot apply the necessary effort to solve even a very elementary problem quite within their understanding. They are absent-minded, easily distracted (they may carry away in their hands a picture, a ring, a tile, or a pyramid), and they are unable to concentrate on anything. They throw one thing away and seize a second or third. These children can neither look nor listen, although they comment on everything that goes on around and intrude all that they see and hear into their conversation.

This group of children show no gross disturbances confined to any one analyzer, but during the performance of tasks addressed to a given analyzer they are apt to wander from the point, to give foolish, incorrect, or impulsive answers, and to incorporate in their statements incidental associations. They may give fragmentary answers in conjunction with the correct performance of a group of tasks. Characteristically they never question their own mistakes and evince complete satisfaction with every mistaken answer.

These children retain their elementary emotional expressiveness, but at the same time, as a result of the disturbance of their cortical neurodynamics, their emotions display an extremely unstable character. These emotional reactions are expressed only while the stimulus remains in the field of their perception.

Their hyperexcitability, distractability, and irritability lead to disturbance of their behavior. Their disorganized conduct and severely impaired capacity for work are responsible for the great difficulties which arise in their education. They quickly forget what they have acquired and must then begin to learn it all over again by heart as if they had never studied it before.

All these symptoms, in contrast to those described earlier, are transient and at times perhaps even paroxysmal in character, being closely dependent on the degree of the child's concentration on the task in which he is engaged.

The structure of the mental deficiency in the early, chronic form of hydrocephalus is thus composed of two series of symptoms: 1) maldevelopment of the cognitive functions, which is due to atrophy of the cerebral cortex and is of a more permanent character, and 2) disturbance of the capacity for work and of behavior, due to disturbances in the cerebrospinal fluid dynamics. The clinical data which we obtained during the study of the structure of the mental deficiency in organic lesions of the brain complicated by hydrocephalus have brought us nearer to an understanding of the distinctive features of the pathogenesis of those forms of oligophrenia in which maldevelopment of the cognitive functions is combined with changes in behavior and a decrease in work capacity.

CHAPTER 4

OLIGOPHRENIC CHILDREN WITH DISTURBANCE OF THE BALANCE BETWEEN THE FUNDAMENTAL NERVOUS PROCESSES, WITH EXCITATION PREDOMINATING OVER INHIBITION

The specific feature of the pathogenesis of this form of oligophrenia is the presence of a disturbance of the circulation of the cerebrospinal fluid in a late stage of the disease. The presence of this additional pathogenic factor leads to specific changes in the cortical neurodynamics, and these, in turn, are responsible for the appearance of a number of additional symptoms in the clinical picture, namely changes in behavior and a decrease in work capacity.

Depending on the character of the disturbance of the cortical neurodynamics, this large group of oligophrenic states can be divided into three subgroups:

1) oligophrenia in which the disturbance of the cortical neurodynamics is characterized by a marked predominance of excitation over inhibition;

2) oligophrenia in which the disturbance of the cortical neurodynamics is characterized by a marked predominance of inhibition over excitation; and

3) oligophrenia in which the disturbance of the cortical neurodynamics is characterized by a marked weakness of both nervous processes.

We shall now turn to the description of that subgroup of oligophrenia in which the disturbance of the cortical neurodynamics is characterized by the predominance of the process of excitation over inhibition. We shall first discuss a few clinical cases.

CASE 1

Vova K., aged 13 years, a boy who is a pupil in the fifth year of study in the imbecile class of a special school. No abnormalities in his hereditary history.

History. The mother of this boy had a total of three pregnancies, in two of which an artificial termination of the pregnancy was induced. Our subject was born from the first pregnancy. The mother was in poor health during the pregnancy. The infant was born at term. Labor was difficult and prolonged, and the child was born in asphyxia, with generalized edema. From earliest childhood the boy showed a severe retardation of development. He walked at the end of his second year, and spoke at three years of age. At the age of $2\frac{1}{2}$ years, Vova fell from a sledge, cried loudly, and soon fell asleep. At the age of $5\frac{1}{2}$ years he had a severe attack of dysentery. From time to time between the ages of two and seven years, the boy had atypical fits during sleep, which could be regarded as an episyndrome superimposed on a residual organic defect. After seven years of age these fits stopped. At the preschool age, in addition to severe general retardation the boy showed certain peculiarities of behavior: he was very restless, irritable, excitable, and extremely disinhibited.

Because of this state of marked disinhibition and his considerable retardation of development, the boy did not attend kindergarten. At nine years of age he was sent to the imbecile class of a special school.

Physical State. The boy's physical development was normal for his age, but considerable dysplasia was observed. The circumference of his head was 54 cm; his trunk was elongated and the chest narrow. On examination of the internal organs the heart sounds were impure and an arrhythmia was present; pulse rate 96 per minute, volume satisfactory. Respiration was vesicular and the rate slightly increased.

State of the Nervous System. The pupils reacted briskly. Convergence was not possible. The facial innervation was symmetrical. No signs of paresis were present. Denervational changes of tone were observed. The tendon reflexes were brisk, with no clear difference between the two sides. The abdominal and plantar reflexes and Mayer's sign were absent. Babinski's sign was more marked on the right than on the left.

The boy switched satisfactorily from one movement to another. In the course of neurological examination the boy showed himself to be extremely easily distracted and fatigued and unable to concentrate when performing the most elementary tasks.

Ophthalmological Examination. Visual acuity of both eyes 1.0. The eyes were steady and the media translucent. Optic fundus: optic papilla pale pink in color, clearly outlined, the veins dilated and tortuous, the margins of the optic papilla were slightly obscure on the left, and the periphery of the region of the macula lutea showed no particular features. Perimetry to white light was normal. During the investigation the boy was very easily distracted and impulsive.

Otorhinolaryngological Examination. Hearing within normal limits.

X-ray Examination of the Skull. Skull increased in size, spherical in in shape, sutures indistinguishable, sella turcica deepened and widened. Well marked digital impressions everywhere. Intensified shadows of the diploic veins and the emissary veins.

Electroencephalography. The α-rhythm was almost completely absent from the recording. Small bursts of irregular α-rhythm were seen in the parietal region, and solitary α-waves in the occipital, temporal, and frontal regions. In the occipital, parietal, and frontal regions slow waves with a frequency of 6-8 per second and of low amplitude were recorded. In the occipital and parietal regions slow waves of the delta type were encountered. A β-rhythm, more marked on the right, was recorded in all regions of the cortex (Fig. 20).

As a rule modification did not occur in response to high-frequency flashes of light. Only in solitary cases could a very persistent and ill-defined modification be observed in response to a flicker frequency of 13 per second. With flicker of higher frequency (21 per second) no modification of the rhythm occurred (Fig. 21).

As shown by the absence of an α-rhythm and the presence in all regions of the cortex of slow waves of different amplitude, the brain lesion was highly diffuse. The ill-defined nature of the modification of the rhythm, especially in response to high frequencies, could indicate a general brain lesion or specific neurodynamic disturbances.

Investigation of the Higher Nervous Activity. During investigation of the higher nervous activity inertia of the nervous processes was disclosed, and this was especially obvious in the system of connections relating to speech. Inertia of the nervous processes and pathological weakness of the process of internal inhibition were also demonstrated by the fact that the verbal evaluation of the stimuli had lost its connection with the application of the direct stimuli themselves and acted as an inert verbal stereotype, independent of the application of direct stimuli. Inertia of the older connections was also shown by the fact that when the names of the stimuli were introduced, the subject drifted into giving the natural series of numbers which he had learned by heart in the course of his education.

The second specific feature of this case was an abnormality of the process of excitation, associated with a tendency to excitatory irradiation, with excitation predominating over the process of inhibition. The achievement of relatively complex forms of differ-

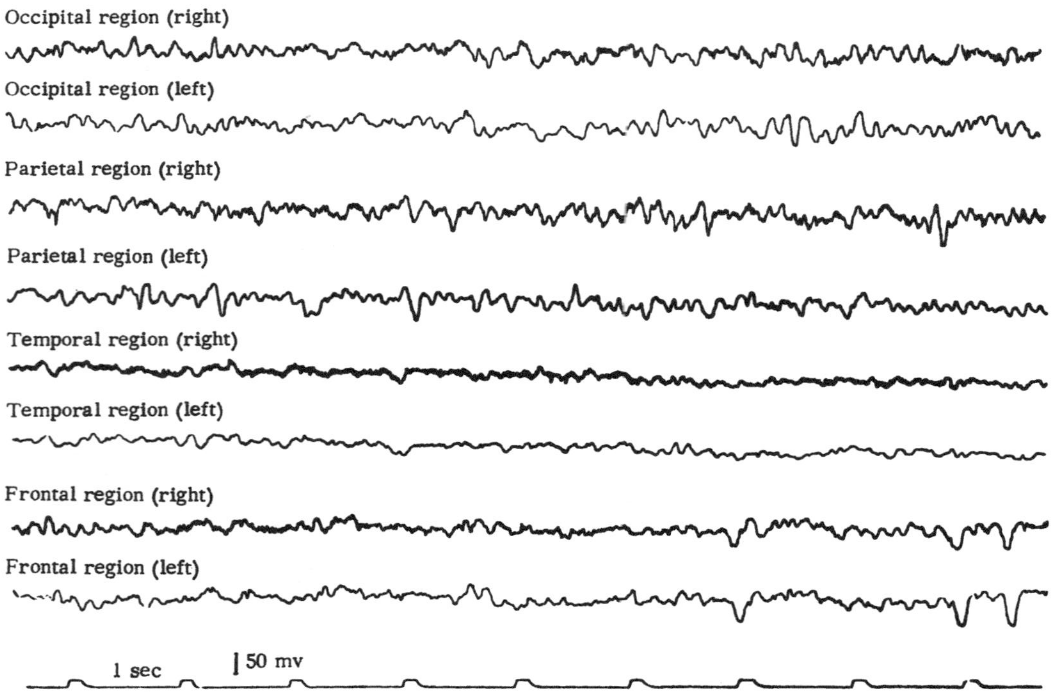

Fig. 20. Vova K., aged 13 years, pupil in the imbecile class (oligophrenia, degree of imbecility). The α-rhythm is recorded in the form of single waves. In all regions of the cortex slow waves and the α-rhythm predominate. Delta-waves are recorded periodically.

entiation was severely hampered, and when finally attained, the system of connections was only sustained by maintaining strictly constant conditions. It was sufficient either to omit the constant speech reinforcement, to alter the order of application of the stimuli, or to change the frequency of their presentation for differentiation to be upset. Constant speech reinforcement probably facilitated the concentration of the nervous processes. When constant reinforcement was omitted considerable irradiation of the process of excitation was observed, leading to disinhibition of differentiation.

Extrastimuli had a marked influence on the function of the developing system of connections. Ringing of bells or questioning by the experimenter led to the collapse of the system of conditioned connections: differentiation was disinhibited and the various positive conditioned reactions were lost.

Mental State

Visual Analyzer. The boy recognized pictures shown to him and named them correctly, but besides the correct names he also gave incorrect, extremely hasty and impulsive answers. Often Vova reacted not to the picture which was shown to him, but to some other picture in his field of vision. When his attention was under control and when his activity was directed into the proper channels he gave the correct names to objects represented on pictures, shown to him either right side up or upside down.

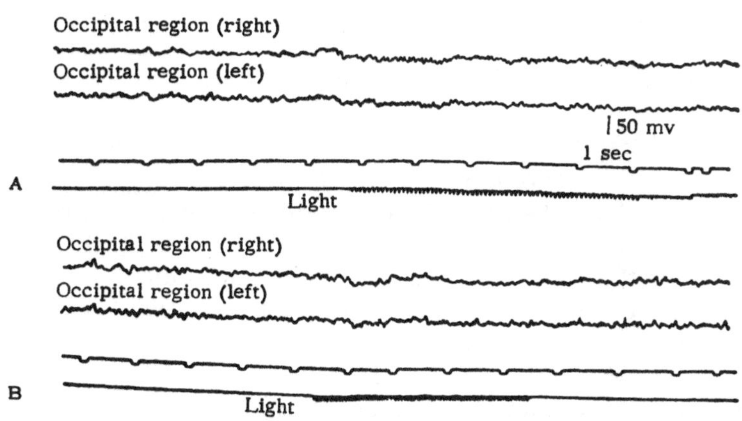

Fig. 21. EEG (of the same subject) during the application of a rhythmic light stimulus. A) Frequency of rhythmic stimulus 13 per second. In the right occipital lead a modification of the cortical rhythm is recorded, which lasts only 1 second. B) Frequency of rhythmic stimulation 21 per second. No modification of the cortical rhythm present.

Spatial Orientation. The boy was orientated in space: he had notions of right and left. When his attention was under control he could assemble an elementary pattern from matches, but when left to his own devices he often failed to do this properly. He could correctly form a triangle or square when given an example, but when the same task was given to him later he was quite incapable of accomplishing it. When more complicated tasks were given to him, considerable difficulties emerged.

Motor and Motor-Speech Analyzers. In tests of postural movement or of dynamic movement this boy revealed all his specific peculiarities: he was extremely impulsive and did not analyze the position of the upper limb which was shown to him, but immediately began to carry out either a part of the pose which was shown to him or a different pose. When, however, his attention was engaged and his activity directed into proper channels, he correctly reproduced the poses he was shown. Vova was much less able to carry out properly the various exercises in dynamic movement. The boy's speech had a slightly nasal intonation, his palate was very narrow, his tongue long and narrow, and his teeth were irregularly formed. The structure of his articulatory apparatus showed certain defects. His speech was very rapid and slurred. He did not finish off his words. When his attention was engaged, however, and the tempo of his speech lowered to some extent, Vova pronounced words and phrases much more distinctly.

Phonemic Hearing. Vova could understand what was said to him, his vocabulary was reasonably good and he could construct a sentence properly. He repeated correlated phonemes correctly, but when the scope of the task was slightly expanded or his general state of disinhibition increased, the number of incorrect answers rose significantly.

No gross localized disturbances of the individual cortical functions were observed, although in the performance of tasks addressed to any analyzer two significant features emerged: a) his disorganization, impulsiveness, and low productivity; b) the difficulties arising when the task itself was made more difficult, because of the low level of development of his entire analytical-synthetic activity.

Cognitive Function and Behavior. The increased excitability, impulsiveness, disinhibition, and inability to concentrate were clearly shown in everything the boy did. Vova was constantly on the move, disinhibited, and somewhat disobedient. In the course of conversation he would pat the doctor or teacher on the arm and ask questions quite unconnected with the subject of the conversation "What is your name?"; "Who are you?"; "What have you got there?"; "Can you read?"; etc.

During the experiments the same impulsivity, hastiness, and thoughtlessness were shown in his answers. He usually started to carry out a task given to him before hearing the end of the instructions. In his classwork the boy still showed restlessness in his motor activity and was easily distracted: he jumped up and down in his place, grabbed tiles and pencils, opened and shut his desk top, fumbled about in his satchel, and took out school belongings. Frequently the boy would intersperse his own talk with word fragments or complete sentences which might come to mind. In the presence of a stranger the boy's general excitation increased even more: he spoke incessantly, laughed without adequate reason, and performed his tasks even less satisfactorily than before.

The process of educating the boy in elementary reading and writing was made very difficult by his extreme inattentiveness. He could only concentrate for very short intervals of time, and in the course of his work he rapidly tired and became distracted, whereupon he ceased to perform the task in which he was engaged.

The boy gave wrong names to the letters he learned, read slowly, and with many mistakes. He would often change the order of syllables or try to read by guessing. He would begin to read more difficult words in the middle or at the end. In class the teacher would have to cover the whole passage except for the word which the boy had to read next, otherwise Vova would join the end of one word to the beginning of the next. When reading, his inability to do sustained work was evident. He would read a passage from his primer even moderately well when his attention was fixed. However at other times he read very badly. It was especially hard, however, to teach the boy to write. Vova wrote carelessly and hurriedly, dividing words into syllables with small strokes. He recognized the sound of each letter and word, but began to write in the middle or even at the end of the word. For example the word "shkola", [school] he wrote as "kolshla," the word "kot" [cat] as "tok," and "rubashka" [shirt] as "kashruba." The boy often omitted vowels and wrote "lk" instead of "luk," and "mk" instead of "mak." Vova usually could not find any of his mistakes himself.

If the boy could be organized, however, and his work tempo somewhat reduced, then with the teacher's help he could perform tasks at a much higher level. When doing written work, the boy appeared to be extremely unstable, and the level of his performance was greatly dependent upon his condition and on the circumstances in which the exercise had to be done.

In individual tasks, with the assistance of the teacher as organizer, and in particular when, by constant speech reinforcement, the concentration of his nervous processes could be improved, the quality of performance of his various tasks increased considerably. Vova had special trouble learning arithmetic. He learned to count up to ten fairly easily, but then this number sequence became a fixed and inert stereotype which he repeated in any kind of exercise.

He learned to count backward from ten with considerable difficulty. He confused counting up to ten with counting backward from ten, the former always displacing the latter. When doing sums Vova did not correlate the number and the object, and he could not start counting from a given number. In all these tasks a stereotyped series clearly emerged. During the solution of problems involving addition and subtraction up to ten, Vova often gave impulsive and incorrect answers. Vova solved his problem with great difficulty and only with the organizing help of his teacher. In the later stages of his education, the disorganized quality of his activities was as obvious as ever. When he tried to repeat a story which had been read to him, he lost the thread and constantly interposed chance associations or things which came into his mind quite unconnected with the story he was trying to tell. By way of illustration we can report the way he retold one particular story. The tale "The Devoted Dog" was read to the boy.

"An old peasant once had a dog. When the dog got old he was no longer a good watch dog, and the peasant wanted to drown him. He took a big stone, called the dog, and went down to the river. Then he got in his boat and rowed to a deep spot, tied the stone to the dog's neck, and threw him into the water. But somehow the stone slipped out and the dog swam to the boat. The old peasant hit the dog with the oar, but the dog still kept swimming. The peasant picked up the oar and tried to hit the dog again, but he lost his balance and fell into the water. The old man could not swim and began to drown. The dog made his way quickly to the old man and seized his master's clothes in his teeth. The dog tried as hard as he could to keep his master on top of the water. Meanwhile, people who were working on the shore saw that somebody was drowning, and many of them rushed to the rescue. A boat went out, and the old man was saved. In tears, he carried the exhausted dog home and took care of him until he was quite well again. Since that day they never parted."

Below we give the story as retold by the boy:

"An old peasant once had a dog and he wanted to drown him. But he shouldn't make fun of animals, he was bad—a rascal! He called the dog and put him in a sack, and then they went down to the river and he fell in himself . . . What do you have in the box? I take books from the library . . . " (The doctor asked the boy to get on with the with the story). Vova proceeded with his narrative: "He put him in a sack, and the dog grabbed his shirt with his teeth and saved him. It was a good dog and he was bad! No, he was good too, because he took the dog home and took care of him. Is that all, do you think? Why am I telling you about this dog? I would rather talk about Tarzan. That was really funny!" (Vova narrates extracts from the film, gesticulates, and laughs.)

These peculiarities of the boy stood out against a background of maldevelopment of the ability to abstract and generalize.

In the picture-classifying experiment, Vova started to carry out the task without listening to the instructions given to him. He worked in a very disorganized manner, and arranged the pictures impulsively and hastily, talking about each picture separately. He tried to classify the pictures into separate groups by working on the concept of pseudocategories, but in the course of his activity it was quite obvious that this activity reflected verbal stereotypes learned by heart, and that his classification was based upon elementary concrete connections. For example, Vova was not in favor of grouping together pictures representing vegetables and pictures representing trees, his explanation being that vegetables grow in the garden but trees in the forest. He did not group a pail with the pots and pans, because it is for carrying water. He removed the saucepan from the other pots and pans, because in his opinion it should not be placed together with them for it is hung up in the kitchen. The knife could not be placed with the pots and pans because it goes into a separate box. Scissors must be kept quite apart, because they are used for cutting nails.

When the groups thus formed were to be extended, elementary concrete connections again appeared: "The picture of a pear goes with a tree." Vova lifted his hand and pressed the picture representing the pear to the flower in the window, and then tried to attach a picture representing a grape in the same place. "The pear grows on a tree and the grape on a bush but the carrot grows in the garden; they can't belong together," said Vova. His replies clearly showed that it was impossible for him to consider an object apart from the situation in which it was found.

The maldevelopment of the ability to abstract and generalize also revealed itself when similarities and differences were established. The boy compared pictures of a cat and a dog in accordance with signs of no significance. In an experiment on reinforced memory, in which the subject had to establish a connection between a word and a picture, he succeeded in coping with this task only in the simplest cases: if, for example, the subject was given the word "mushrooms" and a picture representing a basket, then Vova easily formed a rational connection between the word and the picture: "Mushrooms are gathered in baskets." If the task was made more complicated, the boy then could not solve the problem. When Vova was given the word "well" and shown the picture of a pail, he was unable to form a meaningful connection. It is interesting to note that when Vova identified the essential element connecting these two objects, he connected it with each object separately: "Water is poured into a pail, and water is drawn from a well." He was unable to use the common element which he had identified (water) to form a bond of meaning between the objects.

Whatever task was suggested to the boy, he very clearly revealed the maldevelopment of his capacity for abstraction and generalization. The story "The Unsolved Problem" was read to him:

"The animals were trying to decide what was the best food. The cat said milk, the dog said a bone, the donkey said hay, and the cock said corn."

Vova did not grasp the meaning of this story, and said what he thought was best purely from his own point of view: "The cat was right, milk tastes best."

Vova also experienced great difficulty in describing picture stories: he could distinguish the central figure and even understand the action represented in the picture, but he was quite incapable of establishing an internal connection between the individual elements of the picture and reaching a general understanding of the situation portrayed in the picture.

Clinical Analysis of the Case

The etiology of this case is complex. It may be assumed that there was an intrauterine lesion of the central nervous system, subsequently complicated by a head injury sustained at the age of two years, and by a severe attack of dysentery from which he suffered at the age of $5^1/_2$ years.

The electroencephalography showed an absence of α-rhythm, slow waves of varying amplitude over the entire cortex, with an ill-defined and unstable variation of rhythm, indicating a diffuse lesion of the brain, accompanied by neurodynamic disturbances.

The developmental anomaly arising as a result of the intrauterine diffuse lesion of the brain and leading to maldevelopment of the most complex forms of mental activity provides justification for a diagnosis of oligophrenia.

So far as the qualitative aspect of the structure of the disability is concerned, in this case we have a combination of the fundamental symptom of oligophrenia with nonspecific symptoms in the form of general disinhibition, increased distractability and impulsivity with a marked decrease in the capacity for sustained work. All of this places this case with that form of oligophrenia in which maldevelopment of the cognitive functions takes place against a background of a gross disturbance of the balance between the fundamental nervous processes, with excitation predominating over inhibition. Specific disturbances in the function of different analyzers were not found in this boy. The distinctive feature of the structure of the intellectual defect, namely the combination of a maldevelopment of the cognitive functions with a disturbance of the general behavior and a marked decrease in the capacity for work, corresponds to the distinctive pathophysiological features of this particular case.

Investigation of the higher nervous activity revealed the fundamental pathophysiological mechanism characteristic of the fundamental symptom of oligophrenia, namely inertia of the nervous processes, especially obvious at the level of the second signal system, together with a disturbance of the balance between the fundamental nervous processes in which excitation shows a tendency towards irradiation. The distinctive nature of the pathogenesis is of importance to the development of the disturbance of balance between the fundamental nervous processes in the residual stage of the disease.

The X-ray finding of increased digital markings of the skull, the dilatation of the diploic and emissary veins, together with dilatation of the veins of the optic fundus confirm the presence of residual hydrocephalus. In this case too a connection is clearly demonstrated between the etiopathogenesis, the pathophysiology and the clinical picture.

CASE 2

Tanya K., a girl aged 14 years. This girl is a pupil in the third class of a special school. No complicating factors are found in her heredity.

History. The mother was pregnant four times. The first child, a daughter aged 17 years, was normal and a good student. The second and third pregnancies were terminated by abortion. Our present case was born from the fourth pregnancy. In the eighth month of pregnancy her mother fell, after which she felt ill. Labor took place at term. The child's early development was considerably retarded; she did not begin to speak until she was four years of age. At the age of six months, for no obvious external cause, the girl began to have epileptic fits, associated with states of rigidity. After the age of 18 months these fits ceased. From an early age the girl was very restless and prone to tears, and she slept badly. She was brought up at home. Her mother noticed that she was considerably retarded in her general development at the age of three years. Later, before she reached school age, the girl's restlessness and disinhibition were still more obvious. She could not concentrate on anything, but switched from one thing to another rapidly, and she was garrulous and overfamiliar. In the presence of strangers the girl usually became still more excited: she sang, danced, and chattered a great deal. The girl was not interested in toys, she was a poor listener to stories and did not understand them. With these complaints she was admitted to the first class of a special school.

Physical State. In her physical development the girl was slightly backward for her age. No abnormality of the internal organs was found; only a very slight hypotension was noted.

State of the Nervous System. Investigation of the nervous system showed soft bilateral organic signs of inconstant degree: deviation of the tongue to the left, slight loss of tone in the muscles of the lower limbs, central type disturbances of tone in all muscle groups, and slight instability during Romberg's test. The tendon reflexes were brisk and unequal in amplitude, sometimes more marked on the left, especially in the upper limbs; the abdominal reflexes were brisk, the plantar reflexes greatly increased, and May's sign was absent. Among pathological signs, an inconstant suggestion of a positive Babinski was found.

Ophthalmological Examination. Visual acuity of both eyes 1.0. Optic fundus: disks an intensive pink color, margins indistinct, veins dilated and tortuous. No special findings in the periphery.

Otorhinolaryngological Examination. Hearing within normal limits.

X-ray Examination of the Skull. Microcephaly. Skull dolichocephalic in shape. Base of the skull flattened. Slight calcification along the course of the coronary and lambdoid sutures. Widespread marked digital impressions. Vascular shadows greatly intensified.

Electroencephalography. The electroencephalogram in a state of relative rest indicated a diffuse lesion of the brain as shown by the presence of slow waves, recorded in all regions of the cortex (Fig. 22).

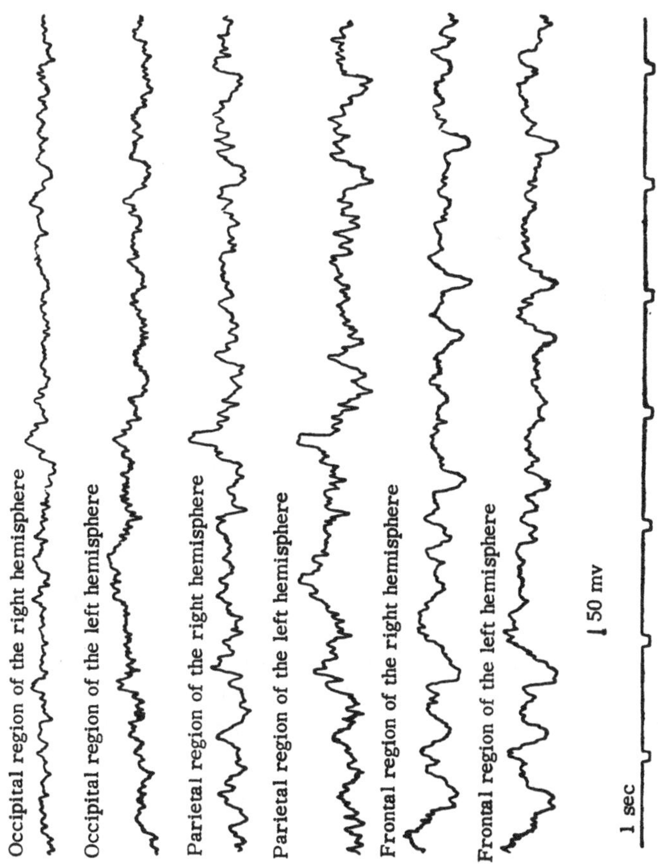

Fig. 22. Tanya K., aged 14 years, girl pupil at a special school (oligophrenia, degree of feeble-mindedness). The EEG shows an absence of the α-rhythm. In all regions of the cortex slow pathological waves are predominant.

The α-rhythm was ill-defined on the EEG.

Stimulation with a rhythmically flashing light with a frequency of 23 per second did not at once cause modification of the cortical rhythm. No modification occurred in response to the first five stimuli; it appeared only after the sixth application of the stimulus. The modification which took place consisted of waves of very low amplitude lasting only about a second when the stimulus acted for six seconds. No modification took place after application of the next few stimuli, and the rhythmic reaction of the cortex in this case was distinguished by its inconstancy for it did not develop in response to every stimulus.

While modification to high and moderate frequencies was so poorly developed in this girl, she showed satisfactory modification in response to light flashes at a frequency of five per second (Fig. 23).

All the properties of the modification described in this case (ill-defined modification at high frequency, inconstancy, slow entry of the cortex into the rhythmic reaction, and rapid emergence from it, as well as the satisfactory modification of the cortical rhythm by low-frequency stimulation) indicate profound changes in the neurodynamics of the cortical neurones.

Investigation of the Higher Nervous Activity. Simple positive conditioned connections, formed by Ivanov-Smolenskii's method, were formed in the first experiments after 6 to 9 combinations. In subsequent experiments one combination was usually sufficient to produce a conditioned reaction.

After preliminary instruction, positive connections were realized at once. The absolute strength of the process of excitation was diminished, as shown primarily by its rapid exhaustion: a decrease in the strength of the reactions was observed during the prolonged application of positive stimuli alone, or when they were presented frequently (especially when the connections were tested one after another, the child ceased to react if the positive stimuli were applied frequently).

Meanwhile excitation showed relative predominance over inhibition. This predominance could be judged from the following facts: a) unaccustomed stimuli (even strong ones) as a rule were generalized with the positive sign; b) frustration in the course of difficult tasks (during overstrain of the process of inhibition) showed a tendency towards excitation (for example, during the repeated application of a negative stimulus differentiation was disinhibited); c) during consecutive tests of the integrity of the more complex

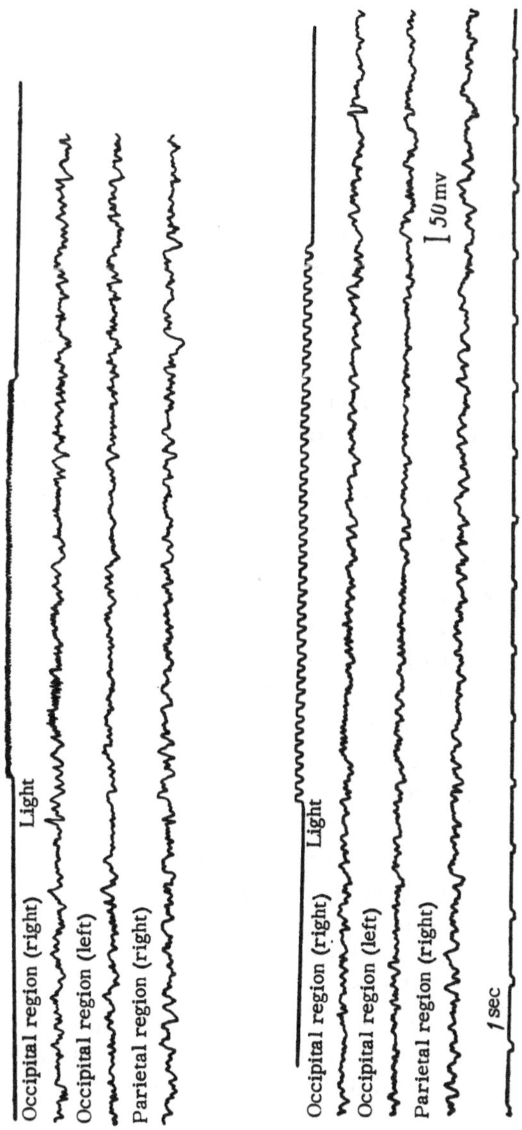

Fig. 23. EEG (of the same subject) during the application of a rhythmic light stimulus. A) Frequency of rhythmic stimulation 23 flashes per second. In the right occipital lead an ill-defined modification of the rhythm is recorded. B) Modification by stimulation at a frequency of 5 per second recorded in the occipital and parietal leads.

differentiations the girl gave positive reactions to all stimuli.

The process of excitation was weakly concentrated and showed a tendency towards irradiation. This was apparent from the following facts: stabilization of the conditioned reactions was extremely ill defined, unaccustomed stimuli were generalized with the positive stimulus, even if they were directed to some other analyzer, and after a few consecutive applications of the positive stimulus, differentiation was disinhibited. This was demonstrated with special clarity during the formation and subsequent modification of complex forms of differentiation. These facts indicate the presence of a strong after-action of the process of excitation.

Active cortical inhibition was considerably weakened. This was shown by weakness of differential inhibition (differentiation of light stimuli by their intensity was produced with difficulty by preliminary instruction; it was impossible to induce differentiation to duration in spite of 393 applications of a positive stimulus and 133 applications of a negative stimulus).

Weakness of internal inhibition was also revealed by the great difficulty or inducing delay during the formation of a reaction to the end of a stimulus (many premature reactions) and also during the production of differentiation of complex stimuli distinguished by their number of identical components (two flashes of light for the positive stimulus and three flashes for the differential stimulus), in which the correct reaction necessitated delay after the second flash while the third flash was being awaited.

The internal inhibition showed a tendency towards irradiation, which was shown by successive inhibition after a few inhibitory stimuli (especially if they were applied frequently). This was revealed most clearly when the connections were tested in sequence. The tendency towards irradiation of inhibition was also shown during the formation of connections by Ivanov-Smolenskii's method, when with a significant increase in the pauses between the positive stimuli no reaction appeared to them without reinforcement, although the connection had previously been established.

During the induction of complex forms of differentiation the degree of irradiation proceeded as far as the development of a state of drowsiness: the girl began to yawn, then laid her head on the table and closed her eyes.

Besides weakness of active inhibition, manifestations of strong external inhibition were observed. The application of an extrastimulus for a few times in succession led to inhibition of the reactions to the positive stimulus. The action of external inhibition was shown especially strongly when it was summated with internal inhibition (if after the extrastimulus the first stimulus was the differential).

Modification of the conditioned meaning of the stimuli in simple systems of connections by the method of speech reinforcement took place easily (after 1-2 combinations), and the influence of training was very conspicuous (a case in which the second stimulus was applied out of place). The modification of more complex connections was more difficult.

In the experiments on the production of motor differentiation, a tendency was shown towards the formation of motor stereotypes. These findings indicate considerable inertia of the nervous processes. Inertia was also revealed in the restoration of old connections when these were tested without reinforcement.

Inertia of a particularly gross degree was apparent in the verbal system. The verbal projection of simple systems of connections was adequate, although it was unstable and easily deformed. Verbalization of erroneous reactions was disturbed. The projection of the formation of more complex systems of connections was profoundly deranged: inertia of the older, previously established verbal connections was found; these were repeated, and represented a substitution of the original projection for the formation of new conditioned reactions and differentiation.

The verbal projection was also profoundly disturbed during the formation of connections after preliminary instruction: during the formation of differentiation to duration, during conflict-producing tasks, and during the formation of reactions in accordance with the principle of alternation the subject's erroneous reactions (the almost complete absence of differentiation) were not reflected in the response, which continued to be a correct repetition of the instruction.

During the formation of connections after preliminary instruction gross disturbances of the regulating function of the verbal system were found. This was shown by the fact that a series of connections was formed with difficulty after instruction (differentiation of light stimuli by their intensity and a delayed reaction). A series of more complex forms of differentiation could not be formed at all after preliminary instruction (differentiation by duration, by the principle of alternation, conflict-producing reactions). On re-examination (one year later) the girl showed considerable changes in her higher nervous activity, in the form of an increased capacity for the formation of difficult forms of differentiation. Whereas during the previous investigation (at the end of 1952) it was impossible to produce differentiation by duration of stimulus, by the principle of alternation ("after every other stimulus") and so on, and differentiation of light stimuli by intensity was only induced with difficulty, upon re-examination (at the end of 1953) all these forms of differentiation could be induced. For example, differentiation to a stimulus differing from the positive stimulus by its duration, was produced after two negative reinforcements of the differential stimulus. In its verbal projection, however, this system was adequately reflected only in the third experiment. For a long time after its formation (before its verbal formulation) differentiation was disinhibited by removal of the reinforcement. Modification in these conditions remained extremely difficult, which demonstrated the gross inertia. A conditioned prolonged reaction to alternate stimuli was produced very slowly (only after three experiments). The reaction "after every other stimulus" became inert after it had been formed, and was reproduced in response to new stimuli. This inertia was also apparent in the working of the second signal system.

Mental State

Visual Analyzer. In addition to correctly recognizing pictures, the girl often gave incorrect, impulsive answers, although she corrected herself. The girl recognized outline diagrams and crossed out figures well, but the same impulsiveness appeared in her answers.

Spatial Orientation. The girl was well orientated in space. She had the concepts of right and left. She pointed correctly to identical arrows. She copied figures from matches at once. In addition to carrying out these tasks correctly, however, the girl often gave incorrect answers because of the ease with which she was distracted.

Motor and Motor-Speech Analyzers. During the investigation of postural movements difficulties arose only in complicated poses. Oral praxis was undisturbed. Imitative synkineses were not well marked. The girl could not cope with the performance of certain tasks related to dynamic movement. If her attention was engaged, the girl showed no disturbances of speech so far as pronunciation was concerned.

Phonemic Hearing. Correlated phonemes were satisfactorily repeated. No displacement of the meaning of words was observed when the experimenter rapidly called out the names of objects. The slight manifestations of amnesia that were observed must be regarded as the consequence of neurodynamic disturbances. The investigation showed the absence of localized cortical disturbances. When carrying out tasks addressed to any given analyzer, the girl showed obvious impulsiveness, lack of concentration on the task, and a noticeable deterioration in her performance during prolonged efforts of perception or when her actions required her to follow an example.

Cognitive Function and Behavior. The predominance of excitation over inhibition was a characteristic feature of the higher nervous activity of this subject, and it was combined with marked weakness of the nervous processes. This property of the process of excitation was clearly demonstrated in the clinical picture. Against this background of general excitation the girl at times did not react to a problem given to her, and failed to carry out assigned tasks. Both in experimental investigations and when carrying out certain tasks at school, she could change with ease from a state of excitation into one of inhibition, and cease all her activities.

The experimental findings showed that excitation clearly predominated over inhibition in this girl. This predominance of excitation was particularly clear and pronounced in the girl's behavior in the first stages of her education at school. Not for a minute could Tanya stay quiet: she fumbled in her satchel, moved things about and played with them, and at times grimaced, laughed out loud, and jumped up and down in her place.

The obvious predominance of excitation in the presence of relative weakness of active inhibition was revealed by the fact that in the course of tasks which she was given the girl could not inhibit the group of irrelevant associations which developed, and she therefore could not confine herself to the task in hand. For example, when she was asked to name five red objects, the girl answered: "A star, flags on the street and on the houses which I saw, and then it is Sunday (the calendar lay on the table), numbers when it is a holiday, a red tie, a carrot, a tomato, red pepper . . . (the enumeration of certain objects was associated with the fact that the girl's glance accidentally fell on one of the show-cases hanging on the wall of the demonstration room of the school, in which she received her instruction). Look at this dirt here, spread over the claws . . . later on I must clean them . . . There is a pail which you have not stood up right. . . I went for a walk in the park and a crow sat in our window."

It can be seen from the above sample of the girl's conversation that she wandered further and further from her task. She showed the same departure from the task at hand in the picture classification experiment: she could group together a series of pictures (vegetables) and call them vegetables, but she could not hold herself in check, and added: "These are vegetables, our mother makes soup from all these vegetables, and this is a cabbage, we chop it up and put on salt, and this is a watch." (The association with a watch arose from the fact that her glance had fallen on the experimenter's wristwatch.)

The girl's extreme impulsiveness, her hastiness and impatience can be explained by the weakness of all forms of cortical inhibition. Tanya could never listen to the teacher's question right to the end, but raised her hand with all possible speed. She would even leave her seat without permission or reason. On one occasion, for instance, when the teacher brought some stuffed birds into the class, she quickly left her desk, went up to the table, handled the birds, and only then went back to her place and sat down.

The ease with which the girl was distracted was also the result of weakness of her active inhibition. During lessons, when asked by the teacher to write down what grows in the forest, she wrote: "The birch, the fir tree, and the oak." Next to this, in another exercise given by the teacher—to write down what lives in the forest, she wrote: "The bear, the rabbit, the fox, and the fir tree," resurrecting the name "fir tree" from the previous exercise.

The same characteristics were revealed during the performance of other tasks, for example when assembling a pyramid. The girl set about the task quickly and impulsively, without listening to the end of the instructions given to her, so that her efforts were unsuccessful. When composing a picture from mosaics, her activities were equally disorganized: she took first one tile, then another, and made no attempt to correlate what was shown with the tiles with what she saw in the picture.

When she was shown picture stories she often would name not the picture which was shown her, but the one next to it. This again showed, on the one hand, the ease with which irradiation of the nervous processes took place in this girl, and on the other hand, how difficult it was to organize a stable orienting reaction in her by means of a simple verbal instruction.

The same characteristic drifting and impulsiveness appeared also when the girl was taught to read and write. Tanya remembered her letters without any special difficulty, but her memory under these circumstances was not permanent. She often forgot letters which she had learned by heart. During reading she skipped from one word to another and would join the beginning of one word with the end of another or, having read a complete word, when repeating it she would not remember the whole word but only one syllable, either initial or terminal. During reading she often lost her place and read words lying close to those chosen for her to read. When writing, the girl showed elements of perseveration, which were evidence of the inertia of her mental processes: instead of the word "kot" she wrote "kok." Transposition or omission of letters was seen. For example, she would write "sobka" instead of "sobaka," "Serezha pasal" instead of "Serezha napisal," or "zelyu" instead of "zemlyu." She made these mistakes both when copying and when writing from dictation. She found it especially difficult to write sentences by dictation. She would turn the sentence round, omit certain words or distort them, and mix up some of the letters in a word. For instance, when the sentence, "Zavtra ya kuplyu ruchku,"* was dictated to her, she wrote "Zavtra rugu." The number of mistakes was very closely dependent on the conditions under which the girl carried out the task. When working individually (under the constant watch of the teacher) the number of these mistakes decreased considerably, but when they were done in the general class work (with many factors to distract her) they were always numerous.

The girl's diminished capacity for sustained work was shown especially clearly when she was learning arithmetic. For a long time she did not know the meaning of a series of numbers and she could not correlate numbers and objects. During the change to elementary arithmetical operations she often gave fortuitous answers, thereby showing a stereotypy of this numerical series. Her calculations also demonstrated the inertia of the numerical stereotypes once they were formed. If the girl established one connection (i.e., 4+5=9;3+6=9;5+4=9), and she was subsequently given an example in which the numbers to be added were changed, her answer would still be 9, invariably reproduced by the previously established connection. If a series of exercises on addition of numbers were given to her in a row, and she was then set a problem in subtraction, the girl would continue to carry out addition of the numbers in the new problem.

Experimental investigations showed the instability of the regulating function of speech, which was also clearly revealed in the girl's play. When playing the game "cats and mice," Tanya was chosen to be "mouse." The game was explained in advance. At first the girl followed the game attentively and ran away from the "cat," but gradually she lost sight of the "cat," forgot her part, and did not realize that because of her the game was spoiled. Laughing merrily she found herself a partner for a game of "chase."

*I shall buy a pen-holder to-morrow.

Obviously the instructions at first sufficed and were also visually reinforced by the fact that the girl saw the "cat," but as soon as the girl playing the part of the "cat" was out of sight, the entire play activity collapsed.

The maldevelopment of her cognitive functions showed up clearly in Tanya. In the picture classifying experiment, for instance, two-situational forms of thinking were predominant in her. She grouped together pictures representing a table, a chair, and a penholder, with the following explanation: "The teacher sits on a chair at the table and writes with a pen." Pictures representing a pail and an inkstand were placed in another group, her explanation being that "you pour into a pail and an inkstand." She was unwilling to group pictures of birds with pictures of animals only because "birds are found in fields and wild animals in the forest." When establishing the differences and similarity between a cat and a dog, she compared the pictures of cat and dog with inconsequential criteria. In an aided memory experiment in which she had to form connections between words and pictures, she managed to form only the most elementary connections. In all these exercises she was often distracted by chance associations, which led her away from the solution of her problems.

The girl experienced great difficulties in the solution of arithmetical problems. She could not establish the required rational connections in these exercises and drifted into the simple and thoughtless manipulation of numbers. For example, the girl was given the problem "In a box there were eight red pencils and five blue pencils. How many more red pencils than blue were in the box?" Tanya could not understand the conditions of the problem, and the word "more" suggested to her that she should add two numbers (8 and 5).

Principal Stages of the Child's Development. Three stages may be distinguished in the development of this girl. The first was before the beginning of her organized education. In this stage her disorganized behavior, her very low capacity for work and her absentmindedness were shown to a very obvious degree. She incorporated in her speech everything that happened to catch her eye or that was said in her hearing, or that came into her mind. At this stage of her development, Tanya could not really occupy herself with any task, although she gave the impression of being busy with something. She chattered continually, but did not finish a job. When she tried to tell a story she jumped from one thought to another, and she was quite incapable of making the most elementary connection; she did not know a single letter and she had no notion of number.

The second stage began at the time the girl received appropriate treatment, and when she also began to receive individual instruction from the teacher. The program of corrective training for this girl was based on the qualitative structural features of her disability. Tanya's inability to organize her activity was the main handicap to her successful education along the lines of the syllabus of the special school. Bearing in mind the girl's individual peculiarities it was essential to create the most favorable conditions for her education and training.

The third stage in the girl's development began at the time of her education in the third class of the special school. At this time substantial changes had already taken place in her development, which were reflected in her more organized behavior, and in her ability to perform certain tasks in accordance with the teacher's verbal instructions. At the same period considerable development of her emotional-volitional functions became apparent, the level of analysis and synthesis in each individual analyzer rose, and a definite improvement was seen in the development of her cognitive functions.

Clinical Analysis of the Case

In this case there are grounds for the assumption that intrauterine injury to the fetus occurred, in connection with trauma sustained by the mother during pregnancy. The epileptic fits, starting at the age of six months and continuing until 18 months, were the consequence of the same intrauterine fetal hemorrhage. The presence of epileptic fits complicated to a greater degree the whole course of the girl's subsequent development (delay in speaking and walking). The neurological symptomatology, the manifestations of which were inconstant, and also the periodically occurring attacks of headache and vertigo, accompanied at times by nausea, suggest disturbances of the circulation of the blood and the cerebrospinal fluid, and this is confirmed by the results of craniography.

These disturbances of the circulation of the cerebrospinal fluid and blood resulted in both weakness of excitation and inhibition and in a disturbance of the balance between these two processes. The changes in the cortical neurodynamics are also illustrated by our electroencephalographic investigations, which indicated the slow entry of the cortex into a rhythmic reaction, and the long latent period and rapid exhaustion of each reaction. Weakness of the fundamental nervous processes and the predominance of excitation over inhibition were established experimentally by investigation of the higher nervous activity. Taken as a whole, the experimental findings are evidence of a lowered capacity of the cortical neurons for sustained work. These neurodynamic features lie at the basis of the distinctive character of the psychopathological symptoms. The combination of maldevelopment of the cognitive functions with the gross neurodynamic disturbances also provide evidence for a diagnosis in this case of oligophrenia in which the qualitative structure of the disability follows a distinctive pattern.

CASE 3*

History. Yura was born after a fourth pregnancy, the course of which was normal although birth was premature, taking place during the seventh month. His early development showed considerable retardation. He began to walk at three and to use words clearly at four years of age. Physically, he was emaciated, with obvious signs of dysplasia (a wrinkled, senile facies). He suffered from the following illnesses: at 7 months from severe and prolonged dyspepsia, at 2 years from diphtheria, at 3 years from scarlet fever. From an early age until he was 13 he suffered from nocturnal enuresis. From the age of 3 or 4 years to the present time, Yura displayed pathological voracity. At the age of 12 years Yura sustained a head injury, which was unaccompanied by any signs of concussion. At an early age Yura attended a nursery, where he was an excitable and restless child. Between 5 and 8 years of age he was at a kindergarten, where attention was also directed to his bad hyperactivity and his retarded development. From eight years of age Yura began to attend a special school for his education, but from the very beginning he showed considerable difficulty in learning and his behavior was disorganized. He was excitable, disinhibited, extremely fidgety, and unproductive. Yura lived at home with his mother, stepfather, brother, and sister.

Nobody in the family gave Yura any systematic training. His mother noticed several bad points about the boy: his fidgetiness, his inability to work. But along with these bad points she also recognized a number of virtues: he very willingly carried out errands not only for his mother but also for neighbors (going to the shop, emptying the garbage, chopping firewood, etc.). His mother, however, blamed the school for all Yura's failures, as he himself did. His mother made no contact with the school, which was bound to play

*In this case we do not describe the principal stages of the child's development, for he has been under our observation for only a year.

an important part in the child's poor compensation of his disability.

Physical State. Yura was slightly backward for his age in his physical development. He showed no abnormality of the internal organs.

State of the Nervous System. There was a slight right-sided hemisyndrome (he could not close his right eye alone, the right nasolabial fold was ill-defined, and the abdominal reflexes on the right were more quickly exhausted). He showed the syndrome of a peripheral type of paresis of the right foot (deformity, reduced muscle power, absent ankle jerk). The tendon reflexes in the right upper limb were diminished and the knee jerk on the right was reduced. The abdominal reflexes and Mayer's sign were increased.

Ophthalmological Examination. Visual acuity was normal. Slight dilatation of the veins in the optic fundus.

Otorhinolaryngological Examination. Hearing within normal limits.

X-ray Examination of the Skull. The skull was spherical in shape. The pattern was obliterated. Flattening of the base of the skull. Sella turcica flattened. Widespread and intensified digital impressions. Marked increase in the vascular shadows.

Electroencephalography. Although the basic rhythm of the electrical activity was preserved in all areas of the cortex, attention was drawn to the hypersynchronized α-rhythm with isolated epileptiform discharges. Along with these, slow waves were seen, mingled with the α-rhythm (Fig. 24). The presence of a hypersynchronized α-rhythm along with epileptiform discharges, in conjunction with the clinical picture, could be interpreted as an indication of an increased level of excitability of the cortex. The presence of slow waves with a specific rhythm indicated that no gross organic lesion of the brain was present.

Investigation of the Higher Nervous Activity. Positive conditioned connections and simple forms of differentiation were established equally quickly (after 3-6 combinations). More complex connections (differentiation by duration, a conditioned reaction to every other stimulus, differentiation between complex stimuli) were formed after ten or more combinations.

Excitation was markedly predominant over inhibition. This predominance of excitation was demonstrated by excessive tension, by an overflow in the direction of excitation, and by disinhibition of differentiation. The process of excitation was adequate in strength and no exhaustion of the conditioned reactions was found in these experiments.

The weakness of his internal inhibition was very obvious in this subject during investigation. The weakness of his delayed and dif-

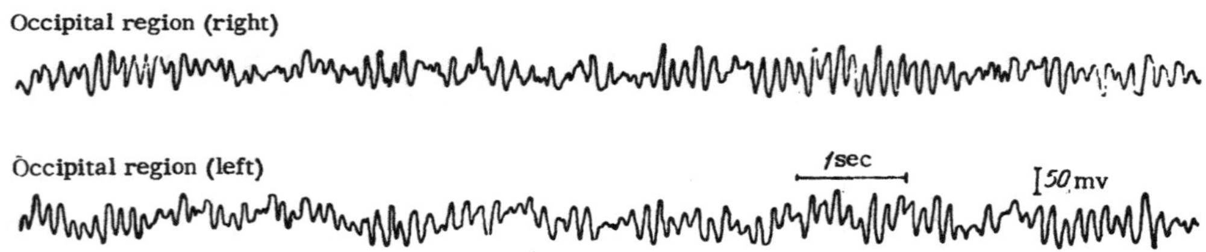

Fig. 24. Yura N., aged 15 years, pupil at a special school (oligophrenia, degree of feeble-mindedness). In the occipital region of the cortex we find a hyper-synchronized α-rhythm of a frequency of 9 per second, in conjunction with epileptiform discharges and slow waves of delta type.

ferential inhibition was especially marked. When stimuli were applied very frequently, the subject worked more accurately and without superfluous tensions. A change to a slow rate interfered with his conditioned reflex activity: excessive tension appeared during pauses.

The weakness of internal inhibition also revealed itself by the great difficulty of production of delay in cases when the subject had to react to the end of a stimulus, and under these conditions many premature reactions were observed. For example, when Yura had to produce a conditioned reaction to a third stimulus, missing two, he did not react to the third stimulus but immediately after the second, which was a manifestation of the weakness of delayed inhibition.

During the production of a conditioned reaction to a complex of two stimuli applied in sequence, Yura reacted to each stimulus separately. The same tendency to react to the individual components of a complex stimulus appeared during the production of a conditioned reaction to a complex of three successive stimuli.

The verbal projection of the production of the simplest systems of connections was adequate but extremely unstable. Chance associations were observed (especially projections of past experiments). The verbal projection of the production of more complex forms of differentiation showed gross inertia of previously formed connections.

Mental State

Visual Analyzer. Yura recognized and correctly named pictures shown to him, whether with right or wrong side up, but besides giving the correct answers he would also give hasty, incorrect, and impulsive answers. Sometimes his answers involved a series of associations which he could not inhibit, and he would recite the names of related objects. For example, when he was shown the picture of a table, Yura called it a "bed," a "chair," a "cupboard," or a "room," and only eventually did he give the correct name of the object represented in the picture.

Sometimes in the course of this examination Yura's answers would reflect elements of pseudo-optic agnosia, as shown by the fact that he recognized only part of an object. For example, when he was shown a picture of some cherries, he was aware of only the green stem, and identified the whole thing as onions. Later he was shown a picture representing an iron, and he persistently called this object a wooden handle. In both these cases there was a fragmentary perception of an individual element and not of the picture as a whole. When his activity was organized, however, and his answering rate became slower as in the case of the next 50 pictures showing various objects, Yura recognized them and gave the correct answers.

Spatial Orientation. Yura was well oriented in space and could correctly point to objects situated on the right and left. He could arrange sticks into most elementary or more complicated figures when given an example to work from. Regardless of the adequate performance of these tasks, he would often reply to questions in an impulsive, incorrect, and foolish manner, or drift away from his appointed task into some quite different activity. Yura could not cope with fairly complicated problems from examples, if the example was covered up after being shown, thus indicating the weakness of his tracing activity.

Motor and Motor-Speech Analyzers. Yura could easily reproduce various poses of the upper limbs demonstrated by the experimenter. He had no difficulty in coping with individual tasks concerned with dynamic movement. His speaking rate was rapid, as a result of which his speech often became indistinct and slurred, but if the rate were slowed, the absence of any form of disturbance of his pronunciation was clearly demonstrated. The boy could repeat, after the experimenter, sentences that were comparatively difficult to pronounce.

Phonemic Hearing. Yura understood completely anything said to him, and he reproduced correlated phonemes almost faultlessly. Errors arose only when the scope of the problem was considerably increased, at which time the boy began to be distracted and drifted away from his appointed task. Yura thus showed no marked defect of the individual cortical functions, and yet at the same time his purposeful activity was disturbed.

Cognitive Function and Behavior. In his behavior Yura was most often excited and disinhibited, with an evidently euphoric tendency in his make-up, and he was disorganized and impulsive. These features were apparent in his external appearance: his shirt collar was unfastened, his belt hung down, his shirt tail hunt out, and his face and hands were usually smeared with chalk and ink. Yura's movements were rapid and impetuous. He exhibited many superfluous movements, grimaces, and tics. In his dealings with adults he was free-and-easy and familiar. He would call the laboratory assistant "Zhena" (wife) and later, "Zhen'ku" (dear little wife), and would pat the doctor familiarly on the arm and reproach him in a joking way for having been kept waiting five minutes.

Yura had no appropriate reaction to his environment. He did not submit to the discipline of the class and his behavior during lessons was unruly. When he was summoned to the blackboard he was not at all embarrassed by the fact that he could not do the problem assigned to him, and he fooled about and grimaced behind the teacher's back. The presence of a stranger in the class during a lesson (the headmaster or the doctor) did not alter Yura's behavior, and sometimes it even increased his tendency to fool around. Yura's behavior was hardly affected by his environment. He was not distressed by the unaccustomed circumstances of his first medical examination. Even then he was just as overfamiliar and uninhibited as ever. When out in the street Yura was just as excitable. When at home he exhibited restlessness, impetuosity, and inability to behave in an organized manner.

Yura's disinhibition and impulsiveness diminished only when he was in very quiet surroundings, for example during conversation with the teacher or doctor. He was unaware of his incorrect behavior or of his misdeeds. Without a trace of embarrassment he told the doctor that he was a bad pupil and got bad marks in arithmetic, and he explained his poor progress as due entirely to the fact that the boys punched him in the back. He got poor marks in Russian because the teacher dictated badly.

Yura was suspended from school for six days on account of his bad behavior, but this punishment made no impression on him. His only explanation of his incorrect behavior was that the other children behaved badly and they all picked on him.

His increased excitability, his disinhibition and his easily distracted nature were very clearly revealed during experimental investigation. The boy was extremely impulsive in his activities. In any form of activity the characteristic feature of his reaction was that he responded only to an individual element of the task. All instructions concerning a task consisting of only one step were carried out easily and quickly by the boy, but the least increase of scope of the problem, i.e., a change to systematized activity, was extremely difficult for him. For example, when arranging tiles to form pictures, Yura set about the task very quickly without waiting for preliminary reflection. In the course of his task he did not correlate the appearance of the tile with that of the picture, and found the appropriate spot for a particular tile with difficulty; having once found it he might at once remove it, or fit it together incorrectly. The boy eventually reached the right solution with great difficulty, by trial and error, but when he again assembled an identical picture he did not profit by his previous experience and repeated the same mistakes. If, however, Yura's activity was organized when carrying out a task of the same degree of difficulty, if his speed was reduced, if the instruction was broken down into its separate parts, then the boy could cope with the task easily and without making any mistakes.

The disturbances of his purposeful activity were shown still more clearly during Yura's education at school. The boy read quickly, often by guessing, without reading to the end and omitting some of the words, but if he was organized, then Yura could read an assigned passage fluently and correctly.

His impulsiveness in writing was revealed by failure to complete words (he wrote "pobezha" instead of "pobezhal," [he ran] and "propa" instead of "propal") [he disappeared] and by omitting letters (instead of "vstal" he wrote "vsal," [he stood up] and instead of "paravoz" [locomotive] he wrote "parovz"). In his writing, Yura exhibited stereotypy, for example the words "narushitel" [mischief-maker] "vdrug" [suddenly], "otmeli" [shallows], "spryatalsya" [behind], and "nastupili" [she stepped] he wrote as follows: "na rushitel," "v drug," "ot meli," "s pryatalsya," and "na stupili." In his writing he also showed perseveration. He always signed his work "Nemkov Yurii Nikolai Nikolaevicha." He wrote extremely hastily and carelessly. His exercise books were dirty, and the pages were torn and soiled. During dictation, in addition to sentences containing incomplete words, omissions, and transpositions, Yura's work also included such correctly written sentences as "The Red Army soldiers went in this car." These omissions in writing, failure to complete words, transpositions, and distortions were encountered both during copying and during writing by dictation.

His impulsive and disorganized actions were revealed still more clearly during counting and solution of arithmetical problems. Yura counted orally very badly. He could add and subtract, even when his activities were of the fragmentary nature which typified this boy, but his ability to cope with multiplication and division was clearly much lower, for these operations demand more complex forms of synthetic activity.

In the solution of arithmetical problems the same hastiness, disorganization and thoughtlessness were apparent. The system of connections required for the task could not be realized by the boy and it did not determine to any degree his later activity. This activity in the process of solving an arithmetical problem consisted of a fragmentary operation with numbers. Yura was assigned the following task: "The brother is 12 years old and the sister 9. By how many years older is the brother than the sister?" Without listening to the end of the description of the problem, he replied quickly, "The brother is 12+9=28 years old."

The experimenter told Yura that he had given the wrong answer, and read the conditions of the problem to him again. Without thinking, Yura interrupted the doctor and said: "I know how old the brother and sister are together, they are 72." The number 72 had stuck in the boy's memory after the solution of a previous problem. Next time, the doctor drew a boy and girl, and below the boy wrote the number 12, and below the girl the number 9. With the aid of this visual guide, Yura quickly gave the correct answer: "By three years." He only had to be asked how he had done this, however, for his whole activity to fall to pieces. For instance, he began to carry out arbitrary operations with the numbers 12, 9, 3, 6, 2, etc., went beyond the limits of the problem and said, "She is a tall one, she is 32 years old, and the brother is bald like he was shaved."

The evident predominance of the process of excitation and its tendency towards irradiation were shown by the fact that Yura could not inhibit incidental connections which he developed, and he constantly wandered away from his allotted task. He was asked to describe a cat and dog with one word, and replied "animals," but immediately drifted away from the problem: "The dog stands on guard, but the cat runs near the house, and the little pig grunts. The dog guards the house but the cat doesn't, but then the cat catches mice."

These peculiarities of Yura's activity and behavior were revealed against a background of considerable maldevelopment of abstract and generalized thinking. When establishing similarity and difference, he did not point to any significant features, but compared the concrete images of a cat and a dog by trivial or nonparallel features. "The dog is brown and the cat grey"; "The cat's tail is grey and the dog's fluffy." Yura's individual answers were more correct, for example: "The dog's nose is long and the cat's like a button"; "The cat is big and the dog too, only it is long." During the lesson, however, Yura could not keep to such answers but drifted at once either into comparing by incidental and unimportant signs (for example, he pointed to the identical flexion of the paw in the cat and the dog) or he ceased to make any comparison.

In the picture classification experiment the boy exhibited the same disorganization, hastiness and impetuosity in his actions and an obvious maldevelopment of the capacity for abstraction and generalization. Yura did not at once understand a task given to him, but rather set about it without waiting until the end of the doctor's instruction, and arranged a few pictures into a pile without examining them. After the instruction had been repeated to him, he grouped together a series of pictures according to dual concrete situational criteria; for example he grouped together pictures showing a little pig, a kitten, and a dog because they only run about in the yard. Pictures representing a ruler, a table, a chair, a pair of scissors, a key, and a knife were grouped together. He called them all furniture, and he said, "I put them together because these things lie on the table." Subsequently he added to this group a pencil, an inkstand, and a pen—all because of the same criterion. Yura used his generic concepts very imprecisely, and they did not help him to differentiate between individual articles. For example, sometimes he included pears among vegetables and sometimes among fruit.

In the experiment on aided memorizing, in which the boy had to form a connection between a word and a picture, it was found that he was capable of forming only a simple connection. For example, he was given the word "mushrooms" and shown a picture of a basket. Yura correctly grouped together the word and the picture which he was shown and said, "The mushrooms are in a basket." Later the boy was given the word "mouse" and shown the picture of a cat. In this case too, Yura easily formed a connection between the word and the picture, saying, "The cat catches mice."

When the problem was made more complicated, Yura experienced considerable difficulty; he had to re-establish the whole concrete situation, to find the intermediate element, which implied dividing the whole task into a series of stages, and only then could the necessary connection be obtained. For example, the boy was given the word "market" and shown a picture representing a shopping basket. Yura said "Mother bought some vegetables at the market."; "Mother bought a shopping basket." Only after these two preliminary steps did he combine the word and picture by a single connection of meaning and say, "Mother bought some vegetables at the market and put them in the shopping basket."

Clinical Analysis of the Case

In this case we are dealing with a residual state after an attack of parainfectious encephalitis. The neurological findings, in the form of a slight residual right-sided hemisyndrome and the syndrome of paresis of the right foot of a peripheral type suggest a residual state after the boy had suffered from an encephalitic form of poliomyelitis.

A series of infectious diseases from which the boy subsequently suffered still further complicated his development.

Developmental disturbances were observed in the very earliest stages of the child's life. From his earliest childhood he was extremely excited, uninhibited and restless. This restlessness was shown especially clearly just before he was of school age. The boy began his education at a special school, where from the very first days the teacher noticed difficulty with his attention, his disinhibition, his increased excitability, and his extreme impulsiveness. All these features were also clearly shown in the later stages of his education and training. This characteristic anomaly of development, on a residual organic basis, in the presence of marked maldevelopment of the boy's capacity for abstraction and generalization, support the diagnosis of oligophrenia in this case.

CASE 4

Serezha Kh., a boy aged 14 years, a pupil in the fifth class at a special school. No abnormal factors in his heredity.

History. The mother of this boy was pregnant three times. From the first pregnancy a son was born, now 25 years old, a deaf-mute after an attack of meningitis at the age of $2^1/_2$ years. From the second pregnancy a son was born, now 23 years old and healthy.

This boy whom we are now considering was a product of the third pregnancy. The pregnancy occurred during evacuation in wartime, when the mother suffered from starvation and had to do hard physical work. Labor was normal and the child cried at once. While on the breast the child grew to be weak, ailing, and drowsy. From the very earliest childhood considerable delay in his development was observed: teeth appeared at two years old; he began to walk and to speak his first words at three years of age. Speech subsequently developed very slowly. At the age of 18 months the boy suffered from an attack of dysentery. During this illness he had a single epileptic fit with prolonged loss of consciousness.

Shortly before reaching school age the boy showed motor restlessness, he was noisy, cried readily and slept badly. Serezha attended neither nursery nor kindergarten. In the preschool period he became still more restless. He could not play with other children, but behaved roughly with small children and took away their toys, at times exhibiting impulsiveness, coarseness, and overfamiliarity. At the age of eight years Serezha joined the first class of an ordinary school, where he studied for a year but did not succeed in learning the elements of reading and writing, and he was therefore transferred to a special school.

Physical State. The boy was slightly backward for his age in his physical development. He exhibited considerable dysplasia. His skull was deformed (circumference of the head 54 cm) with prominent frontal tuberosities, a saddle-shaped nose, a cataract in the right eye, irregular growth of his teeth, and a deformed chest. Internal organs: heart-sounds impure, pulse 90 beats per minute, blood pressure lowered.

State of the Nervous System. The reaction of the left pupil to light was sluggish and to convergence inadequate. During convergence the right eye deviated outward. Nystagmoid jerks were observed when the eyeballs were in their extreme positions. The boy had difficulty in closing the right eye by itself; the right nasolabial fold was ill-defined. The tongue deviated to the left and the uvula to the right. Phonation of the soft palate was adequate. There were no marked motor disturbances, apart from motor stereotypes. The tone was unchanged; the muscle power adequate. The tendon reflexes were brisk. The left knee jerk was more marked than the right. Babinski's sign was positive.

Ophthalmological Examination. Visual acuity of the right eye 0.05, left 0.5-0.6, corneal opacity of the right eye, hypermetropia, no constriction of the visual fields. Optic fundus: margins of the optic papilla of the left eye slightly blurred.

Otorhinolaryngological Examination. On the left side, chronic suppurative otitis media; on the right side adhesive catarrh of the middle ear. Slight deafness of both ears.

X-ray Examination of the Skull. The skull was dolichocephalic. Slight thickening of the bones of the cranial vault. Calcification of the coronary and lambdoid sutures was seen. Well marked digital impressions, especially in the parietal region. Slight shortening of the dorsum sellae. Vascular shadows greatly intensified.

Electroencephalography. The α-rhythm was well marked in the occipital and parietal regions and almost absent in the temporofrontal leads. The α-rhythm was characterized by hypersynchronization and irregularity. Besides the α-rhythm, slow pathological waves were recorded in all regions of the cortex, and were more prominent in the anterior divisions. In addition to the slow waves, in the anterior divisions a β-rhythm was recorded, and this was especially obvious in the temporal region (Fig. 25).

Rhythmic stimulation caused change in EEG frequency of the cortical rhythm when high-frequency flicker was applied. It was

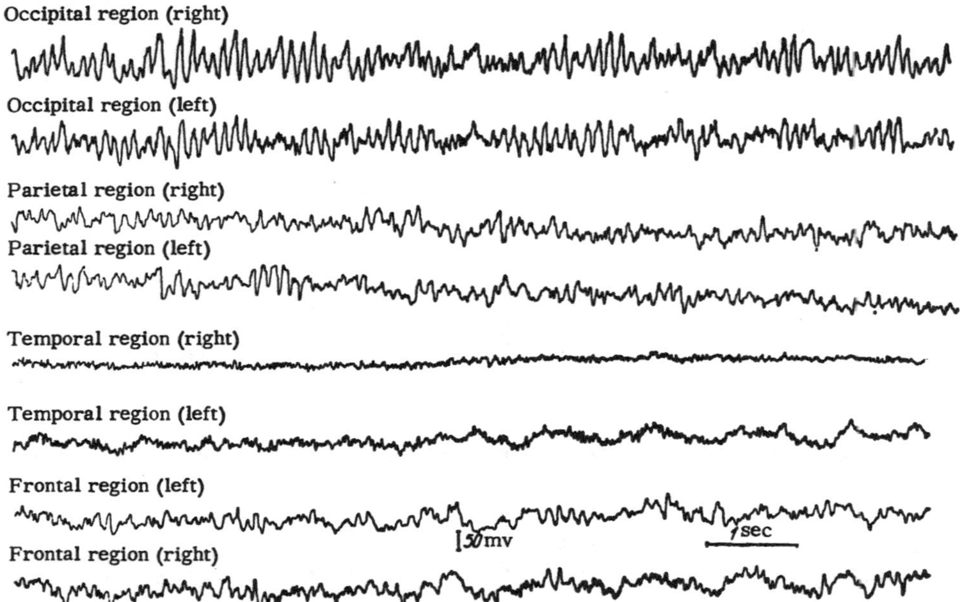

Fig. 25. Serezha Kh., aged 14 years, pupil at a special school (oligophrenia, degree of feeble-mindedness). EEG taken in a state of relative rest. In all regions of the cortex slow pathological waves are recorded. In the occipital regions of the cortex a hypersynchronized α-rhythm is recorded.

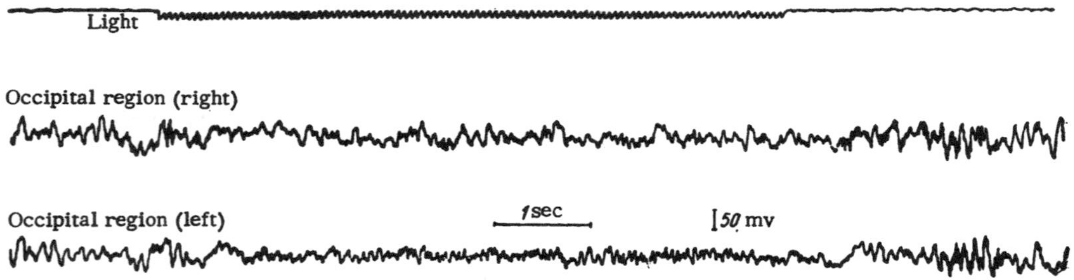

Fig. 26. EEG (of the same subject) during the application of a rhythmic light stimulus. Flicker frequency 16 flashes per second. An ill-defined, irregular change in EEG frequency is recorded in the left occipital region. Slow waves are recorded in the right occipital region.

characteristic that modification of the rhythm was recorded only in small areas of the curve, and was distinguished by its irregularity and its inconstancy. At the same time the rhythmic reaction was found to be rapidly exhausted, and in some cases an increase in the slow waves was seen under the influence of rhythmic stimulation (Fig. 26).

Investigation of the Higher Nervous Activity. Simple positive conditioned connections were established after two and three combinations. The relatively rapid formation of conditioned connections was observed even in complex conditions (a conditioned reaction to every second stimulus appeared after six combinations). No signs of relative weakness of the process of excitation were observed in the investigation, as shown by the rapidity of formation of the conditioned reactions, the absence of decrease in its strength during prolonged experiments, as well as by the absence of any inhibition of the conditioned motor reaction under the influence of extrastimuli.

The excitation showed a tendency towards irradiation. This was manifested primarily by the wide generalization of the stimuli (new stimuli, even those belonging to another analyzer, were generalized with a positive stimulus), and also by disturbance of the stabilization of the conditioned reactions. Signs of weakness of differential inhibition were prominent. In response to most differential stimuli the subject gave inhibited motor conditioned reactions. The process of excitation predominated over inhibition, as was shown by the following:

a) the disturbances of conditioned reflex activity observed in difficult conditions took place almost exclusively on the side of excitation;

b) irradiation of excitation was observed in conditions in which irradiation of inhibition was absent;

c) wide generalization of extrastimuli (even powerful ones) with the positive stimulus.

The typical gross inertia of all oligophrenic children was observed, as manifested by the persistence of old established connections during the formation of new ones in verbal projections, and by the ease of formation of motor stereotypes.

Mental State

Visual Analyzer. During the investigation of analysis and synthesis within the optic analyzer the boy did not recognize pictures of objects shown to him upside down, crossed-out figures; or broken-line drawings of objects.

In the course of his education, however, he made considerable progress in his development, as shown especially by an increase of the level of analysis and synthesis within the limits of the individual analyzers. Serezha easily recognized objects on pictures when shown them right or wrong side up, and could also recognize broken-line drawings, but because he was easily distracted and bored he also produced incorrect answers, or drifted away from his allotted task. The pictures conjured up incidental associations and he often reacted not to the picture which was actually shown to him but to the next one.

Spatial Orientation. Serezha was well orientated in space. He understood the concepts of right and left. He could assemble a pattern from matches or sticks, and he could easily recognize all the letters of the alphabet upside down, but in addition to performing these tasks properly he often would give erroneous, impulsive answers, even in the case of the simplest tasks. In regard to the analysis and synthesis of spatial ideas too, Serezha made considerable progress. In the first stages of his education, for instance, complicated tasks caused him considerable difficulty, but after three or four years of education mistakes appeared in his answers only as a result of distraction, impulsiveness, or lack of organization.

Motor and Motor-Speech Analyzers. In exercises on postural movements, as with dynamic movements, no severe disturbances of the cortical functions were observed, but besides carrying out these tasks correctly, speedily, and accurately, Serezha often did not analyze the position of the upper limb and would reproduce only an individual fragment, or would become totally distracted from the problem and begin to reproduce certain poses but not those which he had been instructed to do. During the investigation only lateral pronunciation of sibilants and whistling sounds was observed, and there was a slight nasal intonation in his speech. At the same time the boy could readily pronounce a difficult sentence.

Phonemic Hearing. Serezha readily understood what was said to him, his vocabulary was adequate, and he constructed sentences correctly. The boy usually repeated correlated phonemes correctly, but sometimes he drifted away from his task and gave incorrect and foolish answers in addition to the right ones. The boy showed no gross disturbances of individual cortical functions, but when carrying out tasks addressed to any analyzer he frequently drifted away from the problem, developed incidental associations and carried out his tasks fragmentarily.

Cognitive Function and Behavior. Contact was readily established with the boy, he readily adapted himself to a new situation and he was easily disinhibited and excited.

During the first year of his education, Serezha's behavior made him one of the most difficult pupils in the class. During lessons he could not keep still for a minute: he grimaced, chatted with his neighbors, teased the other children sitting at their desks, jumped up and down in his place, wandered about the classroom. At times his general level of excitation rose still higher, and Serezha would then throw the school property about and tear his exercise books. During intervals between lessons his excitation increased to an even higher degree: he would start fights with other children and take their possessions. Sometimes he usurped the position of teacher, calling on the other children to be disciplined, without realizing that he was the worst offender of all.

The boy's increased excitability also revealed itself in his motor activity. Although he had no paralysis or pareses, his whole motor activity was extremely disorganized. He exhibited many superfluous and unnecessary movements. Serezha's increased excitability also showed itself in the emotional-volitional sphere, so that all his outpourings were marked by impulsivity. For instance he demanded to be held in high esteem by the teacher, and from the children he required that they should support his election as orderly, monitor, etc.

Serezha's education and training were made extremely difficult by reason mainly of his impulsiveness and the ease with which he became distracted and fatigued. He learned elementary reading and writing with great difficulty. He learned his letters easily, but often became confused and called a letter by the wrong name. He had no particular difficulty in mastering the analysis of sounds and letters, but he often read a word by guessing, without reading it to the end, and sometimes in process of reading he joined the beginning of one word to the end of another. Serezha experienced considerable difficulty in learning to write. He found it difficult to trace the outline of a letter given to him. It was only by supplementary individual tuition that he gradually learned to write. As he progressed with his writing, however, his characteristic mistakes became more and more evident. For instance, when copying he missed out letters, did not finish words, duplicated letters, syllables, and words, and sometimes he reproduced letters which he had previously written. Side by side with this badly executed work, Serezha could write from dictation without making a single mistake, provided that the teacher stood by him and made him work more slowly. In subsequent stages of his education, when the boy's condition was adequately compensated, he still made his characteristic mistakes during writing whether from dictation or copying.

Similar difficulties also arose when the boy was taught to count. He readily learned to count up to ten, but this series of numbers soon became fixed in the form of an inert verbal stereotype. His difficulties in learning to count were due, as in any oligophrenic, to the maldevelopment of his cognitive functions, but along with these difficulties Serezha also had specific difficulties of his own. For instance, he could not count up to a given number, but carried out this task fragmentarily; in solving elementary arithmetical additions and subtractions in the range up to ten, he gave random, impulsive answers, and did not concentrate on his task but drifted away from it. When his attention was organized, however, the quality of his replies immediately improved.

Serezha's diminished capacity for work was greatly in evidence at all stages of his education, and resulted from the ease with which he was distracted and fatigued. When learning to read and write, for instance, he still made his characteristic mistakes. In the fourth year of his education Serezha read fluently and with expression, but as he became excited he attempted to read by guessing, increased his speed, omitted ends of words, and often read a different passage from that selected by the teacher.

The boy's writing remained careless and hasty, whether from dictation or by copying. The standard of all his written work remained extremely uneven. Alongside work containing many mistakes there were exercises without a single error.

All these specific features of the boy were revealed against the background of maldevelopment of the generalizing function of speech. During experimental investigation of his cognitive functions we again discovered a combination of maldevelopment of his cognitive functions with specific manifestations in the cortical neurodynamics. In the picture classification experiment, even in the initial stage Serezha showed his understanding of the instruction, but in doing the task he grouped together only identical objects and frequently became distracted.

Later the boy acquired the ability to make use of ideas which he had learned: he distinguished animals, pots and pans, furniture, etc., but the connections related to these ideas remained extremely vague. For example, in the concept of "fruit," Serezha included pictures illustrating crab, cucumber, and candy, with the explanation that all these were edibles. This immediately gave rise to a series of random associations: "Mother bought me some candy, it was very nice and I ate it, and Vitya bought some candy at a snack-bar." With more extensive picture groups it became obvious that the boy grouped objects together on the basis of their mutual presence in a concrete situation. For instance, he grouped a table and a chair with school equipment, being motivated in so doing by the notion that "the pupils sit here and write, and this (he pointed to the equipment) must all lie on the table, because the inkstand and book must not be put on the floor." He grouped pictures of vegetables together with pictures of pots and pans "because vegetables can be put in a pail, and if they are cut up into little pieces they can also be put into a mug." He classified bottles quite separately "because you can only pour tomato juice into them."

The boy placed a picture representing a fork in a separate group from the pots and pans, and explained that among the pictures of pots and pans there was a mug and only a spoon could be placed in that. In the course of the experiment the boy correctly arranged the pictures in their separate groups, but in his verbal projection he showed absence of true concepts. For example, he grouped together pictures of a pigeon, a duck, a swallow, and a goose; in another group he included trees and flowers. When asked why he grouped these pictures together, however, he replied, "Because trees and flowers grow in the forest, but ducks and geese run about the yard, and swallows and pigeons fly about in the yard."

Throughout the investigation of his cognitive functions, Serezha showed more and more obviously the predominance of his situational connections. One of his characteristic signs was the abundance of situational connections in a series of experiments, which prevented the formation of more abstract connections.

For instance, when he grouped pictures on the basis of ideas he had learned, extension of these groups led to an abundance of situational connections: "You can't put anything with a shopping basket, it is only for carrying. You can put clothes in it, when it is new, when you buy it, then you can't put an overcoat in it because it won't fit." When dividing animals into two groups, wild and domestic, he would not agree to put them together, his reason being that the wolf would bite all the other animals to death. Although he correctly separated the two groups of vegetables and fruit, Serezha would not agree that they could be combined, his argument being that vegetables grow in the ground and fruit on trees.

The boy's cognitive maldevelopment was revealed still more clearly by observation of his comprehension of a story passage. Serezha could not listen attentively enough to the reading of the passage; he did not grasp its theme; he often became distracted and asked many questions without listening to the answers. If the boy was able to concentrate, however, it was readily apparent that a story with a hidden or inner meaning was beyond his comprehension.

The story "The Unsolved Problem" was read to him. Serezha could not draw the proper conclusion, but dwelt on what was nicest from his own point of view: "The cat was right, milk tastes best of all." He was then read the story "Medicine." In reply to the doctor's question whether Tanya had done right, Serezha stated very confidently: "Tanya did not do right, she thought that she would get better, but it was her mother who was ill. She was wrong, she drank it herself, and did not give it to her mother." In this story too, the boy could not come to the right conclusion and definitely regarded Tanya's behavior as bad.

Serezha could tackle successfully an easy series consisting of three pictures: 1) "In the forest they are cutting a Christmas tree"; 2) "They are carrying the Christmas tree from the forest on a sledge"; 3) "The children in the room are dancing around the Christmas tree." He arranged these three pictures in proper order, and when talking about them he linked them into a single theme. In a more complicated series in which no definite story continuity was seen in all the pictures, the boy was unable to join them together in a single theme.

Principal Stages of the Child's Development. In the very earliest stages, Serezha showed not only a disturbance of his development but also a series of symptoms consisting of general motor restlessness, increased irritability, and impulsiveness. During preschool years the extreme disorganization of the boy's behavior was especially marked. The boy was so excitable and uninhibited that he had to be refused admission to kindergarten. At the age of eight years Serezha was admitted to the first grade in regular school, where from the first days of his stay, his disorganized behavior and, later, his complete lack of progress in his lessons, attracted attention. At the end of the term Serezha was transferred to a special school, with a diagnosis of "psychopathic-like behavior."

Properly organized corrective training, which was planned to meet the structural pattern of his disability, led to considerable progress in his development. Educational measures were directed towards the development of inhibitory reactions. The teacher inhibited his impulsive reactions, gave him instructions broken down into details, and in the first stages carried out tasks together with the boy.

At the end of the first year of education an appreciable change in his development could already be seen, mainly apparent in the organization of his behavior and in the development of his emotional-volitional function. Serezha became more restrained and organized, and was less impulsive in his answers and in his conduct. If his excitation sometimes increased, he could inhibit himself now.

At this stage Serezha was more at home in the childrens' meetings, although his agitated appearance and the impatience which he showed when the names of other candidates were called, and the evident joy which appeared when he was nominated were evidence of Serezha's emotions, which he could now control.

Subsequently Serezha behaved in an organized manner at children's meetings, and proposed candididates himself, especially children whom he liked best.

The next, and no less weighty evidence of the development of the boy's emotional-volitional function and personality as a whole was his attitude towards the teacher's opinion of him, and the elements of a critical attitude towards his own work. In the first year of his studies the boy demanded a high appraisal and was quite incapable of correlating the teacher's opinion with the quality of his work. In the second year of his studies he showed well marked emotional experience on the occasion of an unfavorable assessment, and in the third year elements of a critical attitude towards his own work began to appear. For instance, when reciting a fable which he had learned by heart, he told the teacher there and then that he was doing it badly, and he asked permission to repeat it, which he obtained.

In the third year of his studies, Serezha now had a well developed critical attitude towards situations. To the extent to which he could develop his ability to inhibit his impulsiveness, excitability and ease of distraction, improvements took place in his personality, and his emotional-volitional function underwent considerable development.

Serezha also showed considerable progress in regard to the development of the level of his analysis and synthesis within the limits of the various analyzers. Whereas in the first year of his studies complicated tasks addressed to any analyzer aroused difficulties, in the fourth year he could cope with them easily. The maldevelopment of his cognitive functions remained a sufficiently well marked symptom at every stage of the child's development, but nevertheless here too a clear line of development could be distinguished. For instance, in the test of classifying pictures representing various objects the development of concrete situational forms of thinking and the boy's ability to make use of ideas which he had learned were plain to see.

Clinical Analysis of the Case

The etiological factor in this case was congenital syphilis, complicated by head injury and malnutrition during early childhood. The electroencephalographic findings, indicating the presence of slow pathological waves, more marked in the anterior divisions, taken in conjunction with the residual and scattered neurological symptomatology, confirm the presence of a diffuse lesion of the cerebral cortex.

The early diffuse lesion of the brain, leading to a disturbance of development from earliest childhood, and the presence of maldevelopment of the capacity for abstraction and generalization, are evidence in favor of the diagnosis of oligophrenia. The qualitative structural pattern in this particular case is determined not only by the maldevelopment of the generalizing function of speech, but also by the marked disturbances of the cortical neurodynamics.

Clinical studies suggested that the disturbance of the cortical neurodynamics took the form of predominance of excitation over inhibition. Experimental investigation of the higher nervous activity showed disturbance of both the mobility of the nervous processes and of the balance between the fundamental nervous processes, with the predominance of excitation over inhibition.

The presence of disturbances of the balance between the fundamental nervous processes in a stage of the disease at which the active pathological process had long ago ceased, was associated with an additional etiological factor in this particular case, namely a closed head injury sustained at the age of eight months. The specific inflammatory intrauterine disease, complicated by the head injury, led not only to a diffuse lesion of the cerebral cortex but also to a residual hydrocephalus.

The presence of hydrocephalus was also confirmed by the craniographic findings. X-ray examination of the skull showed well marked digital impressions which, as we have repeatedly shown, indicate a disturbance of the cerebrospinal fluid circulation.

The combination of maldevelopment of the cognitive functions with the special features of the cortical neurodynamics are evidence in favor of including this case as a variant of oligophrenia of the sort we have discussed. A careful study of the structure of his disability in the initial stages of his education permitted the organization of correct medical treatment and educational measures. Medical treatment was directed toward the improvement of the flow of cerebrospinal fluid. For this purpose, twice a year Serezha received a course of hypertonic infusions. In addition he received systematic small doses of bromides, which strengthened his inhibitory processes. These measures were applied in conjunction with educational measures, which were also directed toward the development of inhibitory reactions in the boy, and they were followed by considerable compensation of his condition.

ANALYSIS OF ALL THE RESULTS OBTAINED

Special Features of Early Development. Besides the general retardation of development in children belonging to this subgroup, a series of specific features appears very early. At nursery age, these children are restless, irritable, capricious, and frequently suffer from disturbances of sleep and appetite. During their preschool years, in addition to those distinctive features of development which are typical of any form of oligophrenia (limited vocabulary, lowered interest in stories and pictures, tendency towards stereotyped and primitive play), various specific features are evident which are characteristic of oligophrenics of this particular group. These specific features are most commonly revealed in the general disinhibition of these children, which forms the basis for their obvious inability to concentrate. They are easily distracted, cannot concentrate for long when either listening or looking. These children are noisy, garrulous, overfamiliar in their dealings with others, irritable, and capricious. They do not submit to the rules of the game, and do not play their part in the game as they should. Most children of this group were educated in the ordinary school before being transferred to the special school, and there they showed a group of specific features in addition to the features common to all oligophrenics (difficulty in learning to read, write, and count). The disinhibition of these children was particularly prominent in the ordinary school, and their ready distractibility and inability to concentrate were also clearly evident. In class the children were excited, disinhibited, and disorganized. The inability of these children to carry out sustained, purposeful activity was very obvious.

X-ray Examination of the Skull. A specific feature of the pathogenesis of this form of oligophrenia is the presence of residual hydrocephalus at a late stage of the disease. In these cases the hydrocephalus evidently lies at the basis of the chronic disturbance of the balance between the fundamental nervous processes. The presence of hydrocephalus in all the cases which we studied was confirmed by craniographic investigations (Figs. 27-30).

The craniographic findings indicate changes in the configuration of the skull, thinning of the bones, and digital impressions. The results of pneumoencephalography indicate the enlargement and dilatation of the ventricles of the brain and changes in the pattern of the subarachnoid spaces. Disturbance of the flow of blood and cerebrospinal fluid in the brain in this variant of the defect (in contrast to other variants) is shown by the presence of a group of general cerebral symptoms. These symptoms include episodic attacks of headache and vertigo, in some cases psychosensory disturbances, and rapidly developing fatigue and exhaustion.

Neurological Investigation. The neurological manifestations in oligophrenics in whom the balance between excitation and inhibition is disturbed are diverse in nature, but most frequently changes are seen in the tone of all muscle groups, slight disturbances of coordination of movements and static activity, briskness of the tendon reflexes, which are often unequal in amplitude, and the presence of pathological reflexes. The neurological manifestations as a whole are diffuse and extremely unstable.

Investigation of the Electrical Activity of the Brain. Investigation of the electrical activity of the brain in children with this variant of oligophrenia shows a relatively more severe abnormality of the EEG than is found in the basic form of oligophrenia. As a rule no α-rhythm is present in the EEG; along with slow, pathological waves of low amplitude typical delta waves are seen. As an example we show the EEG of the boy Alesha F. (Fig. 31), which shows a complete absence of the α-rhythm and the presence of typical delta waves.

The gross nature of the changes in the electrical activity of the brain do not correspond to the severity of the defect, from which it may be concluded that these changes should be interpreted as an index of the neurodynamic disturbances. This point of view is confirmed especially clearly by investigations of the EEG taken during application of functional loading. Stimulation with flickering light

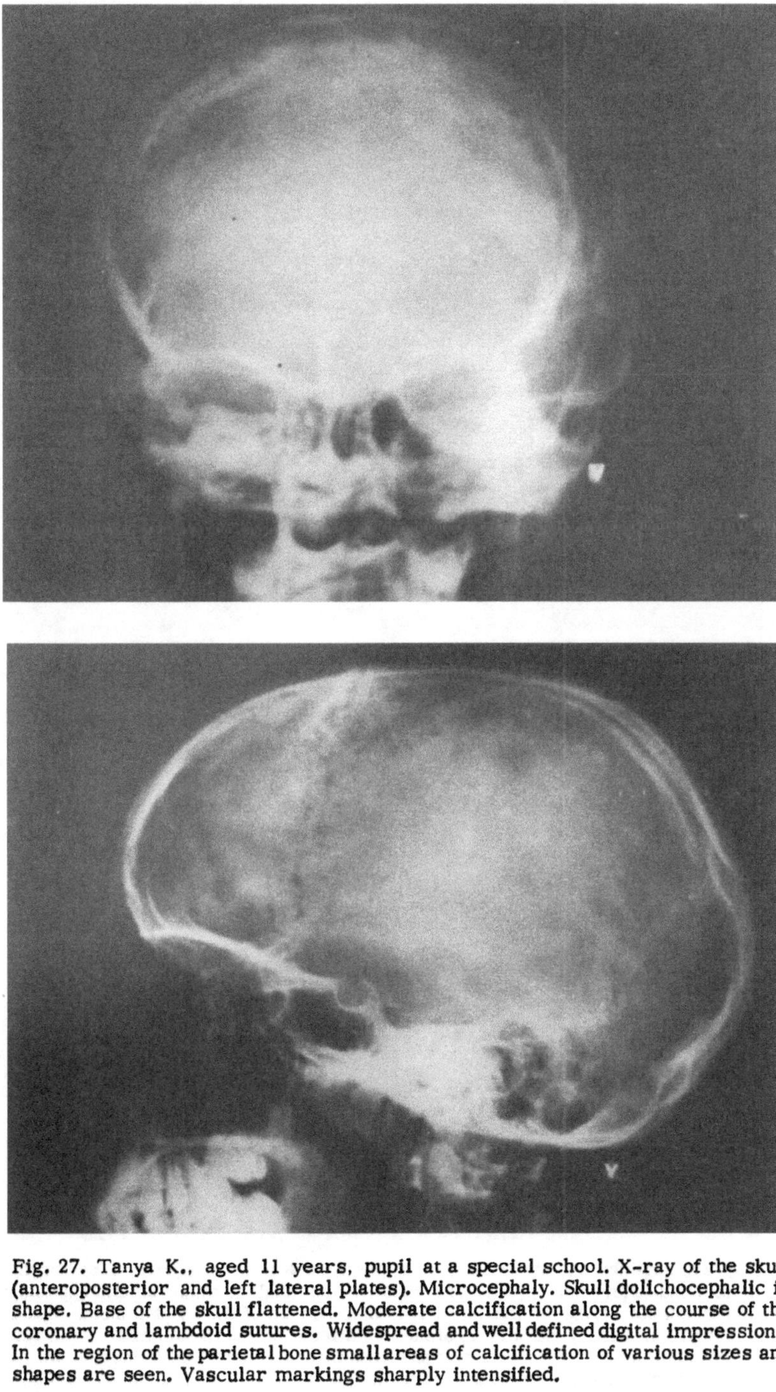

Fig. 27. Tanya K., aged 11 years, pupil at a special school. X-ray of the skull (anteroposterior and left lateral plates). Microcephaly. Skull dolichocephalic in shape. Base of the skull flattened. Moderate calcification along the course of the coronary and lambdoid sutures. Widespread and well defined digital impressions. In the region of the parietal bone small areas of calcification of various sizes and shapes are seen. Vascular markings sharply intensified.

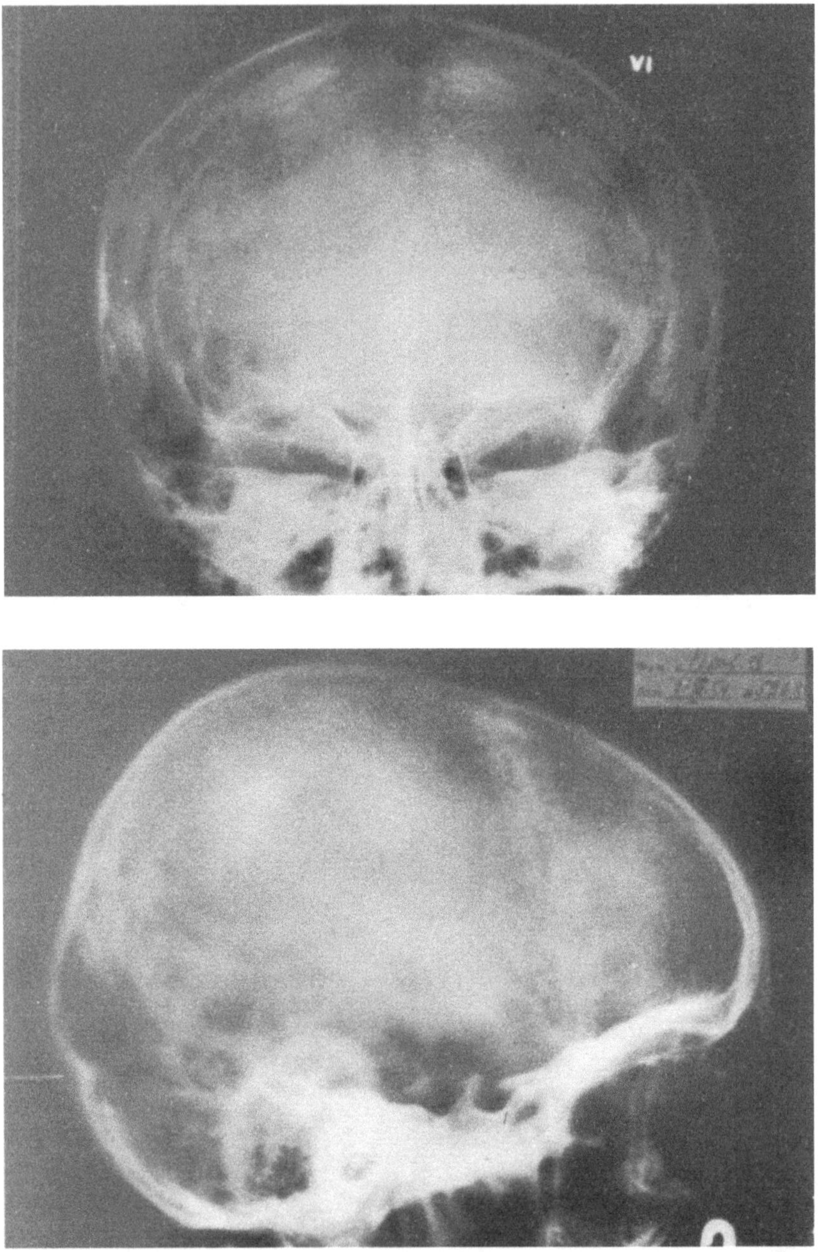

Fig. 28. Serezha S., aged 12 years, pupil at a special school. X-ray of the skull (anteroposterior and right lateral plates). The skull is enlarged and approximately turret-shaped. Base of the skull flattened, bones of the vault thinned. The cranial sutures can hardly be distinguished. Pattern of the inner table of the skull obliterated. Shadows of the transverse and sagittal sinuses slightly increased. Shadows of the Pacchionian granulations increased in density.

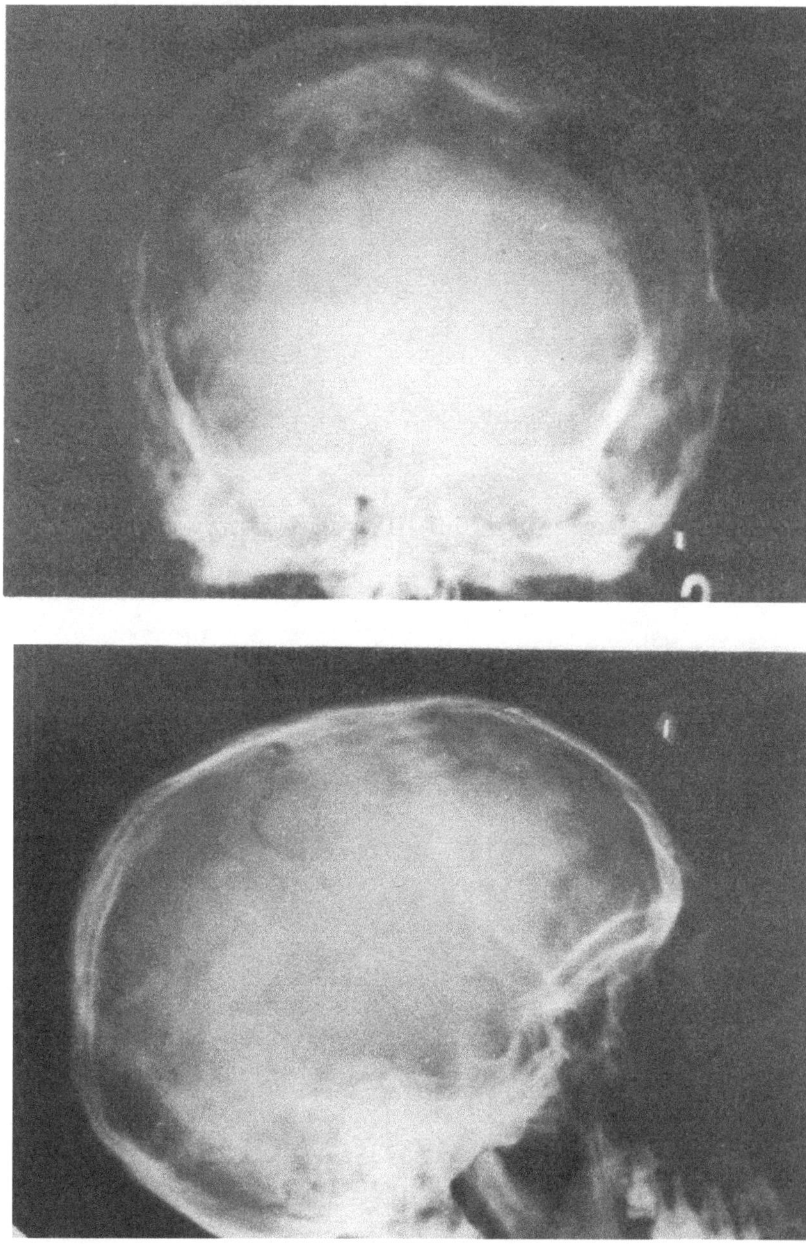

Fig. 29. Vova K., aged 14 years, pupil in the imbecile class at a special school. X-ray of the skull (anteroposterior and right lateral plates). The skull is enlarged and spherical in shape. In all regions the digital impressions are obliterated and the shadows of the diploic veins increased in density. The cranial sutures cannot be distinguished. Sella turcica deepened and widened.

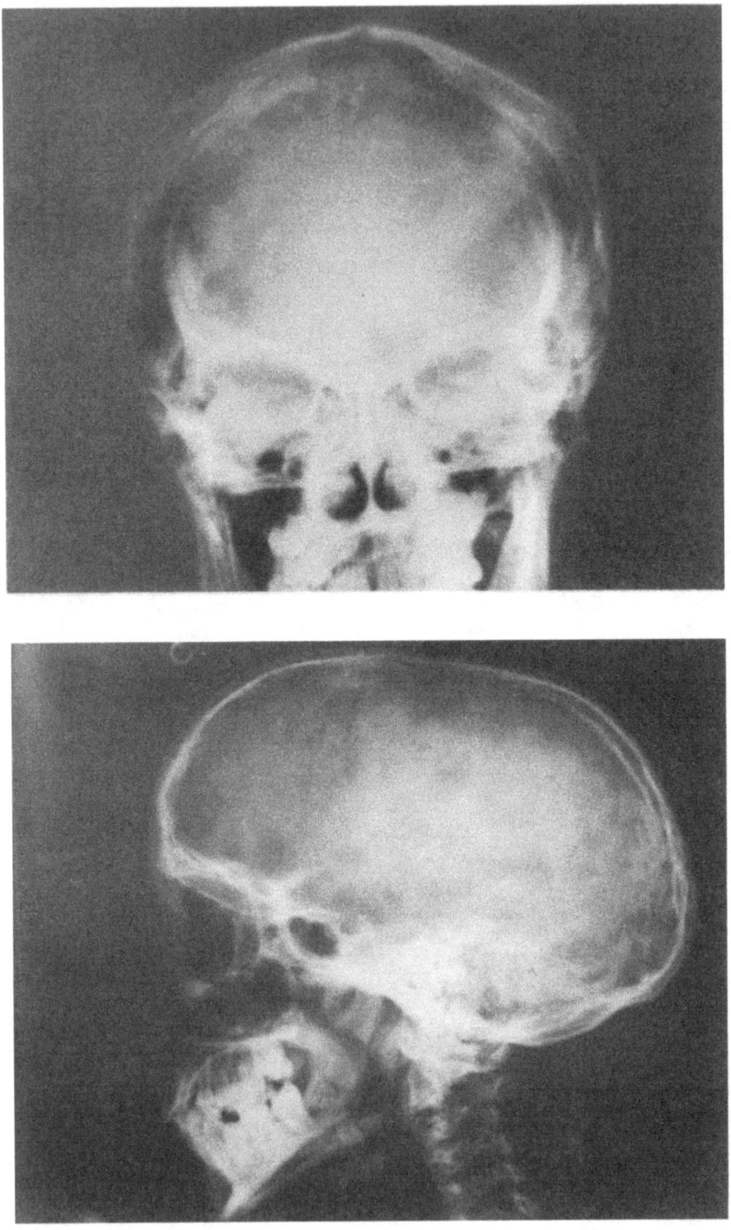

Fig. 30. Valya S., aged 12 years, pupil at a special school. X-rays of the skull (anteroposterior and left lateral plates). Skull dolichocephalic in shape. Well marked digital impressions, especially in the parieto-occipital region. Lambdoid suture ill-defined. Shadows of the Pacchionian granulations increased.

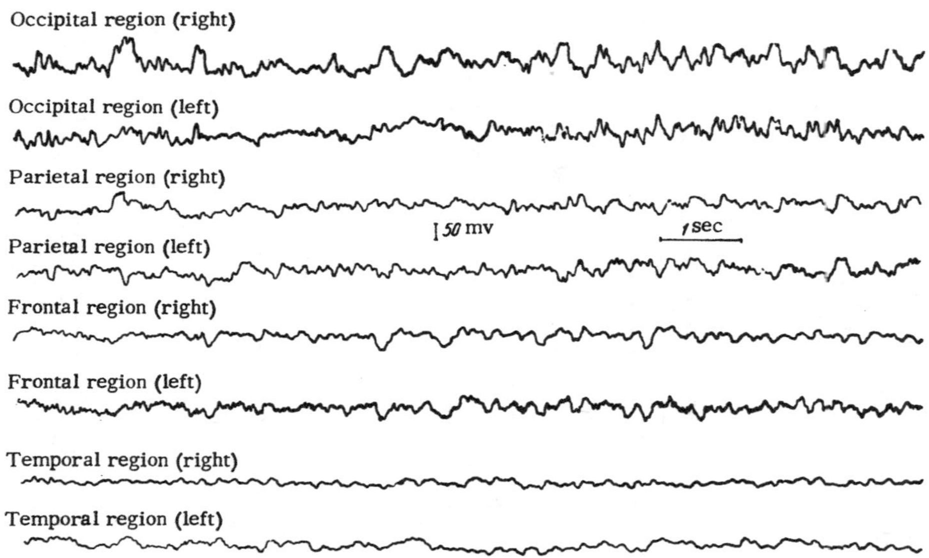

Fig. 31. Alesha F., aged 13 years, pupil at a special school (oligophrenia, degree of feeble-mindedness). Grossly abnormal EEG, as shown by absence of α-rhythm and the presence of diffuse pathological delta waves in all regions of the cortex.

reveals an ill-defined modification of the cortical rhythm in response to a high frequency, inconstancy and slowness of development of a rhythmic reaction by the cortex and rapid recovery (Fig. 32, A). Modification of the cortical rhythm by low-frequency stimuli are also seen (Fig. 32, B) and a characteristic parabiotic reaction in the form of the appearance of slow waves in response to high-frequency flashes of light (Fig. 32, C). This modification of the cortical rhythm indicates gross changes in the neurodynamics of the cortical neurons.

Characteristics of the Higher Nervous Activity. Investigations of the higher nervous activity of the subgroup which we are now studying, conducted by V. I. Lubovskii, showed that the dynamics of their nervous processes have several essential features which stand out against the background of general maldevelopment of the higher nervous activity characteristic of any form of oligophrenia.

A conditioned motor reaction is produced in these children usually after 1 to 3 combinations (only in isolated cases was a larger

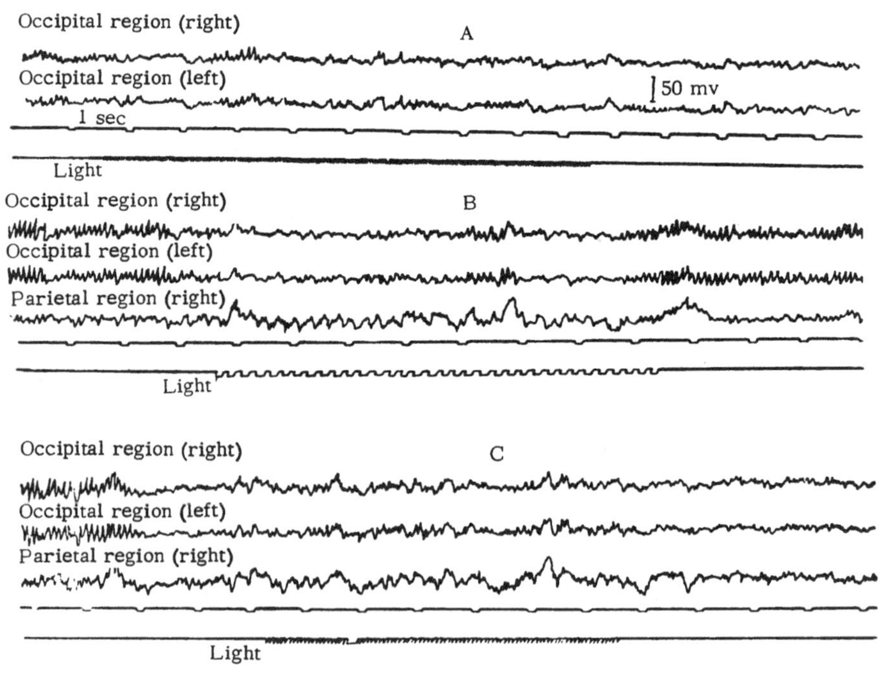

Fig. 32. Lyusya K., aged 15 years. Electroencephalogram during the application of a light stimulus. A) Flicker frequency 20 per second. In the occipital leads an ill-defined modification of the rhythm is recorded. B) Modification to a flicker frequency of 4 per second recorded in the occipital and parietal leads. C) Rhythmic light stimulation causes the appearance of slow waves in the EEG.

number of combinations required—up to nine); in repeated experiments under the influence of exercise the conditioned reaction appears in most cases after one combination. Such rapidity of the formation of connections confirms the presence of a relatively high level of excitation. The process of excitation is far weaker than normal, however, in these children. It is exhausted more easily, as is shown by the decrease in the strength of the reaction during the prolonged application of positive stimuli, and also by the extenuation of the conditioned reactions during the frequent application of positive stimuli (especially when the connections are tested without reinforcement).

In certain oligophrenics of this subgroup, in whom the clinical manifestations were less severe, laboratory experiments revealed excitation to be less marked.

In the case of every child without exception, we could detect signs of well marked irradiation of the process of excitation, as revealed primarily by the extensive generalization of positive stimuli during their initial application. In these children we also noted a considerable number of intersignal reactions (weakness of the process of inhibition was also shown here) and by the manifestations of a considerable after-effect of excitation, as a result of which these children often give a positive reaction to a differential stimulus, especially after several applications.

Active cortical inhibition is severely weakened in these children. The weakness of differential inhibition clearly emerges in experimental conditions, where it takes the form of delayed formation and consolidation of all relatively complex forms of differentiation (by intensity, by duration, etc.).

The weakness of active inhibition is shown especially clearly during investigation by the method of preliminary instruction. The formation of all relatively complex forms of differentiation by instruction is made far more difficult, and in some cases it is impossible. Delayed inhibition is also considerably disturbed, as was discovered during the production of delayed reactions.

During the formation of relatively difficult forms of differentiation it was found that inhibition irradiates in the cortex extraordinarily easily, leading to the development of a state of drowsiness. Thus while the usual behavior of these children is clearly marked by increased mobility and excitability, in certain experimental conditions, on the contrary, they are sleepy and inhibited.

As also in children with other clinical variants of oligophrenia, these children show gross inertia of their nervous processes, which is shown especially strongly in the verbal system (inertia of old established verbal connections).

In all the children of this subgroup the process of excitation predominates over the process of inhibition. This is demonstrated partly by the above-mentioned experimental findings (the abundance of intersignal reactions, the extensive generalization of stimuli with the positive stimulus, etc.). This is also shown by the behavior of modification of the conditioned meaning of stimuli, and also by the fact that "frustrations" during the more difficult tasks usually take place on the side of excitation. It is thus a characteristic feature that the disturbance of the neurodynamics in these oligophrenic children consists primarily of weakness of the inhibitory processes and the predominance of excitation, which in turn shows a tendency towards pathologically wide irradiation, and is itself weakened. The inadequacy of the regulating function of the second signal system is clearly shown.

The pathophysiological features listed above lie at the basis of the distinctive clinical picture of this particular subgroup of oligophrenia.

Investigation of the Individual Cortical Functions. Investigation of the cortical functions shows no gross defects within the limits of the various analyzers. Optic analysis and synthesis in these children are usually preserved; they rapidly recognize objects shown to them, drawings of objects in broken lines, geometrical figures, and crossed-out pictures. In addition to correct recognition, however, they may also give wrong and impulsive answers. For instance, these children often react not to the picture which is being shown to them, but to a neighboring picture. The answers given by these children show the development of random associations in the process of their recognition of pictures.

During the investigation of visual perception in children with this particular variant of oligophrenia, we observed phenomena of pseudo-optic agnosis, when the children apparently recognized only part of an object shown to them.

These erroneous answers of the type of pseudo-optic agnosia arise paroxysmally and alternate with correct answers. Elements of pseudo-optic agnosia disappear in conditions in which the child concentrates on his task.

When these children are called upon to name the various articles represented in a picture, manifestations of pseudoamnesic aphasia also arise. In addition to the correct name of an object the child attempts to give a description of the object by its name.

For example, when a picture was presented showing a wine glass, the boy said, "Its name has flown right out of my head, but it is for drinking wine . . . a wine glass!" On being shown the picture of a comb he said, "Oh dear, I've forgotten this too. I have a red one like it which mother bought for me."

The child was shown a picture of a goat, he looked at it for a long time, and then said, "I've forgotten what it is called, but it gives milk, . . . no, it's a ewe . . . that's what it's called, a ewe. No, it's a 'strekoza' 'no, no, it's a 'koza.'"*

The appearance of these amnesic phenomena takes place only paroxysmally, and in children in a state of increased excitability, and their alternation with correct answers and, finally, the disappearance of this type of incorrect answers in a state of compensation give full justification to their being regarded as pseudoamnesic.

During the investigation of spatial orientation in these children, no gross abnormality is found. Together with correctly carrying out their tasks, however, these children also give random and impulsive answers. During the investigation of postural movements difficulties are found only in complicated tasks. Their oral praxis is not disturbed.

No special disturbances are found in the auditory and motor-speech analyzers in these children. All the children of this subgroup well understand what is said to them and readily construct sentences which are grammatically correct, and their pronunciation is pure. These children usually have a larger vocabulary than other oligophrenic children, they possess a greater wealth of grammatical speech construction, and they distinguish correlated phonemes well, demonstrating that their auditory perception of individual sounds is well preserved. They are capable of differentiating between the quality of verbal stimuli, however, only at the beginning of a task. The children then drift into motor-speech stereotypes. During investigation of rhythms these children at first correctly execute a task, but rapidly become fatigued and develop perseveration. The investigation consequently shows absence of gross changes within the limits of a given analyzer, and at the same time discloses specific peculiarities in the activity of these children.

Characteristics of the Cognitive Functions. During the education and training of these children in the special school it is important to study their cognitive activity. Like other oligophrenics, children of this subgroup show features common to all – maldevelopment of the capacity for abstraction and generalization, but at the same time

*"Strekoza" is Russian for dragonfly, "koza" is Russian for goat. The confusion was caused by the same spelling and pronunciation of syllables "koza."

investigations readily reveal characteristic features of their cognitive functions which distinguish the children of this subgroup from the remaining oligophrenic children.

These aspects of their cognitive functions are shown primarily in the dynamics of their intellectual processes, in their difficulty in keeping their activity within the bounds of their appointed task, and in their inability to inhibit chance associations. These features stand out in any experimental psychological investigation, when they disturb the normal course of the experiment. A few examples may be cited.

In the picture classification experiment, which is one of the principal methods of investigation of the cognitive functions of oligophrenic children, as a rule the subjects do not listen to the whole of the instructions given to them, but rapidly set about arranging the pictures haphazardly, easily developing numerous chance associations regarding each picture. Only after repetition of the instruction or reduction in the scope of the problem do these children manage to complete the basic task, exemplifying the typical oligophrenic defect of abstraction and generalization. These defects usually take the form of particularly concrete forms of classification, their unbreakable attachment to a visual situation, or execution of a task in a purely verbal way. All these features distinguish the subgroup of oligophrenic children which we are describing from uninhibited children with reactive disorders or psychopaths, who also have difficulty in retaining a verbal directive, but who never show such primitive, and usually narrowly concrete forms of classification as are characteristic of oligophrenic children. Generic concepts are employed by these children usually very imprecisely, and they do not use them as a basis for the classification of objects. This vagueness of generic concepts is a characteristic sign of any form of oligophrenia; however, for the subgroup under discussion we should note the fact that during the classification of pictures they develop a large number of connections, each of which draws them away from the solution of their allotted task.

For example, one of these subjects, who was assigned the task of classifying pictures, said, "This is a cherry, it is a fruit, but we can't put the plum there because jam is made from it." "The pail cannot be placed with the pots and pans, because there are toy buckets and big ones." In a special experiment in which the child had to establish the similarity and difference between a cat and a dog, these children, like most oligophrenic children, do not compare the cat and dog according to important signs. In this experiment too, however, at times the children do not confine themselves to comparing individual signs, and they often lose sight of the requested comparison altogether, drifting away from it by developing a series of random associations. As a typical example we may cite an extract from the records of an experiment in which a 12-year-old oligophrenic child was given the task of saying what was the difference between a cat and a dog and what they had in common: "The dog has a long body, the dog has different parts; the dog has a tail and without a tail it would not be a dog, unless its tail had been cut off earlier. We have a dog and it has a big tail." This extract shows how quickly the basic task (the comparison of two objects) is replaced by side associations. After being distracted in this way, the subject generally ceases to compare the objects presented, or begins to compare them by random signs.

Similar results may also be obtained in an experiment to investigate aided memorizing, in which the child has to use the picture which he is given as an aid to memorizing a necessary word and to establish a bond of meaning between the word and the picture. In children of the subgroup which we are considering, all the common oligophrenic defects are revealed (the dual concrete nature of the connections, the impossibility of using them as means to any special end), together with specific features. The formation of relationships is complicated by the development of chance associations which the children cannot inhibit and which interfere with the accomplishment of their allotted task. Besides the maldevelopment of their cognitive functions, other characteristic signs of the oligophrenic children of this group are thus their inability to retain the task in mind and the relative ease with which they drift away from it.

Characteristics of the Emotional-Volitional Function. The fundamental defect in oligophrenic children of this particular subgroup, i.e., the maldevelopment of complex forms of cognitive activity, stands out against a background of a disturbance of the emotional-volitional function. These children's behavior can be distinguished by the fact that they are easily excitable, their motor functions disinhibited, and they are irritable and easily distracted. During lessons these children jump up and down from their seat, open and close their desks, fumble in their satchels from which they remove various school things, look around, nudge their neighbors, laugh and grimace, jump up from their seats and go to sit in some else's place, and sometimes even run in and out of the classroom. During recess the general disinhibition and excitation of these children are still further increased. These oligophrenic children are not usually inhibited when in strange surroundings.

The emotions of these children are extremely unstable, labile, and changeable. Besides their increased excitability, some of them show a tendency towards acute affective outbursts. In addition to their disorganized behavior, these children also show a greatly diminished capacity for work. Their inability to concentrate on a task, and their distraction in the course of its execution are shown in even the most elementary forms of activity, quite within their grasp.

These children cannot carry out an appointed task because they are incapable of making the necessary effort of will.

Characteristics of the Motor Activity. Investigations of the motor activity of these children revealed no marked disturbances of the motor analyzer. In contrast to children showing appreciable defects of the cortical coordination of movements, in these children as a rule no appreciable signs of motor clumsiness nor disturbances indicative of apraxia can be observed. During physical education, however, and also when engaged in manual work, they exhibit a series of typical defects in the organization of movements, which make the management of these periods of instruction difficult. As a rule the main disability handicapping these children is their motor restlessness, with the presence of many superfluous movements. They show a tendency to a speeding up of the tempo of all their movements. The motor activity of these children is characterized by hastiness, disinhibition, and disturbance of the sequence of their movements. When engaged upon individual tasks in the program of remedial exercises, one of our subjects found it impossible to combine the three or four elements of the task in the correct order. For example, one child was given the task to a) sit still for 3 seconds, b) get up from the chair and clap his hands 8 times, c) go to another chair, bring it out from under the table, and d) sit on it for the next 8 seconds. He could accomplish only one element, and his efforts to do the others were frustrated.

The accurate execution of the task is prevented by the hastiness, impetuousness, and the extremely rapid tempo. These features were no less apparent during the next task. The boy sat at a table, and in front of him, in the center of the table, was a box of matches. His fingers lay motionless on the front edge of the table. He was required to do the following with each hand separately, in turn: a) take the box, b) abduct his arm and place the box on one side of the table near the edge, c) replace the box in its former place, and d) replace his hand in its original position.

A task of this sort is easily done by oligophrenics who have no gross disturbance of the balance between excitation and inhibition.

In our subject, when engaged in this task, no motor stereotype was formed for a long time. Then, to help him, verbal instructions were given to him one step at a time. At a reduced speed, he was able to carry out these movements correctly once or twice, after which his tempo began to accelerate and his movements became rapid and impetuous, lost their distinction from each other, and became merged. He took the box and immediately put it on one side, saying, "I took it." In response to the second command he at once threw the box on to the table and withdrew his hand. He seized the box with both hands at once or, on the contrary, he continued to carry out all his actions with the same hand.

Consequently, in the performance of the easiest and perfectly practicable tasks, these children show a disturbance of purposeful activity. They set about any task, for example the assembling of a pyramid, very quickly and without a preliminary attempt to familiarize themselves with the material, which interferes with their performance. When they make mosaic pictures, they set about doing the task quickly, taking first one tile and then another, without correlating what they see on the picture with what is on the tile, resulting in a rapid loss of organized and purposeful activity.

Specific Features of the Children of This Subgroup Becoming Apparent in the Course of Education

A. Specific Mistakes in Writing and Reading. Weakness of excitation and of all forms of cortical inhibition were also revealed when these children were taught to read and write. In the first stages of their education it is very difficult to attract the child's attention to the letters, although the teacher tries by every means to do so. The children gaze around them and say all sorts of things having no relation to the job in hand.

In the next level of education, after the child has been successfully taught a series of letters, the child again reveals by his replies this inability to concentrate on the task. The child names a familiar letter, placed before him, by the name of any other letter which he knows.

If a familiar series of letters is arranged before the child and he is asked to select a particular letter, he then begins to rearrange them all and to select any but the one chosen by the teacher.

These children pronounce a syllable with difficulty, calling out each letter separately. After prolonged and special methods of instruction, they master the process of fusion of sounds into a simple syllable (formed directly from two letters, for example, "ma," "sha," "ra," etc.).

The formation of a reversed syllable or of a direct syllable with the complication of a third element often leads to the collapse of the child's whole activity. The transition to reading by syllables is difficult for these children, for often they read words by guesswork or by their similarity to the letters of a previous word. Having read in his primer the word "Masha," [Mary] he reads the next word ("mama") in the same way, i.e., "Masha;" he reads the word "mala" [small] properly, but he again reads the next word ("myla") [washed] like the first. During reading, these children often forget letters with which they are familiar, and slip from one line to another.

During their reading they often combine the beginning of one word with the end of another, or having spelled out a whole word, when they repeat it they reproduce only one syllable. For example, a girl belonging to this subgroup reads the word "gladila" [ironed]. When the teacher asks her what she has read, she says: "Igla" [needle]. She spells out the word "utyug" [iron], and when the teacher asks her what she has read, she says: "Yug" [no meaning]. Often in these cases a tendency is shown to read words differing slightly from the word selected for reading. For instance, a pupil in the third class has to read the word "yubka" [skirt], and instead of that he reads the next word "Yulya" [Julia].

The letters of the alphabet have a definite disposition in space. Some letters are symmetrical mirror image forms, while the letters "y," "k," "b," and "d" have an asymmetrical structure, and in order to write them it is necessary to have a well-preserved and clear orientation in space.

In oligophrenic children of this subgroup the visual organization of writing does not encounter any special difficulties. Of the children in this subgroup whom we studied, only in one were we able to detect any difficulty in the visual organization of writing, but this was overcome comparatively easily. Nor did we observe in these children any difficulties in learning to write associated with a disturbance of phonemic hearing, although at the same time difficulties did arise in these children in the very earliest stages of learning to write.

It is very difficult to attract the attention of such a child to the performance of a writing task: the teacher asks the pupil to join two dots by a stroke, and in response to this the child haphazardly draws lines on a sheet of paper, going right across the whole sheet. Later the child tries to carry out this task, but again he overshoots the limits of the line.

These children write the elements of individual letters very carelessly, and sometimes they may write letters relatively correctly two or three times, but then they gradually drift away from their appointed task and do not write what they have been given. This is shown by the fact that the children either attach superfluous elements to letters or omit essential elements: in the first case the letter "n" is changed into "m," the letter "u" into "w," "o" into "a"; in the second case, on the other hand, "m," by omitting an element, is changed into "n," "w" into "u," and "a" into "o." Sometimes in the course of writing letters the children, having once written a letter properly, will attach elements of another letter, usually elements which have happened momentarily to catch their attention. The extensive period spent practicing the differentiation and accurate pronunciation of phonemes before starting on their primers, and the teacher's particular attention to the analysis of these sound components enable these children to learn to read and write according to the special school's syllabus, despite the difficulties which have been described.

The whole complex process of writing, however, does not merely consist of the elements noted above. The child who writes a sentence from dictation has to remember it, it must be clearly distinguished from other irrelevant stimuli; when writing he must keep the sentence in its proper order, he must know what he has already written and what he still has to write. Without all these factors, every interruption in writing would disturb the necessary sequence of the act of writing.

At a certain stage of their education, the children under our observation learned to distinguish the sounds of regular speech and to easily remember the outlines of the separate letters. They made mistakes in writing, however, because having listened to the sentence or word they would begin to transpose elements from the end of the word or sentence, or else they repeatedly wrote a syllable, word, or letter which they had previously written.

In writing, then, these children show a tendency to rush ahead; there is a stronger kinesthetic afferent influence from consonants, so vowels are dropped because of their weaker afferent representation. This propulsive tendency leads to the loss of clarity of each separate word, so that several words are merged into one. If a sentence is copied repeatedly it is found that it may be grossly distorted the first time, written almost correctly the second, and the third time the same mistakes arise over again: anticipation, transposition, omission of vowels. This is all evidence that the child is not yet capable of regulating his activity. He characteristically drifts away constantly from his allotted task. Or in another sentence a tendency may be shown to arrange the words properly, but the arrangement of the words is lost because the child cannot inhibit the tendency to anticipate. During the second attempt to write the same sentence, the series of characteristic mistakes stands out sharply. These pupils make a lightening approach to their work, write quickly, carelessly, and hastily, hand in their work first without checking it, and when writing from dictation or copying they make a series of characteristic mistakes (superfluous strokes, omission and transposition of letters in words, and of words in sentences, anticipation of consonants, and omission of vowels).

The child has to write from dictation the word "trus" [coward] but writes "stu," he has to write the word "koshka" [cat] but the first time he writes "okka," i.e., he transposes the sound "o" from the middle to the beginning of the word, perseverates the sound "k," omits the sound "sh," and writes a final "a." When the experimenter suggests that he write the same word again, he remembers all the sounds but transposes them, and writes "okkash." The third time he writes "kokash," and finally, he writes it properly – "koshka." The words " v lesu" [in the woods] he writes "sleu."

When writing, these children often omit vowels, for example instead of "Olya myla listo" [Olya was washing her face] they write "Olf mla ltso," or instead of "Ya zhivu doma" [I live at home] they write "Ya zhddoma" (Figs. 33 and 34).

At the basis of these mistakes (fusion of several words into one, perseveration, transposition of letters and words) lies a weakness of all forms of cortical inhibition, and in particular of delayed inhibition. By virtue of the weakness of their delayed inhibition the child cannot refrain from writing the succeeding elements (anticipating). The weakness of inhibition in these children is apparent in the motor link, as a result of which superfluous elements are found in their letters. The defect of inhibition is also shown in their writing by the fact that these children cannot write along a line, but their hand moves in a circle whose radius is the forearm and whose center is the elbow, which leads to slipping from the line.

Similar mistakes (omission of letters, substitution of some letters for others, inclusion of superfluous letters in a word, transposition of letters) were found by Gur'yanov and Shcherbak during their investigations of 7-year-old children just learning to read and write.

Omission of letters is observed in 7-year-olds during the whole of the ABC level, but at its end this is appreciably decreased. In words of one syllable the middle vowels are most frequently dropped. For example, instead of the word "shar" they write "shr," instead

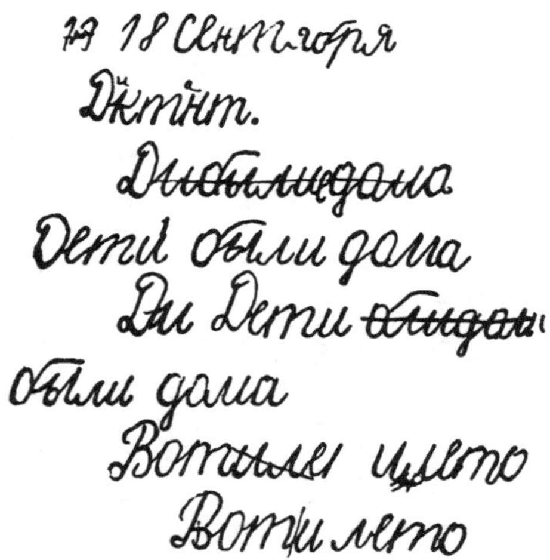

Actually written	Should have written	English equivalent
18 Sentyabrya	correct	18 September
Dktnt	Diktant	Dictation
Dibyliedoma	Deti byli doma	The children were at home
Deti byli doma	correct	The children were at home
Di Deti blidoma	Deti byli doma	The children were at home
byli doma	correct	They were at home
Votile ileto	Vot i leto	Now it's summer
Voti leto	Vot i leto	Now it's summer

Fig. 33. Subject S., aged 11 years, pupil at a special school (oligophrenia, feeble-minded or moron level). Marked disturbances of writing in the form of omission of letters and merging of words together.

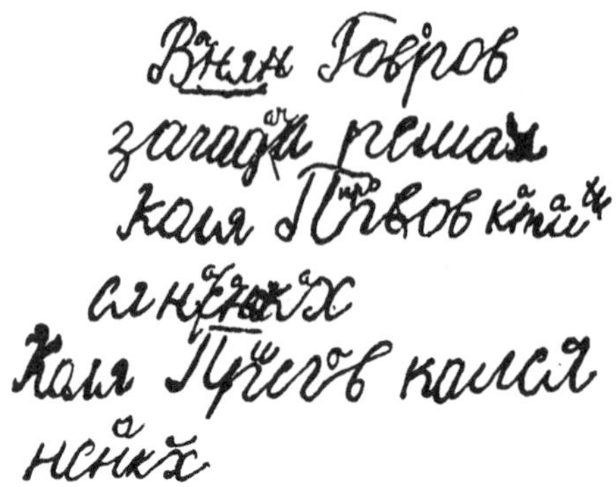

Fig. 34. Tanya K., aged 11-1/2, pupil at a special school (oligophrenia, feeble-minded or moron level). Marked disturbances in writing in the form of omission and transposition of letters, and contamination.

of the word "sad" [garden] they write "sd," etc. They write superfluous letters in the words. In these conditions the children write "saad" instead of "sad," "ruuuka" instead of "ruka," [hand] "blulka" instead of "bulka," [roll] etc. From an analysis of these mistakes, Gur'yanov and Shcherbak conclude that if omissions alternate with correct writing, if vowels and consonants are found in different combinations, and if the pupil can at the same time analyze the given sounds, this is evidence of insufficient attention during the analysis preceding the writing, and of poor memorizing of the letters composing the word. Inadequate attention is seen still more clearly in the transposition of the letters in a word. "The transposition of letters in a word," write these authors, "shows that the pupil has correctly determined the sound content of the word, but has lost sight of the sequence of the sounds, having perhaps been distracted by the solution of other graphic or technical tasks. In such cases pupils sometimes write 'shri' instead of 'shar,' "sku" instead of 'suk,' [branch] and 'bluka' instead of bulka'" [roll].*

The presence of similar mistakes in 7-year-old children in the early stages of learning to write is explained by these investigators by the inadequate attention shown by these children. The pathophysiological basis of this inadequacy of attention is a weakness of all forms of active cortical inhibition. We know that, at the age of seven years, active inhibition has not yet reached an adequate level of development. For 7-year-old children writing is a complex form of activity which leads to overstrain of the process of inhibition in them. Hence a disturbance of the process of inhibition arises on account of its overstrain.

Similar mistakes in the form of perseverations, transpositions,

*E. V. Gur'yanov and M. K. Scherbak, The Psychology and Technique of Education in Writing in the ABC Period, p. 70, Izd. APN RSFSR, Moscow, 1950.

and contaminations were observed by Bogoroditskii in persons in a state of fatigue or slight intoxication. He wrote, "Adjacent letters are transposed, which takes place in consequence of the fact that ideas of letters are not present in the mind in the order in which they should be reproduced, for example "vsoikh" – "svoikh" [pl. possessive pronoun].*

Similar mistakes arise during oral speech in normal children in the first stages of development of their speech, and are called anticipatory (i.e., "okno" [window] is said as "kono"), omission (i.e., "moloko" [milk] is said as "moko"), perseveration, contamination (running two compound syllables into one), or transposition. At the basis of these mistakes in early childhood lies the maldevelopment of all forms of cortical inhibition. In normal children, however, these mistakes are easily overcome, and during the process of learning to read and write they are of no real significance.

We can thus see that in all cases in which a weakness of cortical inhibition is seen, whether this be the underdevelopment of cortical inhibition in small children at an early stage of mastery of oral speech, or the overstraining of the process of inhibition in 7-year-old children when learning to write, or yet again the disturbance of the process of inhibition in pathological conditions (intoxication, fatigue), or finally, the weakness of all forms of cortical inhibition in the case of this particular variant of oligophrenia, we have identical mistakes, which lead to transient disturbances in writing in the form of transpositions, perseverations, omissions; the common pathophysiological mechanism causes common clinical manifestations.

B. Characteristic Difficulties in the Solution of Arithmetical Problems and Tasks. The weakness of all forms of cortical inhibition also reveals itself in the process of teaching mentally retarded children of this subgroup to count. At first in school this is very hard for these children. For a long time they cannot grasp the concept of numbers. They cannot detect an omission in a numerical series. Furthermore, they cannot correlate numbers and objects.

The counting of numbers (counting sticks) was rendered more difficult by their impulsiveness, their extreme impatience, and their inability to size up the problem. The children usually grabbed the sticks haphazardly, disturbing the order in which they were offered. They often accompanied this chaotic activity with expressions which were quite unrelated to the task assigned to them. The

*V. A. Bogoroditskii, Essays on Linguistics and the Russian Language, pp. 89-90, Uchpedgiz, Moscow, 1939.

execution of this elementary task could be prevented by any other stimulus which caught the child's eye.

If the teacher was able to inhibit the purposeless movement and the irrelevant verbal expressions, the children could perform an elementary arithmetical problem only if it was accompanied by a step by step series of instructions. If the teacher gave only a preliminary instruction, then the whole of the child's activity collapsed, even within these elementary limits.

These specific features of the children's activity were conspicuous at every stage of their education. For instance, if the child were presented with ten counting sticks arranged in front of him and asked to take a certain number of them, in spite of the fact that the child understood the teacher's instructions and correctly repeated them, nevertheless he did not perform the task correctly. The child had only to reach out for the sticks for his entire organized activity to collapse: he grabbed any number of sticks, sometimes all of them at once.

In tasks in which the child was asked to accompany certain arithmetical operations with words, for example to count the sticks lying in front of him and to call out the numbers, loss of continuity between speech and action developed and it became impossible to combine them correctly. This loss arose from the increased tempo of performance. Their speech rate increased, either anticipating motor action or, conversely, hasty rearrangement of the sticks preceded the corresponding verbal description.

With proper corrective training it was possible to teach these children some elements of arithmetic, although complicated problems still revealed the child's inadequacy. For instance, if the child were asked to take a certain number of sticks from a row placed in front of him, because of his impulsiveness he could not carry out the task. In the worst instance he took them all, one by one, and at best he left some, although not the number he was supposed to leave.

Graphic representations of individual numbers caused no particular difficulties in these children: they recognized and distinguished them comparatively easily. They could not accurately transfer to a more complicated task (to match a number with the corresponding number of sticks). The child correctly called out the number shown to him on a card, correctly repeated how many sticks he must take, but when he set about doing this he grabbed any number of sticks, without carrying out the task that had been set.

When changing to addition and subtraction of numbers up to ten, children of this group give rapid, thoughtless and random answers, usually by offering stereotypes of the natural series, for example: 2 + 1 = 3; 1 + 2 = 4; 3 + 1 = 5; 7 + 2 = 6; 3 + 2 = 7. In all these answers the numerical evaluation is quickly divorced from the computation, and acquires the character of an automatic series. The stereotypes of the natural series are not overcome in cases when the experimenter says that the answer is wrong. Sometimes the answers given by these children show a tendency to replace the correct solution of an example with an inert perseverating answer.

In subsequent stages of education these features appear during mental arithmetic. If, for example, a child is given the problem of mentally subtracting 18 from 100, quickly and without thinking he gives the following answers: 72, 62, 42, 32, i.e., the mental calculation is replaced by the reproduction of an automatic series.

The disturbance of purposeful activity shows itself especially clearly in these oligophrenics when they solve arithmetical problems. They are not aware of a system of connections in the problem and it does not determine their subsequent activity. Their activity arises in the process of solving the problem, as a fragmentary operation with numbers.

One of our subjects (a pupil in the sixth class of a special school) was given the following problem: "Five cups cost 40 rubles. How much do two cups cost?" In this problem there is a hidden link in the form of the unasked question "How much does one cup cost?" The subject gave an answer very quickly: "10 rubles". He explained his answer by saying that one cup costs five rubles and two cups cost ten rubles. In response to the suggestion to think how much two cups cost, he did not set about solving the problem, but confidently gave the answer that they cost 10 rubles. In response to the experimenter's suggestion to explain how he reached this solution, the boy rapidly answered: "Take 20 from 40, which gives 10, and we know that two cups cost 10 rubles." The experimenter told the subject that his answer to the problem was wrong, but the subject continued to assert that two cups cost 10 rubles. Some doubt then developed in his mind, and he declared: "I was wrong, very wrong" — and thereupon added: "One cup costs 10 rubles, and two cups cost 10 rubles; one cup = 5 rubles; 5 + 5 = 10; 4 cups = 20 rubles, 5 cups = 25 rubles." He repeated the conditions of the problem correctly, but gave the wrong answer, saying that 5 cups cost 30 rubles: "1 cup = 5 rubles, 5 cups = 30 rubles, and 10 rubles are left over."

The subject thus sets about the solution of the problem very quickly, without any preliminary steps to size up the task. He establishes no system of connections which would lay down the lines of a subsequent solution, but gives an impulsive solution by means of the transfer of one of the elements of the conditions of the problem into a ready-made answer. He at once changes 5 cups into 5 rubles, and then easily multiplies $5 \times 2 = 10$, and tacks on the stereotyped answer: "two cups cost 10 rubles." All his subsequent reasoning is replaced by this stereotyped answer, and he now operates with a ready-made, inert stereotype. The doubts arising in the process of solution of the problem are readily overcome by the same inert stereotype. Then comes a simple calculation, based on the stereotyped answer. He remembers the conditions of the problem confidently, but they are dissociated from his actions. Subsequently, under the influence of the inert stereotype, the conditions of the experiment themselves are distorted.

Thus in spite of the fact that the subject retains the conditions of the problem, he does not develop the necessary system of connections. Instead, he blurts out an impulsive answer, which consists of the substitution of an inert stereotype, which replaces any subsequent solution. All attempts to elicit a rational operation are thwarted by repetition of the stereotype and by calculations within its limits.

The same problem was presented to this subject on the visual plane. The visual expression of the conditions of the problem did not help him to solve it. Connections are not created within the conditions, the superfluous connections are not inhibited, but a fragmentary connection appears and becomes inert. All the remaining operations are carried out within the limits of this fragmentary connection.*

Ways of Compensation. Results from our dynamic investigation suggest that children of this subgroup of oligophrenia, as all oligophrenics, show a maldevelopment of the higher forms of generalization and abstraction, together with a disturbance of sustained, purposeful activity.

The inability of these oligophrenics to carry out sustained purposeful activity is shown in any task, from the most elementary to the most complex. This inability determines the pattern of behavior of these children in the classroom during different lessons, with different teachers, at home and in experimental conditions. It is the principal obstacle to the success of their special education.

*In this section we do not discuss the differential diagnosis, which will be given in relation to all three subgroups of oligophrenic children in whom the neurodynamics are disturbed.

Should this fundamental defect be diagnosed in time, however, and a suitable system of measures be devised to overcome it, then such a child may make appreciable headway with his education. The plan of the corrective training program for such children must be based upon the qualitative structural pattern of the defect. As a first measure, therefore, their activity is organized by utilization of all possible educational devises.

Since such a child will be easily distracted from a task by any stimulus, it is important to remove all stimuli not concerned with the particular type of activity. For example, during lessons the teacher did not leave a single object on the desk, and the child received the necessary visual aids only when he had completed his task. The children tried to carry out the task but could not do so on account of the ease with which they were distracted. When they were learning to read and write it was found that they quickly lose what they have acquired: however well they learn their letters today, by the next lesson they will have forgotten them. This makes it absolutely essential to consolidate carefully both by sight and by sound the letters they have learned, by means of tactile methods and by comparison of one letter with another. The transition to syllabic reading revealed several characteristic difficulties: excessive hastiness and the tendency to rush ahead caused these children to join the beginning of one word to the end of another, which greatly complicated this form of reading. Bearing this fact in mind, the teacher covered the whole text except the word which the child had to read. This method proved very effective and enabled the children to learn to read successfully.

When they were learning arithmetic, these children showed their impulsiveness particularly clearly. During the performance of complex activity the child must inhibit his spontaneous reactions and make a preliminary appraisal of his allotted task. The inhibition of spontaneous impulsive reactions must be the subject of special training methods used with children of this subgroup.

A second and no less important measure is the organization of the child's activity by the combined performance of a task. When organizing the behavior of such a child, the teacher must at first carry out the task together with the child. Noting that these children are often hampered in their work by other children, the teacher says quietly to the child, "Let the child who has been called on do his work, and you and I will do it after him. Wait for him to finish." The child stands by the teacher; he wants to get to work, but he keeps himself under control, and impatiently waits until the child called on has done his work. At the end of the day, when the progress and conduct of the children are reviewed, the teacher must then make a point of emphasizing before the whole class, "Children, you have seen how S. has waited patiently until he was called on, did not interrupt, did not jump up and down in his seat and keep the other children from doing their work. He has become a good pupil." When the child demands that he be called on at once, the teacher says, "Be patient for just a few more seconds, I will certainly ask you, but the other children also want to be asked; there is only one of me, but there are many of you."

If the child succeeds in restraining himself even for a few seconds, the teacher fixes the attention of the whole class on this fact. At first such children are able to wait only a minute or two, but gradually the number of minutes increases considerably.

This method enables them to control their behavior still more in the future. Special rhythm exercises and remedial exercises as well as school lessons were used to produce inhibitory reactions.

When doing a given task the children could not make the required effort and organize their behavior in accordance with the preliminary instruction of the teacher. They were repeatedly distracted from the solution of their allotted tasks by an abundance of irrelevant associations. If the instruction were broken down and constantly reinforced, the development of these irrelevant associations was considerably reduced and work capacity was restored.

At first the teacher's instructions regulated the child's activity, but subsequently the child's own speech was incorporated for this purpose. This self-control, by speech, of the performance of a given task restricted the child's talkativeness and his tendency to drift from a task, and thereby made his activities still more organized. All these measures were employed by the teacher during work by the class as a whole, during individual tuition, and also at home.

The result of these teaching methods was that the children became more organized. Tanya, for example, who during her first year at school was one of the most difficult pupils in the class, and who by her disinhibition and impulsiveness interfered not only with her own work but also with that of the whole class, by the end of the first year became less excitable and impulsive and could listen to the teacher's instructions from start to finish. She learned to wait until the teacher came to her and gave her the help that she required. Tanya subsequently conformed completely to the school rules. If occasionally in the course of a lesson Tanya tried to tell something of her life-story, this would not now involve some irrelevant associations or expressions of random stimuli, as previously, but rather some event which had made an obvious emotional impact on her.

A concern about the teacher's estimation, and a self-awareness and self-evaluation testify to the great progress in the general development of these children. In accordance with the emergence of their ability to organize their activity, their attainment of a definite level of knowledge and skill, the development of an interest in school activities, and a critical attitude towards their work, the teacher could then begin to organize more complex activities. In particular it was important to teach the children not only to do a particular job, but also to see that it was done properly.

It will be remembered that due to their characteristics, these children often performed a given task at a lower than optimum standard. First they checked their work with the teacher. Later they checked their own work under more general supervision. In this way the teacher introduced an additional stimulus: the children were warned they would not be marked off for mistakes which they discovered themselves.

As a result of proper instruction, after a year these children progressed considerably. They became less irritable, they had learned self-restraint, and they could listen to instructions through to the end. They learned to wait until the teacher came to them to give required help, they did not display their former hastiness in their work but were able to accomplish a task under the supervision of the teacher.

At the beginning of the third year of education the behavior of these children had improved so much that comparison of their first and third year characteristics would lead one to believe that they were different children. Subsequently their educational level was further improved. Their behavior improved considerably, and they became more responsible. They carried out their school duties, overcame problems in their work and became much more productive when working alone. The combination of corrective training with medical treatment led to considerable progress in the development of these children. The medical treatment consisted of systematic courses of hypertonic infusions, general tonics, Pavlov's mixture, and small doses of bromides.

We found compensation of the above-described defect only when the teacher carefully studied each child and planned his work to meet his unique structural defect, utilizing the positive aspects of the child's personality.

CHAPTER 5

OLIGOPHRENIC CHILDREN WITH DISTURBANCE OF THE BALANCE BETWEEN THE FUNDAMENTAL NERVOUS PROCESSES, WITH INHIBITION PREDOMINATING OVER EXCITATION

In this subgroup of children we include those oligophrenics in whom the disturbance of the balance between the fundamental nervous processes is characterized by the predominance of inhibition over excitation. These children, too, as all oligophrenics, have a low capacity for abstraction and generalization. Their specific features are inhibition, lethargy, and slowness, which are revealed in their behavior and their motor and cognitive functions. This chapter is written on the basis of a prolonged study of 18 cases. We will turn now to a description of the results of this study.

CASE 1

Mila U., aged 13 years, a girl pupil in the second class at a special school. When she started at the school she showed the following: lethargy, passiveness (indifference in relation to persons around her), and considerable mental retardation. There were no abnormal factors in her heredity.

History. Mila's mother had been pregnant eight times, resulting in five artificial abortions and three deliveries. A daughter, age 24, is healthy and normal, and works as a teacher; a daughter, age 19, is a student at a technological institute; the third daughter is our present case, Mila, born from the seventh pregnancy, the course of which was normal. Labor was difficult and took place in the country, with the assistance of a midwife, during wartime evacuation. The child was born in asphyxia. During her first days of life the girl had two convulsions accompanied by vomiting. Her feeding was inadequate during her first year and she suffered from a severe form of malnutrition. From an early age the girl showed considerable developmental retardation. She began to hold her head up at nine months; she cut her first teeth at one year; she began to sit only at 3 years of age and to walk at 4 years; she began to say her first words at the end of the fourth year. From early childhood the girl was lethargic and inactive: she reacted neither to sounds nor to bright objects, and until the age of three years she spent most of her time in bed asleep.

At preschool age the girl was just as lethargic, passive and indifferent: she did not play with other children and was not attracted to them. She rarely made a request of an adult. At the age of six years Mila was admitted to hospital with scarlet fever. The unaccustomed surroundings caused her to become even more severely inhibited. Mila did not react to the environment and at times refused to eat.

At the beginning of school age the girl remained just as lethargic and lacking in initiative. She was interested in nothing, unable to look after herself and she did not play with other children. At the age of nine years she was sent to the imbecile class of a special school, where she remained an extremely inhibited girl, indifferent to the teacher's estimation of her work. She never asked questions of the teacher and never showed any interest in the children.

During her instruction in the imbecile class she was extremely unproductive. Only at the end of four years of schooling did she master the earliest elements of reading and the most elementary skill in writing and counting. She had no interest in her studies.

Physical State. The girl's physical development was normal for her age. Her skull was hydrocephalic (circumference about 52 cm). No gross abnormality of the internal organs.

State of the Nervous System. Full range of movement of the eyeballs, but accompanied by movements of the head. The right nasolabial fold was ill-defined, the tongue deviated to the right in the mouth, but when protruded deviated only slightly to the right. During phonation the right pharyngeal fold contracted less than the left. No reflex from the uvula was present. The chest was flattened, and wasting of the left deltoid, the left suprascapularis and the supraspinatus muscles was observed. The mammary glands were asymmetrical. The girl offered poor resistance during testing of the muscle groups. Paresis could therefore be judged only by the presence of atrophy and of paretic poses. Severe changes of tone of denervatory type were present. During the investigation of tone in the knee joints, immediately after the stereotype of extension and flexion of the left knee, the girl carried out the same movements on the right without being asked to do so. When instructed not to move her leg the stereotyped movements ceased and a perceptible contraction of the quadriceps muscles took place, more obvious on the left. The tone of the plantar-flexors was greater on the left. Pseudo-Kernig's sign on the left. Investigation of the power of the muscle groups in the legs was quite impossible. The dragging of the lateral edge of the left foot, the limitation of dorsiflexion (greater on the left), and the absence of isolated movement of the digits on both sides (more marked on the left), the impossibility of holding the foot oustretched, the paretic tremor of the foot — all these were evidence of a previous low paraplegia, mainly affecting the left foot. The marked bilateral pes planus could also be a result of the weakness of the quadriceps muscles. The tendon reflexes were more marked in the left arm. High knee jerks were observed, with extension of the zone in an upward direction. Elicitation of the left knee jerk caused the development of a motor stereotype resembling the pendulum type of reflex, and differing from this only by the fact that it could be stopped by command. During the investigation clonic jerks were observed in both feet. Babinski's sign was hardly perceptible on the left. The abdominal reflexes, which were fairly weak on the right and weak on the left, were quickly exhausted. Mayer's sign was absent on both sides. When sensation was tested in respect of position and movement, a vocal stereotype quickly developed, which interfered with the assessment of the position sense. The girl showed vasomotor disturbances, more marked in the legs (cyanosis of both prepatellar areas, and of the soles of the feet, erythremic and cyanotic changes in the digits). Residual manifestations of a tetraparesis were thus present, in which the cranial nerves were more affected on the right and the nerves of the limbs more affected on the left. The distribution of the paresis, i.e., its predominance in the proximal segments of the arms and legs, was evidence that the motor lesion was located in the cortex.

Despite the extent of spread of the lesion in the motor sphere, the residual paretic phenomena were apparent only as a result of special investigations. This fact suggests that the girl had suffered from subarachnoid and parenchymatous hemorrhages at the point of communication between the middle and anterior cerebral arteries.

Ophthalmological Examination. Visual acuity in both eyes normal. Some dilatation of the veins observed in the optic fundus.

Otorhinolaryngological Examination. Hearing normal.

X-ray Examination of the Skull. Microcephaly. Skull approximately turret-shaped. Base of the skull flattened. Along the course of the coronary and lambdoid sutures there was moderate calcification. Widespread and well marked digital impressions. Vascular shadows greatly intensified.

Electroencephalography. The alpha-rhythm was irregular, ill-defined and recorded only in the occipital areas of the cortex. In all regions slow waves with a frequency of 2-4 per second were dominant. In addition to the slow waves a beta-rhythm was recorded, which at times reached a high amplitude (up to 50 mm), mainly in the occipital regions (Fig. 35).

The electroencephalogram showed considerable abnormalities, in the form of the almost complete absence of an alpha-rhythm and the presence of diffuse slow waves. The sharp decrease in the amplitude of the electrical activity in the anterior regions of the cerebral cortex, like the presence of slow waves, possibly indicated the inhibited state of the cortex. The change from an alpha-rhythm to a rhythm of the same amplitude but a frequency of 20 per second indicated special neurodynamic changes.

Investigation of the Higher Nervous Activity by the Method of Plethysmography.*In the first experiments well-marked waves of the third order were seen, together with respiratory and cardiac arrhythmias. These were manifestations of the weakness of the cortical regulation. With any change in the conditions of the experiment, causing external inhibition, all the phenomena mentioned above were intensified and stood out particularly clearly. The drawn-out character of both the conditioned and the unconditioned vascular reactions (duration of the reaction 1-2 minutes as compared with the normal 10-30 seconds) indicated both the predominance of a state of inhibition in the cortex and considerable inertia of the nervous processes.

Against this general background of inhibition foci of pathological inertia developed. In the course of an experiment to produce two conditioned reflexes—to a metronome 120 a sensation of cold, and to the word "cabbage" the same—it was found that the first conditioned connection caused an adequate vasoconstrictor reaction, but the second connection gave a distorted, vasodilator reaction. Mila stated that after the word "cabbage" it was a hot iron that was applied to her hand, and not ice as in fact it really was.

The formation of conditioned reflexes in response to other verbal stimuli evoked an adequate reaction. It may be accepted that this pathological connection was laid down in the child's past experience, and was very stable. It was again shown when the experiment was repeated after $2^1/_2$ years. This connection could not be

*Only a few children of this subgroup were investigated by plethysmography.

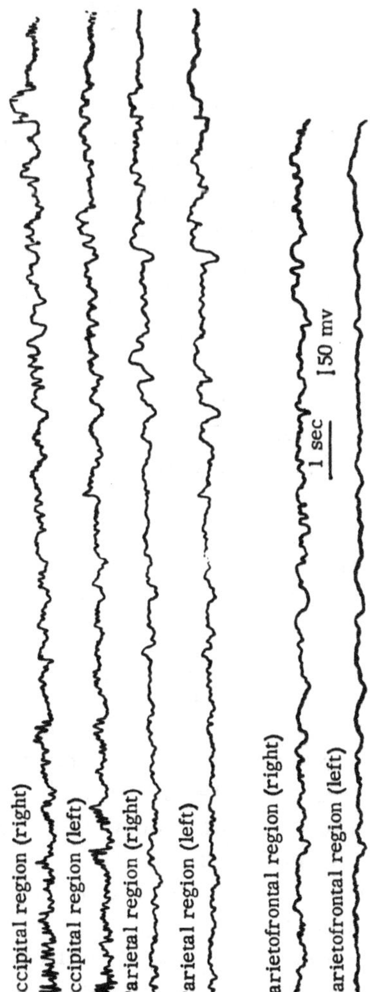

Fig. 35. Mila U., aged 13 years, pupil at a special school (oligophrenia, degree of imbecility). Marked abnormalities of the electrical activity: slow pathological waves predominant in all regions of the cortex.

disturbed even when the girl was shown an unconditioned stimulus (ice).

The girl also showed a tendency towards echolalia and echopraxia, together with increased suggestiveness, during investigation of the vascular reactions. The application of an indifferent stimulus, the warning word "warm" or "cold," produced a vascular reaction corresponding to the verbal stimulus. If the application of a cold stimulus was accompanied by the words "hot iron," a vasodilator reaction arose, whereas the same stimulus unaccompanied by words elicited an adequate reaction. The results obtained indicated the predominance of inhibition in the cerebral cortex, the marked inertia of the connections and the appearance of persistent foci of pathological inertia.

Investigation of the Higher Nervous Activity. The girl was first investigated in 1953. Her reaction to a direct command did not appear at once, it was poorly stabilized and it was distinguished by its low magnitude (although the power of the hand was good). The first conditioned reaction to a light stimulus (a red light) was formed very slowly. It was shown at first in the form of a movement of the hand towards the push-button (after 18 combinations). A conditioned reaction in the form of pressure on the push-button appeared only after 90 combinations. Subsequent conditioned reactions to other stimuli were formed rapidly. Simple differentiation by color and intensity were formed extremely quickly (after the first combination). Differentiation was stable and was maintained from one experiment to the next. Simple differentiation was still intact even after an interval of two weeks.

Modification of the conditioned significance of the stimuli took place rapidly. The rate of transformation of an inhibitory into a positive stimulus was slower than in the opposite direction. No reactions took place to the word denoting the positive stimulus. These could be produced by a combination of the word with this stimulus, but were quickly inhibited. The verbal projection of the simplest experiments was adequate, but certain differences in the stimuli (for example, differences in intensity) could not be verbalized. It must be mentioned that supplementary questions readily caused the development of irrelevant associations. During the application of light stimuli of different intensity, disturbance of the strength relationships was observed (phasic phenomena). The reactions to conditioned stimuli were of very low magnitude. They were strengthened when an additional stimulus of moderate strength (a soft sound, an increase in the general level of illumination, etc.)

was applied briefly or in the background simultaneously with the conditioned stimulus.

The development of complex forms of differentiation was severely retarded. For instance, differentiation in accordance with the principle of alternation (to every other stimulus) was formed after more than 40 applications of the stimulus.

The girl gave the verbal projection of this operation in a primitive form. In each experiment there were no reactions to the first stimuli (or if present they were very weak), and then they gradually became strengthened. Reinvestigation showed that the individual elements of the connections laid down in the previous experiments were maintained. These elements of the old connections were apparent in the verbal projection. Motor reactions in response to a command were drawn out, and included pressing on the button between stimuli and reactions of the perseveration type. Stabilization of the conditioned reaction was very ill-defined (for all practical purposes it was absent). The conditioned reaction to a simple light stimulus appeared after one combination.

During the development of differentiation a wide generalization of the stimuli beyond the limits of one analyzer was observed. After the development of differentiation generalization took place only within the limits of one analyzer. Simple differentiation to color was produced after one combination, and differentiation to intensity after three combinations.

Modification of the conditioned significance of the stimuli in a simple system of connections took place after 1-2 combinations: in a system including differentiation by intensity a more rapid transformation of the positive stimulus into a negative was observed than vice versa. Extrastimuli caused inhibition of the conditioned reactions. In certain cases their application led to disinhibition of differentiation. "Dynamic transmission" was disturbed: during the substitution of the corresponding words for the direct stimuli, the girl also reacted positively to the word designating the differential stimulus.

Complex forms of differentiation were developed slowly (differentiation to duration after 12 combinations was consolidated very slowly, and the conditioned reaction to every other stimulus was first shown after 23 combinations, but was not maintained in a stable form). Modification of complex systems of connections took place much more slowly than simple. It was found that positive stimuli were changed into inhibitory more quickly than vice versa.

The verbal projection of the development of the simplest systems of connections was adequate, although irrelevant associations were observed (especially in the projections of past experiments). In the projections of the development of the more complex forms of differentiation (especially differentiation by duration), the gross inertia of the previously formed verbal connections was revealed clearly.

Negative induction was well marked. This was shown extremely clearly during the formation of two reactions (motor and vocal) to one stimulus; under these circumstances first one and then the other reaction was extinguished. Disturbance of the strength relationships was observed during the action of light stimuli of different strength. During the investigation of the reactions to sounds of different strength (which was carried out later, after many experiments), in one experiment paradoxical relationships were observed, and in another the relationships were balancing in character, while in the third group they were normal with a balancing tendency.

The considerable weakness of internal inhibition was revealed not only by the difficulty in the production of complex forms of differentiation, but also by the fact that if two differential stimuli were applied in succession after differentiation had already been established, then as a rule a conditioned reaction was observed to the second stimulus. This was shown also by the disinhibition of differentiation when reinforcement was removed. By preliminary instruction simple conditioned connections were easily formed and were readily modified. In some cases, however, it was found that a conditioned reaction did not appear after the first stimulus, but in response to the second or third. The conditioned reactions to individual positive stimuli failed to develop, and in a prolonged experiment whole series of conditioned reactions were missing. The formation of relatively complex connections by preliminary instruction was grossly disturbed. These were formed gradually, the instruction did not operate at once, and differentiation was not established after the first application of the inhibitory stimulus, but after the second or third. During modification by preliminary instruction the inhibitory stimulus became positive after the third application, and the positive stimulus acquired an inhibitory significance. After modification by preliminary instruction there was a tendency for the old connection to return. It frequently happened that, after the formation of an appropriate system of connections by instruction, the girl gave an inadequate verbal response.

Mental State

Optic Analyzer. During the investigation of the optic analyzer, the girl recognized pictures shown to her and named them correctly, but she gave her answers very slowly and then only after additional stimulation. Sometimes her answers were wrong, showing that she had developed a complex of associations which she could not inhibit. In the same experiment she revealed a tendency towards perseveration. For instance, the girl was shown a picture of a cow, which she named correctly, but when further pictures were shown to her (chicken, table, pen, exercise book), she again said "cow."

When the pictures were shown to her a second time she named them all correctly; this shows convincingly that her answers were perseverative in nature.

Spatial Orientation. Mila was capable of the most elementary forms of spatial orientation: she could correctly point to her own right and left hand, but she had much more difficulty in pointing to her classmate's right and left hand; she often followed the mirror image. She could only carry out these simple tasks, however, with additional stimulation by the experimenter. When shown an example the girl could form the simplest figures from sticks (a triangle, a square, a letter "T," a little house, etc.). With the experimenter's help she could also form more complicated figures.

Motor and Motor-Speech Analyzers. The girl experienced similar difficulty performing postural movements. Her dynamic movements were particularly deranged, but with additional stimulation and encouragement she managed to do them.

The girl's speech at times was scanning, and because of her lethargy and passivity her speech became slurred, indistinct, inexpressive, and slow. At the same time she had no difficulty in the pronunciation of words and phrases (she could freely repeat to the experimenter sentences which were comparatively difficult to pronounce).

Phonemic Hearing. The girl's understanding of everyday speech was complete. She understood correlated phonemes correctly.

Though there were no gross defects within the limits of the individual analyzers, she carried out every alloted task slowly, and then only after additional stimulation. At times her reactions completely disappeared. These characteristic features were shown particularly clearly during her school work.

Cognitive Function and Behavior. The girl could easily count up to 20, but when counting backward she experienced difficulty and showed a well-marked tendency to reverse herself and count up the scale. She could only count backward when given organizing help by the teacher. Mila had an elementary idea of numbers. She could give any required number of sticks (up to ten), but only if she was organized, directed, and stimulated.

Mila could also do simple problems in addition and subtraction up to ten, but only with concrete objects as aids (sticks, counters). In the absence of such material aids she could solve problems involving numbers up to ten but only by adding or subtracting one at a time. However, the girl could not make independent use of her counting ability. If she was asked to solve a problem without the help of the teacher, she would replace any of the numbers and usually write the number 18 instead, acting on impulse. With organizing help she could solve such problems without a single mistake.

The girl's specific characteristics became apparent when she was learning arithmetical operations. She showed a tendency toward perseveration and inertia (the compulsive writing of the number 18), and was unable to make use of her knowledge of arithmetic for herself. It has been mentioned above that her productivity was considerably increased when she carried out the identical task with the teacher's organizing help and encouragement.

The same features were also apparent in her writing: when copying she contaminated words, i.e., joined several words together, did not finish words, transposed, repeated items, and omitted individual elements of the letters and even of whole words. The teacher's assistance, directed towards the organization of her activity, corrected her writing; Mila could do her work under these conditions almost perfectly. The same dependence on a certain amount of activation was also revealed in other elementary tasks. For instance, if Mila was asked to insert various geometrical shapes into corresponding holes, she could not do so unaided, and made a number of inept attempts. With organization and stimulation, however, i.e., with increased activation, she managed to accomplish this task almost without a mistake.

From the findings described above it may be deduced that the marked reduction in Mila's productivity was due not only to the inadequate development of her cognitive functions, but also to a depression of her cortical function.

To confirm this, the caffein test was performed. Before receiving an injection of caffein she was given a few tasks to carry out. First she was asked to solve six problems in addition and subtraction up to ten. To all six problems the girl gave the incorrect perseverative answer "18." She was then given problems of equal difficulty, but with some slight additional help from the teacher.

The girl made a number of mistakes. When, besides receiving additional encouragement, the girl was further asked to call off the numbers herself which she used in her arithmetical operations, the number of her mistakes decreased.

Mila was then asked to count up to 20 and back. The girl did this task, too, with a great many mistakes. When she copied a few simple sentences without help, her writing showed serious defects: transpositions, perseverations, and contamination. The girl took dictation with preliminary analysis of each separate word slightly better than she copied, but here too she made mistakes. After the injection of caffein the girl's activity improved considerably: she correctly performed all tests of the same difficulty as those previously given to her. The girl's writing also improved greatly.

The injection of caffein thus showed convincingly that the marked decrease in the girl's capacity for work was due to the predominance of a state of inhibition in the cerebral cortex This state of inhibition may be expressed to a varying degree. In its severest form the girl was lethargic and inactive and she could not carry out tasks given to her that were within her grasp; with a somewhat less severe degree of inhibition, in the process of carrying out certain tasks the girl showed very clearly perseverations and stereotypes (the stereotyped reproduction of the same number during the solution of arithmetical problems and of identical patterns during drawing). In one such experiment the doctor, to encourage Mila, patted her on the arm. In response to this Mila became enlivened, repeated the same action to the doctor, attempted to embrace the doctor and began to repeat in a stereotyped manner "Mariya Semenovna — a braided hairdo, what a braid you have." This stereotyped connection was very persistent and extremely inert, and she reproduced it whenever she saw the doctor.

The girl's lethargy, passivity, and inhibition were clearly apparent in her general behavior. For instance, Mila would come into the classroom silently and with no form of greeting, and sit down in her usual place. If she was not encouraged or stimulated, or if no problems were given to her, then she might stay for a long time perfectly indifferent, immobile, and inactive. Inhibition and lethargy appeared in the girl's whole demeanor, and especially in her motor activity: her face was frozen and lacking in expression, and her poses and movements were monotonous and extremely slow. If Mila was asked to repeat some action of the hands, the tempo of her movement was slowed, the movements themselves were weakened and limited in range, and gradually ceased. The girl showed no animation even when at play. Occasionally, for instance, she joined in a game of lotto; the card was in front of her and she lifted her hand correctly when the picture on her card was called. When the girl sitting next to her grabbed her card and added it to her own, Mila showed no reaction whatever, but remained lethargic and indifferent, as usual.

Observation of the girl revealed the extreme monotony of her behavior: lethargy and passivity in conjunction with absolute submission. The teacher never once heard from her words such as "I don't want" or "I won't," nor on the other hand, requests for something. In experimental conditions, in conversation with the doctor, when the girl was slightly encouraged and stimulated into activity, she showed some signs of a peculiar animation: the repetition of a particular word as in echolalia, or the patting of the doctor on the shoulder.

These characteristic features of the girl's behavior were revealed against the background of incomplete development of her cognitive functions.

By herself she was unable to arrange pictures in a certain order. She had difficulty in rejecting a superfluous picture. If she was helped a little, by means of leading questions, Mila was able to distinguish a nonmatching picture, but she could not explain why she rejected it. The inertia of the connections, once they were formed, was shown very obviously in this experiment. The girl was shown four pictures, representing a horse, a cow, a goat, and a spoon. She correctly distinguished the picture of the spoon as the one which did not match, but gave the following explanation: "They all run, but the spoon stands still." This inert connection ("They all run, but the spoon stands still.") was then reproduced by the girl during all the subsequent experiments.

When changing to another task, in which she had to give cards representing flowers to the experimenter and to keep cards representing furniture herself, Mila reproduced the stereotype of the previous experiment, i.e., she rejected the fourth (superfluous) card. If Mila was encouraged, organized and stimulated, then her performance was improved.

In an experiment to reject a fourth superfluous card she was shown pictures of a carrot, a cabbage, a cucumber, and a mouse. The girl was asked to name the pictures separately. She named the first two correctly, but when shown the third picture, representing a cucumber, she exclaimed, "A cucumber, I ate a cucumber"; when shown the fourth picture, which represented a mouse, she named the picture and reproduced an old inert connection as she did so:

"It washes itself and cleans its teeth." She was then asked to distinguish the one picture which did not match the others. She correctly chose the picture of the mouse. When asked why she had chosen this picture, the girl at first replied: "Because it isn't necessary," and then reproduced the old inert connection formed during the previous response: "The carrot stands, the cabbage stands, but the mouse isn't necessary, the cucumber stands, lies, and it sleeps." Gradually, by means of leading questions, it was possible to obtain from her a doubly concrete but more accurate explanation: "The carrot grows, the cabbage grows, but the mouse doesn't grow."

When the girl was organized and stimulated in her activity, she could be led up to a more generalized formulation. She was able to say that "the carrot, cabbage, and cucumber are vegetables," that "the bicycle must be rejected because it is not a vegetable," and that "the squirrel is not wanted because the carrot is a vegetable but the squirrel is not a vegetable." During the experiment she also succeeded in transferring this elementary generalization to other groups. For example, she was given pictures of a squirrel, a cat, a fox, and a house. The girl's first answer was: "The squirrel is not needed." Slight stimulation in the form of the instruction, "Think, look first at what is there" was sufficient, however, to make the girl give the proper answer. "The house is not needed, and the rest are wild animals."

In the picture classification experiment, when the girl had to arrange the pictures according to existing examples, she grouped a picture of a certain object in a suitable category, but could not explain why she had put it in this group. In the experiment with a simple series of pictures telling a story, she understood the task given to her and with the doctor's help she was able to establish the proper order. In a more difficult series the girl at first examined each picture separately, described it briefly, and sometimes reproduced old stereotyped connections as she did so. By means of leading and stimulating questions it was possible to discover that the girl could establish a bond of meaning between individual pictures. She herself then arranged the pictures in a certain order, and her remarks reflected the basic theme of the series. When the girl was given a series of consecutive pictures she was able to arrange them in a certain order by herself, making very slight mistakes which were easily rectified when the experimenter stimulated her.

During the experiment she repeatedly revived the old stereotyped connection: "Mariya Semenovna — a braid, doctor — a braid," she said, and stretched out her hand to the doctor.

Principal Stages of the Child's Development. In the first stage of her development the combination of maldevelopment with general lethargy could already be clearly recognized. From her history there are grounds for assuming diffuse and profound inhibition of the cerebral cortex, for until the age of three years the girl slept a large part of the day and all night. Only at the beginning of school age was there some progress in her development, for she slept much less, although she still remained very inhibited.

The next stage in her development can be taken to be the period of her education in the imbecile class of the special school. The combination of intellectual maldevelopment with severe inhibition led to a considerable backwardness in her studies. During her first year she made no progress. Only after her second year of education could some progress in her development be discerned as her inhibition diminished, but not until the end of the third year of her stay at the school did Mila master elementary reading, writing, and arithmetic.

In the clinical diagnostic unit of the medicopedagogic consultation service of the Institute of Defectology, where the syllabus of education for this child was planned on the basis of the qualitative structure of her disability, some progress was made in her development. Mila became more active, more lively and slightly more productive in her school work.

Clinical Analysis of the Case

The principal etiological factor in this case must be considered to be the asphyxia at birth. The two convulsions which the girl had in the first few days of life were the consequence of this paranatal asphyxia. The subsequent development of the child was complicated by malnutrition from which she suffered during the first year of her life.

In this case the fundamental pathogenetic factor of oligophrenia, namely the diffuse lesion of the cerebral cortex, is well marked. In favor of the diffuse lesion of the cerebral cortex there are the neurological findings (residual paretic manifestations, revealed only by special investigations, the distribution of the paresis, i.e., mainly present in the proximal segments of the upper and lower limbs) and the results of electroencephalographic investigation.

The diffuse lesion of the cerebral cortex is combined with

residual hydrocephalus. The presence of hydrocephalus is confirmed by the craniographic findings and digital impressions. These distinctive pathogenetic features are also responsible for the specific features of the higher nervous activity. The experimental findings obtained during the investigation of the higher nervous activity by the motor-speech method, like those obtained by the method of plethysmography, clearly revealed a considerable inertia of the nervous processes, as well as a marked predominance of a state of inhibition in the cerebral cortex.

These etiological, pathogenetic, and pathophysiological features are responsible for the qualitative characteristics of the structure of the disability, which, in this case, is determined by the presence of the fundamental symptom of oligophrenia, i.e., the incomplete development of the cognitive functions. In addition to this fundamental symptom a series of supplementary symptoms is observed, determining the specific features of this particular case. These supplementary symptoms include extreme inhibition, sluggishness, lethargy, and passivity. This case may accordingly be included with the variant of oligophrenia which we have described.

CASE 2

Zina K., aged 14 years. Pupil in the fifth class of a special school. No abnormal factors in her heredity.

History. Zina's mother was twice pregnant. The elder daughter was normal, and died in adult life from a severe physical illness of uncertain etiology. Zina was born from the second pregnancy, which followed a difficult course with general toxemic manifestations. The girl was born in prolonged asphyxia. From her very earliest childhood her mother noticed that her development was retarded. She held her head up only after the age of one year, and was late in cutting her teeth. At 18 months she suffered from some disease of uncertain etiology accompanied by cerebral manifestations (convulsions, loss of consciousness), after which her development was still more severely disturbed. Zina began to walk at the end of her third year of life, at which time she could say a few disconnected words. At preschool age the girl was noticeably lethargic and passive. She did not attend nursery or kindergarten. As school age approached, the girl's peculiarities became still more clearly demonstrated. She spoke little and badly, she was lethargic and passive, she had no feelings towards other children and no interest in toys, and she slept a great deal.

At eight years of age Zina began to study at a village school, where after spending three years in the first class she had not learned even the rudiments of reading and writing; she remained lethargic, inhibited, and passive, would not reply to the teacher's questions, did not play with other children and differed very markedly from other children in her behavior. In 1951 she was accepted in the first class of a special school.

Physical State. Microcephalic skull, head circumference 48.5 cm. The girl was backward in physical development and indeed showed physical weakness, but the internal organs were normal.

State of the Nervous System. The pupils reacted briskly to light. Slight nystagmoid movements when the eyes were turned to the side, convergence poor, the tongue deviated slightly to the left and the uvula to the right. Slight weakness of the right upper limb.

Zina could hop well on either foot and her toe movements in both feet were good. Muscle tone was normal but gross innervational disturbances were observed. During attempts to relax the muscles motor stereotypes were observed. The tendon reflexes in the upper limbs were brisk and equal, but those in the lower limbs could not be elicited. The abdominal reflexes were brisk and the plantar reflexes very sluggish. Neurological examination indicated minimal and diffuse symptomatology, more marked on the right.

Ophthalmological Examination. Visual acuity in the right eye 1.0, in the left 0.8. Sight not improved by glasses. Optic fundus: on the right the optic disk was pink, its outline was well defined and the caliber of the blood vessels normal; on the left the borders of the optic disk were ill defined, but the vessels were also normal in caliber. The periphery, in the region of the macula lutea, was normal. On the left there were traces of a previous attack of optic neuritis. Perimetry to white light was normal.

Otorhinolaryngological Examination. Hearing within normal limits.

X-ray Examination of the Skull. Microcephaly. Base of the skull flattened. Pattern of the inner table of the skull obliterated. Well-marked digital impressions observed. Calcification along the course of the coronary suture. Sagittal suture widened.

Electroencephalography. Diffuse and gross pathological changes in the brain were observed, in the form of absence of the alpha-rhythm and the predominance of rapid waves in all regions of the cortex (Fig. 36). Modification to both high-frequency and low-frequency flashes of light was absent. The absence of slow waves on the EEG and the presence of rapid waves suggested neurodynamic disturbances.

Investigation of the Higher Nervous Activity. This girl was given two series of experimental tests. The motor reactions in response to a command were very weak, and at the beginning of the examination they were drawn out and poorly stabilized. The first conditioned reactions were formed in the first examination after two combinations, and in the second after thirteen. Once it had appeared, the conditioned reaction was gradually strengthened. Wide generalization of the newly introduced stimuli was observed (not confined to one analyzer). Simple differentiation to color was formed with slight delay (in the first investigation after eight combinations).

After the formation of differentiation some increase in the strength of the conditioned reflex to a positive stimulus was observed. Modification of simple systems of connections took place quickly (the differential stimulus was converted into a positive after two combinations). The positive stimulus changed into an inhibitory stimulus more rapidly than vice versa.

Differentiation by intensity was first obtained after five combinations and was consolidated very slowly. Negative reinforcement

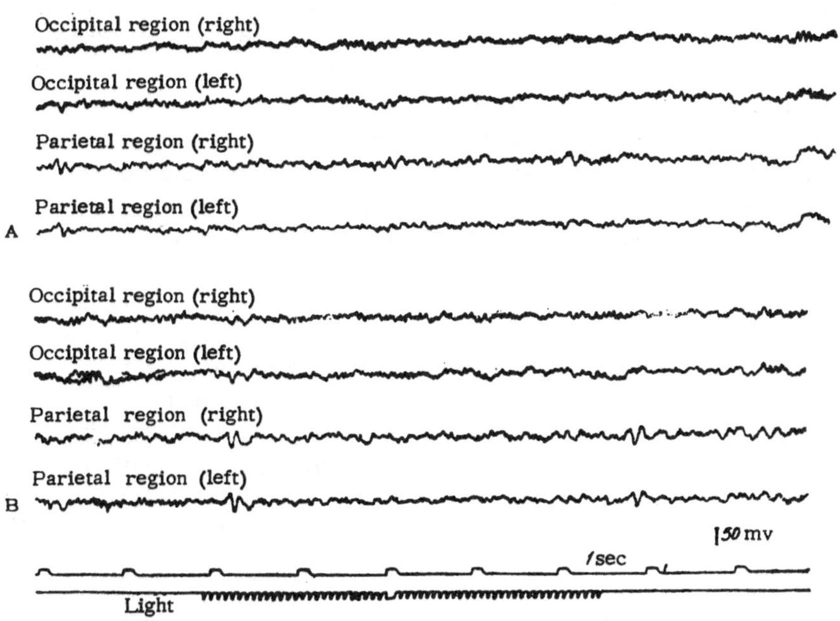

Fig. 36. Zina K., aged 14 years, a pupil at a special school (oligophrenia, degree of feeblemindedness). A) In all regions of the cerebral cortex a beta-rhythm is predominant; the alpha-rhythm is ill-defined. B) The application of a flickering light stimulus. Changes in EEG frequency of the cortical rhythm to a flicker frequency of 12 per second are absent.

of the differential stimuli caused inhibition of the conditioned reaction to a positive stimulus for a very long time. An adequate response to differentiation by intensity was obtained only after prolonged consolidation. Differentiation by duration first appeared after two combinations, was then disinhibited and reappeared only after 13 combinations.

Old, inert verbal connections were subsequently projected. Differentiation by intensity and by duration were not maintained to the next examination. When reinforcement was removed some of the conditioned reactions failed to appear. The removal of reinforcement after modification led to restoration of the old connections. The request to name the stimuli in accordance with the verbal projection led to the disinhibition of differentiation. Differentiation was restored with difficulty.

Differentiation by duration in response to another stimulus was formed and verbalized relatively rapidly. This girl showed a whole series of pathological changes in neurodynamics typical of oligophrenic children as a whole (inertia of the nervous processes, pathologically wide irradiation, weakening of internal inhibition, strong negative induction). Several facts indicate that the general pattern of this girl's neurodynamics is dominated by the process of inhibition. This is demonstrated by the decrease in the strength of the conditioned reactions, the drawn out nature of these reactions, some slowing of the formation of conditioned reactions, a more rapid conversion of positive stimuli into inhibitory than the converse, the strong successive inhibition, and, finally, the lapse of some conditioned reactions after the removal of reinforcement.

Mental State

Optic Analyzer. Zina recognized pictures representing various objects only when they were shown to her slowly, and the girl gave her replies only after additional stimulation. In the initial stages of her education Zina did not recognize pictures of objects upside down (outline or crossed-out figures), but subsequently, with additional stimulation, the girl was able to cope with these tasks.

Spatial Orientation. Zina was capable of spatial orientation. She grasped the notion of right and left, and correctly copied figures made from sticks, but she could only carry out such tasks in the presence of additional stimulation. At times she was inhibited and ceased to perform the task, but if once her hand were made to move one of the sticks, Zina would begin to arrange them into a figure. In the initial stages of her education Zina could cope only with the easiest tasks, but later she was able to produce more complicated figures.

Motor and Motor-Speech Analyzers. The girl showed no gross disturbances of praxis, but she could only perform certain tasks with great difficulty, often with perseveration of previous tasks.

Zina had to be stimulated for each task. The clarity with which she pronounced words and sentences was dependent upon her general condition. Because of her high degree of inhibition and her lethargy the girl usually pronounced words indistinguishably, and her speech was soft and lacking in expression.

Phonemic Hearing. The girl's understanding of everyday speech was complete. Zina often made mistakes when repeating correlated phonemes, especially when the scope of the task was extended.

Cognitive Function and Behavior. Lethargy, extreme inhibition, and the impossibility of starting on any form of activity were the girl's most characteristic features. In all her movements she clearly showed lack of confidence and uncertainty. When walking she often took the wrong direction. She had difficulty in setting herself in motion. She would stop while the other children continued to perform some task or other, or she would continue in some action when the rest had stopped. The girl's extreme inhibition also showed itself in her behavior. She attended her lessons punctually. During her lessons she was very tense and taciturn. She never asked the teacher anything of her own accord and was very slow to answer questions.

Zina was a difficult child to approach. Her general state of inhibition was particularly bad when she was in new surroundings or when a stranger was present. In such cases she usually stopped the task in which she was engaged. The girl's persistent silence, her general tenseness, and her involuntary facial grimaces were suggestive of a negativistic reaction. These states may be distinguished from negativism, however, by the fact that the girl was comparatively easily brought out of her condition, and if another person began to carry out a task together with her, then in the future she could do it by herself.

These features were demonstrated especially clearly in the initial stages of her education. The girl mastered reading and writing with great difficulty. She easily forgot letters which she had learned, and confused them with others that looked similar. When writing separate words from dictation she often omitted the vowels: for example, instead of the word "dom" [house] she wrote "dm," instead of "kot" [cat] she wrote "kt," and instead of the word "kust" [bush] she wrote "kst."

During her subsequent education various mistakes appeared:

1) perseveration (for example, instead of the word "obedayut" [they ate dinner] she wrote "obbeedayut," instead of "obruch" [hoop] she wrote "obbruch," and instead of the word "deti" [children] she wrote "dettti");

2) omission of letters (for example, instead of the word "stul" [chair] she wrote "sul," instead of the word "litsu" [face] she wrote "liu," and instead of the word "koren" [root] she wrote "korn").

3) failure to complete letters and words (for example, instead of the sentence "Uchenik risuet kartinku" [The pupil draws pictures] the girl wrote "Uchenik risue...," instead of the word "kartofel" [potato] she wrote "karto," and instead of the word "Grisha" [Gregory] she wrote "Gshrg");

4) transposition of elements in a word or sentence (for example, instead of the word "malyar" [painter] she wrote "marlyar," instead of the word "nastupilo" [it came] she wrote "nasuiilp," and instead of the word "brat" [brother] she wrote "barat").

Throughout the whole period of her education, especially in writing, Zina showed very clearly how differences in the level of her performance depended upon her condition. With increasing inhibition the number of mistakes which she made increased sharply. The quality of her work also depended on the circumstances in which she carried out her task. In individual work, for instance, when the teacher encouraged the girl and stimulated her, she was able to write from dictation without a mistake.

Fifteen minutes after receiving an injection of caffein the girl was given dictation, which she wrote without a single mistake, and in the course of the work she was more active and lively than usual.

The distinctive features of the girl's neurodynamics were revealed against the background of gross maldevelopment of her cognitive functions. The girl's inability to speak in abstract or general terms was most obviously revealed when she was required to classify pictures.

In the initial stages of her education she understood only the word "arrange" in the instruction she received, and with this understanding she arranged the pictures singly. Zina could not take advantage of help during the test. In later stages of her education the girl managed to group together a few pictures, but did not employ essential signs in making her classification (she used color, size, etc.).

In the third year of her education the girl, to some degree, developed situational thinking, and at this stage she was able to group together a number of objects related to a single situation. The girl also showed the same maldevelopment of cognitive function when comparing and contrasting objects. When she compared pictures of a cat and a dog, she did so by unimportant signs.

Difficulties specific for oligophrenia children were revealed by Zina in her understanding of passages read to her from stories. The story "What Serezha Thought" was read to her. In spite of the fact that Zina remembered the content of the story, she was unable to reach any conclusion or to establish the necessary bonds of meaning between the various parts of the story that had been read to her, and she merely reproduced isolated fragments of it.

In reply to the experimenter's question "What did Serezha think?" the girl reproduced stereotyped connections from her own past experience. "The dishes must be washed and the room tidied every day."

Zina experienced difficulty in interpreting picture stories. She was often unable to do more than enumerate what she saw in the picture. She found it still more difficult when she had to arrange the pictures in a certain order in which they were connected by a common theme. Zina often regarded each separate picture as a completed episode. The maldevelopment of her cognitive functions was clearly demonstrated in the course of the child's studies at the special school. Analysis of the sound meaning of each letter and the fusion of sound-letters into complexes presented difficult problems to her. Even when she had mastered these problems, Zina still did not grasp the meaning of what she had read. She experienced particularly great difficulty in learning to count. After three years of study in the first class of the village school, the girl could only count up to five, and could not count backwards at all. Subsequently she experienced great difficulty in addition and subtraction, and she could only solve such problems on her fingers. She learned her multiplication and division tables well, and she was able to add and subtract numbers up to 100 and multiply and divide up to 50, although in so doing she often used her fingers and mechanical aids to counting. She needed assistance to perform difficult tasks such as subtraction of one two-figure number from another two-figure number involving carrying ten.

She solved arithmetic problems better when they were written on the blackboard or in an exercise book, for she memorized them poorly and forgot individual elements of the problem. The change from one form of solution to another was very difficult for the girl.

The maldevelopment of her cognitive activity showed itself especially clearly during the solution of arithmetical problems. In the fourth year of her education in the course of her lessons the girl was given the following problem to solve: "Ninety-six kilograms of cucumbers were gathered from a garden, 80 kg pickled and the remainder were divided equally among four workmen. How many kilograms of cucumbers did each man receive?" After the preliminary analysis of this problem and a careful exposition of the various steps, the girl was asked to solve it by herself. Here is a sample of her work:

1. "How many cucumbers were taken? 96 kg − 80 kg = 6 kg."

2. "How many cucumbers did each man receive? 80 kg ÷ 4 kg = 20 kg."

The formulation of the first problem had no relation to the task assigned, and was none other than a stereotyped connection brought into this problem from others which she had solved previously. The girl's action was properly chosen, but it did not follow from the formulation of the problem. She made a mistake in her subtraction and lost ten. The girl copied the second question from her problem book and correctly chose the arithmetical operation, but the numbers which she used showed that she did not understand the course of solution of the problem. Later she was given an equally difficult problem to solve. "A boy read a book in two days. The first day he read 22 pages, and the second day even 9 pages more. How many pages were there in the book? Solution:

1. "How many pages did the boy read in two days? 22 pages + 2 pages = 24 pages."

2. "How many pages were there in the book? 24 pages + 9 pages = 33 pages."

The girl formulated the first question incorrectly, using the formula of a previous stereotype. The girl chose the correct course of action, but made a mistake in the arithmetical operation. She copied the next question as stated in her problem book, but chose the wrong action. She did not solve the problem as a whole because she could not elaborate the complex system of bonds of meaning between the formulation of the problem, the numerical data, and the nomenclature.

After the solution of these problems, the girl was given a task consisting of one question. "Some children gathered 28 cucumbers from a garden, the same number from another garden and 17 cucumbers from a third. How many cucumbers altogether did the children gather?" We give below a specimen of her solution:

1. "How many cucumbers were taken from the third garden? 28 + 17 = 45 cucumbers."

2. "How many cucumbers altogether did the children take? 45 + 17 = 62 cucumbers. The children took 62 cucumbers altogether."

It is interesting to direct attention to the formulation of the first question. The girl solved this problem after she had practiced the solution of problems with a hidden content. As a result of this, Zina applied the type of solution used in the previous and more complicated problems to this simple problem, and she accordingly formulated the first question as follows: "How many cucumbers were taken from the third garden?" The incorrect formulation of the problem was also due to the problem itself in that the numbers had been replaced by words, "the same number from another garden."

The inertia of a system of verbal connections, once it had been formed, stood out very clearly against the background of gross maldevelopment of the cognitive functions. When during a clinical conversation the connection of naming the months in the normal and reverse order was firmly established, if she was asked to name the days of the week she would stubbornly continue to recite the names of the months, and if asked to name the seasons of the year she would give the days of the week.

In the picture classification experiment Zina for a long time solved this new problem in the way she had learned to figure out the previous task (the rejection of the fourth superfluous picture).

The specific feature of this case was the predominance of a state of inhibition of the cerebral cortex. The state of inhibition bore a very variable and unstable character, and was dependent on the conditions in which the child's activities were carried on. In the ordinary surroundings Zina was less inhibited and more productive, but in unusual surroundings her level of inhibition rose sharply.

Principal Stages of the Child's Development. The disturbance of her development was very well marked even at the earliest stages of this girl's life, and was characterized not only by the imperfect development of the most complex functions (walking and speech), but also by specific features in the form of lethargy and inhibition, absence of reaction to her environment and drowsiness.

At the beginning of her school career the girl obviously failed to make adequate progress in her development. It might be considered that the stay of this extremely backward and inhibited girl among normal children at an ordinary school was a factor which retarded her development. During the attendance at the special school she showed not only a profound degree of mental retardation but also extreme inhibition, timidity, and a tendency towards marked negativistic reactions. Her timidity, anxiety, and marked negativistic reactions, which were relatively easily overcome by a proper approach by the teacher, should be regarded as a characteristic reaction to the girl's long unsuccessful education in the first class of the ordinary school.

Only at the end of the second year of her education, as a result of properly organized educational measures, in conjunction with suitable treatment, was visible progress observed in the child's development. Zina became more lively and active and her negativistic reactions were perceptibly diminished. Whereas previously any attempts to assist the girl had aroused in her a series of marked negativistic reactions, she now accepted this help. Later she developed an interest in the teacher's evaluation of her, but at the same time the progress in the development of her cognitive functions was very limited. Zina learned reading, writing, and elementary arithmetic, but she had a very poor grasp of what she had read and she was quite incapable of solving arithmetical problems. This severe maldevelopment of the girl's cognitive functions led to difficulties in her education, and the teachers' committee of the school repeatedly discussed whether or not to transfer her to the imbecile class. In addition to receiving properly organized assistance with her general class work, the girl also had the benefit of individual tuition.

Zina showed interest in her work and showed appropriate attitudes towards her teacher's evaluation. The girl became more approachable in her dealings with other children and with adults. She became more organized and purposeful. Besides the improvement in her general condition and the development of her emotions, the girl mastered with great difficulty, but did nevertheless gradually master her assigned school work. At the end of her fourth year of education the girl's general progress was still more obvious. Zina was well disciplined, relaxed and obeyed all the school rules. Her negativistic reaction had completely disappeared. The girl even behaved more actively. We may note that in her third school year Zina would go into the dining room and go up to the waitress, but could not tell her what she wanted. Now Zina could enter the dining room, and ask the waitress for everything she needed. Formerly, if the girl had filled her exercise book she did not go up to the teacher and ask for a new one. Now, if her exercise book was full she raised her hand and asked for another.

At the end of the second year of her education Zina began to be concerned about what others thought of her, but what she felt one can only guess because she would blush and be embarrassed, tears would come to her eyes, but she would never express her dissatisfaction with the teacher's report. Now, if she received a bad report and considered that it was lower than the quality of her work deserved, she would go up to the teacher and ask why her report was so bad. Whereas in the first years of her education the tempo of the girl's work was very slow and she would succeed in completing only part of a task, in her fourth year she was almost equal to the rest of the class in her working rate. She was interested in all forms of activity within her capacity. In the bookbinding department she was one of the best pupils and won prizes nearly every month.

The girl's cognitive functions showed appreciable development, as was very clearly revealed in the picture classification experiment. Whereas in the first years of her education she understood the instructions literally and did not grasp the idea of classifying the objects represented on the pictures, at the beginning of the third year of her education she grouped these objects together, although not in accordance with important signs, and by the end of the third year of her education she had developed concrete situational forms of thinking. When she subsequently performed similar tasks she was able to relate previously acquired abstract concepts to concrete situational forms of thinking. The whole of our analysis indicates considerable progress in the girl's development.

Clinical Analysis of the Case

The presence in the psychopathological picture of the fundamental symptom of oligophrenic mental deficiency in the form of maldevelopment of the capacity for abstraction and generalization, and the development of this symptom on the basis of an early organic lesion of the central nervous system together justify the diagnosis of oligophrenia. It must be pointed out that the principal etiological factor in this case is taken to be the prolonged and severe asphyxia at birth.

The physical disease of uncertain etiology from which the girl suffered at the age of 18 months, accompanied by convulsions and loss of consciousness, must be regarded as the reaction of a defective brain to severe infection. Although we consider this disease to be the reaction of an already defective brain, it was nevertheless an additional etiological factor complicating still further the subsequent development of the child.

Analysis of the distinctive features of the psychopathological picture, namely the combination of considerable maldevelopment of the cognitive functions with the absence of gross localized defects, together with the absence of primary, gross abnormalities of the emotional-volitional function, give grounds for estimating the degree of spread of the pathological process, viz., we believe that in this case there was a mainly diffuse, superficial lesion of the cerebral hemispheres.

The neurological symptomatology also confirmed the presence of a primarily cortical lesion. In this particular case the diffuse lesion of the cerebral cortex was complicated by a residual hydrocephalus, the presence of which was also confirmed by the skull x-ray findings. It was this additional pathogenetic factor which was responsible for the more complex and gross changes in the cortical neurodynamics.

Experimental investigation of the higher nervous activity showed that this girl demonstrated a number of special characteristics in addition to the changes of cortical neurodynamics common to all oligophrenic children. These specific characteristics include an evident predominance of inhibition over excitation. In view of the above findings we are justified in classifying this case as an example of the type of oligophrenia which we have delimited.

CASE 3

Natasha E., a girl aged 15 years. No abnormal hereditary factors.

History. The mother was twice pregnant. The son born of the first pregnancy died at the age of one year from umbilical sepsis. The girl we are now discussing was born of the second pregnancy. One month before term the mother had a slight hemorrhage. Labor was at term. The child was born in asphyxia. In earliest childhood the girl was already observed to be very lethargic. She nursed poorly. At three months Natasha had a severe attack of influenza, after which she became still more lethargic and reacted neither to bright objects nor to loud sounds. At the age of seven months she had a severe and prolonged attack of dysentery. Her early development was somewhat retarded. Her teeth appeared at six months, and she began to walk at the beginning of the second year, to speak single words at 18 months and to use sentences at the age of two years.

Natasha was brought up at home under her mother's care; her mother noticed a considerable retardation in development. The girl was so sluggish, passive, indifferent and inactive that her mother had to do nearly everything for her. For instance, the girl could only look after herself with difficulty, the main problem being that she always had to be prodded into activity. Her slowness and lethargy were especially apparent in her movements and behavior.

At preschool age slight progress in her development was observed, but she nevertheless could not carry out the most elementary task if no stimulation was applied. She occasionally showed an interest in children of her own age, but she was unable to play with them and she usually remained in the role of passive spectator. The girl preferred monotonous forms of activity: winding thread, stringing beads, and arranging sticks. Natasha loved to hear stories and tales, but even then would remain equally lethargic and passive.

At seven years of age she began to attend the first class of regular school, but could not adapt herself to this new experience, and after three months was removed by her mother. From seven to eight years of age Natasha was tutored by her mother and a teacher. With individual training she remembered letters comparatively easily and learned to form them into words, and then without much difficulty began to read and write. This progress in her education did not lead, however, to the development of interest in her work.

She easily learned to count up the scale, but counting backwards was very difficult for her. She could not correlate numbers and objects for a long time.

After a year of study at home, the girl was again returned to the first class of regular school. She managed well in Russian, but in arithmetic she was very backward and could not do the problems. After spending two years in the first class of regular school, Natasha was promoted to the second class, but soon afterwards developed endomyocarditis; upon recovery she again studied at home. In her mother's words, the girl remained just as lethargic, passive and slow at home. At the age of ten Natasha was again sent to the second grade of regular school, but three months later was transferred to a special school. Actually, though, until she was 14 years old she studied at home with a special teacher. Only at 14 years was Natasha accepted in the fourth class of the special school.

Physical State. Circumference of the head was 50 cm; face was small and pale, tongue thick, teeth eroded. Her physical development was retarded for her age. Her chest was narrow and flat, her shoulder blades were slightly winged. The hands and palms were narrow, moist and weak. Her skin was pale, with hypertrichosis along the spine and extremities, and the turgor of the skin was reduced. The respiratory movements of the lungs were weak. The borders of the heart were widened, the apex beat was diffuse and visible in the sixth intercostal space. Accentuation of the sounds in the vessels. Moderate tachycardia. Pulse 98 beats per minute, poor volume. Blood pressure 115/65 on the right and 110/60 on the left. No abnormalities of digestion. Sexual development complete: the child had menstruated since the age of eleven. Physically she was greatly weakened. The heart defect was compensated.

State of the Nervous System. The pupils were wide, the reaction to convergence brisk, to light sluggish. At extreme lateral gaze a rapidly disappearing nystagmus was noted. There was a very slight flattening of the right nasolabial fold. She could not wink the right eye. A divergent strabismus was present.

Both hands and feet were slightly atrophic and weak, the distal portions being most affected. The fine movements of the hands were severely disturbed, hand grasp was adequate, and resistance to passive movement was good. Her legs were weaker than her arms, with variable weakness of the right lower extremity. Range of movement of her feet was restricted. She stood and hopped badly on both sides. Hypotonia and slight innervational disturbances were observed. The tendon reflexes of the upper limbs were slightly diminished and equal on both sides. The knee jerks were lively, especially on the right. Mayer's sign was absent, and the palm-chin reflex was also absent. A bilateral positive Babinski was found. Oppenheim's sign was more marked on the left than on the right. The abdominal reflexes were absent on the right, and on the left they were consistently brisk. Barre's sign was diminished on the right.

Vasomotor lability was observed. Her hands felt cold. When the girl was asked to raise both hands above her head, her hands would become pale and her face reddened. Investigation of deep sensation showed no disturbances, but during the analysis of superficial sensation the girl gave stereotyped interpretations.

In this particular case the neurological symptomatology was diffuse and mainly cortical in character (the differential character of the paresis, the innervational changes of tone, the stereotyped discrimination of superficial stimuli). A series of signs was present indicating that the brainstem was involved (strabismus, nystagmus, sluggishness of the pupillary reactions, the nasal intonation of the voice and the weakness of phonation). Several symptoms indicated that the left cerebral hemisphere was more deeply involved than the right.

Ophthalmological Examination. Visual acuity of both eyes 1.0. Optic fundus: optic disk clearly outlined and pale pink, dilated veins in the region of the macula lutea, with no changes observed at the periphery.

Otorhinolaryngological Examination. Hearing within normal limits.

X-ray Examination of the Skull. Skull diminished in size. Base of the skull flattened. Anterior clinoid processes ill defined. Cranial sutures poorly differentiated. In all regions of the skull digital impressions were seen. Vascular shadows intensified (diploic veins and transverse sinus). The x-ray findings suggested the presence of residual manifestations of hypertension and hydrocephalus.

Electroencephalography. The alpha-rhythm was absent from the electroencephalogram. In all regions of the cortex slow waves of low amplitude were recorded, in some ways resembling a slow alpha-rhythm in configuration. The curve of the electrical activity of the brain was slightly depressed (Fig. 37). The depression of the electrical activity of the brain and the predominance of low-voltage slow waves on the electroencephalogram may be interpreted as an indication of the predominance of inhibitory processes in the cortex and is evidence of the presence of neurodynamic disturbances.

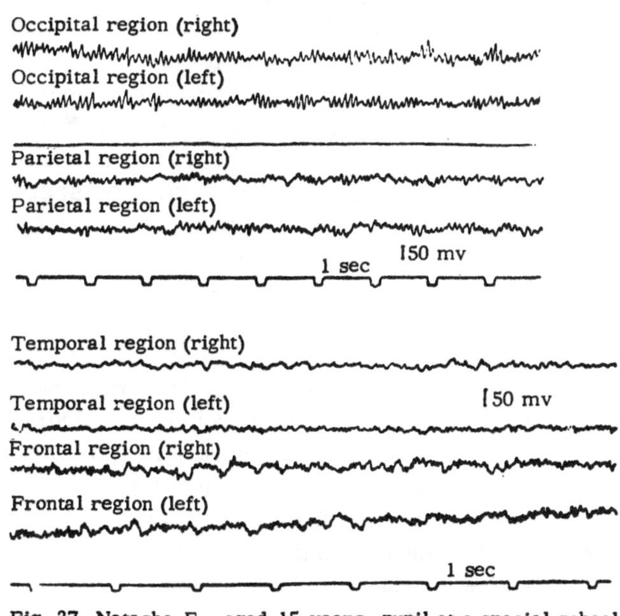

Fig. 37. Natasha E., aged 15 years, pupil at a special school (oligophrenia, feeble-minded degree). In all regions of the cortex slow waves of low amplitude are recorded, with superimposed beta-rhythm.

Investigation of the Higher Nervous Activity. Conditioned reactions to simple light and sound stimuli were formed on the average after two combinations. Simple differentiation (to color and to intensity) was produced after two or three combinations. This at once became stable to negative reinforcement introduced during the formation of differentiation, and led to inhibition of the conditioned reactions to positive stimuli.

In the initial stage of consolidation of the first conditioned reaction generalization of new stimuli with the positive stimulus was observed within the limits of a single analyzer. After the consolidation of differentiation even those stimuli which were very close to the positive stimulus were not generalized with it.

The verbal projection of the production of conditioned reactions to simple stimuli and to simple differentiation was adequate. Differentiation was stable and lasted for several days. During the modification of simple systems of connections the change in the significance of the formerly differential signals into positive signals took place slowly (at the first modification after 17 combinations, but it did not take place during the first combination of the conditioned reaction, even in response to a command). Positive stimuli changed to inhibitory ones after a single combination. The production of more complex forms of differentiation (differentiation by duration) was severely retarded. Relatively stable differentiations were produced only after 16 combinations.

Verbal projection showed the inertia of the old verbal connections (projection of a previously formed differentiation to intensity which could not be overcome even by prolonged consolidation of the new connection and by a series of special measures). This inertia was revealed both during the production of differentiation to duration and during the formation of a conditioned reaction to alternate stimuli.

Nonverbalized differentiation to duration could not be modified in spite of scores of combinations. Complex systems of connections were strongly affected by the action of extrastimuli, which led to inhibition of the conditioned reactions. During work with more complicated forms of differentiation (at the beginning of each experiment, after interruptions in the course of the experiment and after verbal projections) the conditioned reactions were absent for a short time. The introduction of reinforcement was necessary for them to be restored.

Nonverbalized and relatively complex forms of differentiation, even when consolidated, were readily disinhibited after removal of the reinforcement. In the presence of reinforcement, even in the form of the words "that's right," differentiation could be reproduced for a long time. Disinhibited differentiation was soon restored after the introduction of reinforcement.

Natasha's higher nervous activity was characterized by a series of pathological features common to all oligophrenic children (wide generalization of stimuli in the initial stage of development of conditioned reactions, weakness of internal inhibition leading to the slower formation of relatively complicated forms of differentiation, gross inertia of the old verbal connections and strong external inhibition).

Several signs indicated the predominance of the process of inhibition in the general picture of the higher nervous activity. This was revealed by: the considerable successive inhibition after the introduction of negative reinforcement, which was particularly strong and prolonged during the formation of complex forms of differentiation; the absence of primary generalization of even closely related stimuli after consolidation of differentiation; the markedly delayed modification of the value of the differential stimulus into positive inhibition — conditioned reactions to positive stimuli at the beginning of a new experiment and after each break in the experiment.

Mental State

Optic Analyzer. The girl recognized pictures of different objects, but often gave her answers slowly and only after additional stimulation. In addition to correctly recognizing many pictures shown to her, she would suddenly stop recognizing objects with which she was familiar. For example, among a series of pictures the girl did not recognize the picture of a carrot, but looked at it for a long time, turned it in every direction, peered at it closely and put it back. Two minutes later she easily recognized the same picture of the carrot; she then repeated the same behavior in relation to the picture of a barrel. Natasha looked at the picture for a long time, turned it in all directions and said that it was a drum, whereupon she pointed to the top of the barrel and then easily recognized this picture. She recognized without any particular difficulty outline drawings of objects or crossed-out figures, and also pictures shown to her upside down.

Spatial Orientation. The girl could orientate herself in space, and knew right from left. She copied stick figures correctly, but did this very slowly. Additional stimulation was essential. She experienced difficulties when the task was made more complicated. Natasha had no particular difficulty in arranging pictures from tiles, but she could only do this with additional stimulation.

Motor and Motor-Speech Analyzers. The girl's movements were extremely slow, clumsy and poorly defined, as clearly demonstrated when she carried out the most elementary tasks. The girl particularly needed additional stimulation in the performance of isolated movements and actions. In postural movements the girl manifestated some apraxia, which she could overcome. Natasha found it especially difficult when she was instructed to perform ordered movements with both hands. She could do this only if the movement was accompanied by conversation. She had no difficulty in the pronunciation of individual words and she could repeat difficult sentences relatively well.

Phonemic Hearing. Natasha fully understood what was said to her. She repeated corrolated phonemes satisfactorily, even when the scope was extended to some degree, but in this case additional stimulation was required.

Though there were no gross localized cortical disturbances, in a task involving any analyzer this girl clearly displayed lethargy, passivity, and slowness, and at times her reactions to a stimulus disappeared altogether, even with the application of additional stimulation.

Cognitive Function and Behavior. The girl's motor activity clearly revealed her individual peculiarities. Her deportment was rigid: her spine was overerect, with a slight inclination forward, the head and shoulders hung down, the hands were immovably pressed to the body and were tense. The girl's posture was inexpressive and inflexible. Occasionally she would turn her head to the side. She would sit for more than an hour in the children's matinee absolutely motionless. Her face was frozen, and only a scarcely perceptible suspicion of a smile might sometimes lighten and enliven her eyes.

Natasha was under our observation for a year. She was punctual for her lessons. In class she was well disciplined and attentive. The individual traits of this girl appeared within a few days of her attendance at the school. She was very slow to start on a task and appeared to be somewhat helpless: she could not take her textbooks or exercise books from her school bag, and when leaving she would not gather up her school supplies but would often leave it all on her desk.

She could never remember her homework, so that her mother

had to phone the teacher to find out. At first the girl remained tense and confused and at times she forgot to eat her lunch.

Natasha would begin a task only after additional stimulation. She apparently did not react to instructions at first, and she began to follow them only after they had been repeated two or three times. When doing a particular job she had to be additionally stimulated, otherwise she would stop working. Natasha could solve arithmetical problems involving all four operations and utilizing numbers up to 100 without particular difficulty, but when she was in a state of inhibition she could not do simpler problems. For example, the girl was asked to solve the following problem orally: "What is 21 minus 17?" Her replv was 13. When the problem was repeated she could not solve it correctly and she stubbornly wrote the number 13 again. No form of stimulation could enable Natasha to find the right answer. After three minutes, when the problem was written down for her, she was able to solve it correctly. Natasha was then given the problem of subtracting two from 20. Usually the girl readily performed tasks of similar nature, but with an increase in her level of inhibition, instead of solving this problem she counted backwards from 20. In doing so she became confused and did not realize that she had given the wrong answer. The girl remembered the task she had been given and correctly repeated it, but when carrying it out she again drifted to counting backwards, which she had learned by heart. She often finished by repeating the number 20 many times. This number 20 which stuck in her mind prevented her from accomplishing her tasks when the instructions were broken down into separate stages. When actively encouraged, Natasha attempted to subtract with the aid of her fingers, but this too was impossible. For instance, she subtracted 2 from 14 and obtained 20. "Oh, this twenty again, it comes up everywhere; no, I can't," exclaimed the girl.

If she was asked to subtract 2 not from 20 but from 10, then she could do the problem. When, after solving this problem, she was again asked to subtract 2 from 20, however, she once more went through the stereotype of counting backward from 20.

During the solution of arithmetical problems well within her capacity, the girl would show temporary lapses of activity, which would take the following form. At first, due to her unstable memory, she would make mistakes when repeating the items of the problem, and then she would forget individual links and try to achieve a fragmentary solution. Subsequently she would calculate by unsuitable methods, and then finally she would say repeatedly, in a stereotyped fashion, any particular number which happened to stick in her mind.

These incorrect solutions could result from her failure to master the various arithmetical methods, but this explanation is not supported by analysis of the available evidence. At times the girl could solve all these problems correctly, and then, on the other hand, with increasing inhibition, she would make a number of characteristic mistakes when carrying out comparatively easy tasks.

Natasha was a good pupil in Russian. She wrote in a correct style and knew how to use grammatical rules she had learned. At the same time she made a series of characteristic mistakes, i.e., omissions, failure to complete words, transpositions, and perseverations. When answering questions on Russian she would repeat individual words in a stereotyped way. This was shown clearly in the following example of her work.

She was given the task of choosing words related to the word "len'" [laziness]. The other children chose the following words: "len;" "lenyus'" [I am lazy], "lentyai" [lazybones], "lenivitsa" [a lazy girl] and "razlenilsya" [he grew very lazy]. The teacher wrote these words on the blackboard and the work was all explained. The words written on the blackboard were then erased and the pupils had to do the problem by themselves. Among the words which Natasha had written correctly she had repeated the word "liniya" [a line] six times, i.e., her activity had become disorganized as a result of the perseverative repetition of the word "liniya."

Clinical conversation with the girl clearly revealed both her general intellectual inadequacy and her lethargy and passivity. For example, in reply to the question where she lived, the girl said: "On the block where the 'Gastronom' [the grocery store] is." Natasha knew her address, but in order to obtain the correct answer from her some additional stimulation was required. Natasha did not understand a question if its formulation was insufficiently concrete. If she was asked to name the season of the year, she would stubbornly give a list of the months.

If the question on the seasons was put into concrete terms, then she could overcome her inertia and answer the question correctly. If she were then asked to list the days of the week, she would recite the months, i.e., inert, stereotyped connections would once again appear. If the question were repeated, Natasha would say with some confusion: "The days of the week, what can the 'day of the week' be?" She could not translate her experience into concrete terms, and after every pause she would again begin to recite the names of the months. Repetition of the question increased the girl's confusion: "What can these 'days of the week' be? Are there really 'days of the week'?" The doctor had only to say the word "Monday," however, for the girl to recite easily all the days of the week (either in normal or reverse order).

For a long time the girl could not adapt herself to her new school environment, but remained confused and extremely inhibited. Natasha obeyed all the teacher's orders, but showed no spontaneous activity. She never raised her hand and often answered the teacher's questions incorrectly.

The impression was thus created that the girl was indifferent to her surroundings, and especially to the teacher's estimation of her ability. The impression of her indifference was deceptive, however, for Natasha, on returning home, often would tell her mother all that happened in school, go over her failures, be upset when she had received a bad mark and happy at her success. All these features of the girl's behavior were portrayed against the background of maldevelopment of her cognitive functions.

The picture classification experiment demonstrated clearly the maldevelopment of the girl's capacity for abstraction and generalization. She listened attentively to the instructions, but only after additional stimulation did she start to carry out the task.

She grouped identical pictures together, either on the principle of their color or on the basis of doubly concrete connections; for example she grouped the picture of a fork with the picture of a knife, her explanation being that, "You eat with a fork but you also need a knife for cutting." When grouping together pictures of trees, she separated one picture which represented a Christmas tree. She could not agree to group this picture with the others because she explained that a Christmas tree needed a room and trimmings. When the picture classification experiment was repeated she demonstrated considerable inertia of the connections once formed. For instance, when grouping together the pictures of a knife and a fork she was motivated by the fact that these objects are placed together on the table. Natasha subsequently applied this formula during the whole of her picture classification experiment (for example, "the shopping basket and satchel go together," "the overcoat, hat, and galoshes go together," and "the frying pan and saucepan go together").

In the course of the picture classification experiment her low capacity for abstraction and generalization, the inertia of established connections and the passivity of her cognitive functions were clearly demonstrated. The latter also showed itself in the difficulties which the girl had when reading story passages. Oseeva's story "The Sons" was read to Natasha. She worked on it in school and at home.

Natasha was asked the question, "Why did the old man see only the son?" She replied, "Because he took the pails and helped his mother." She was then asked the supplementary question, "Why didn't the old man see the other sons?" Natasha replied, "Because they were hiding."

It is clear from these answers that Natasha could not establish the necessary bond of reasoning between the individual parts of the story, which prevented her from understanding the theme of the story as a whole and from reaching the proper conclusion.

The girl was then read the story "The Unsolved Problem." Natasha listened to this story to the end, and after additional stimulation, in reply to questions could retell it, but she could not form conclusions.

The girl had great difficulty in interpreting picture stories. In the easiest series, with additional stimulation, she could establish the necessary connection between the pictures, but if the task were slightly more complicated she could not cope with it. She would look upon each picture as a complete episode in itself, without establishing the common theme.

Definite changes were revealed by prolonged observation of the girl in the course of her education and training. At times Natasha was more composed and active, required less stimulation, and made few mistakes when writing from dictation, when copying or when solving arithmetical problems. At times the general level of her inhibition rose, and the girl became lethargic, unproductive, and made more mistakes. Natasha was very sensitive to changes in her surroundings. At home, when working individually, she was most productive and demonstrated her relatively well-preserved emotional make-up. In new and unfamiliar surroundings she was inhibited, confused, and exhibited a sharp decrease in her work capacity.

Organized teaching, befitting the girl's individual problems, in conjunction with medical treatment, produced positive results. Natasha became appreciably more active during lessons, and occasionally raised her hand and asked questions, and timidly indicated that she wanted to answer. She began to mix more with the other children in the class. The tempo of her work improved slightly.

Principal Stages of the Child's Development. Before she reached school age the combination of a general backwardness in her development with well marked lethargy and slowness of all her mental processes was already quite obvious. The corrective training carried out properly by her mother yielded good results and led to some progress in her development. Immediately before going to school Natasha could respond to a number of instructions, and loved to listen to stories and tales. When carrying out various tasks the girl slowed a tendency to stereotyped reactions and perseveration.

The girl's attendance at an ordinary school at the age of seven years clearly had an adverse effect on her development and led to an increased lethargy and decreased productivity. Tutoring at home by a teacher who specialized in handicapped children not only enabled Natasha to make considerable progress in her development but she also learned skills such as reading, writing and arithmetic: at the age of $8\frac{1}{2}$ years the girl's condition was so well compensated that she was able to return to the ordinary school, but she continued to do poorly in arithmetic. Because of a severe and prolonged physical illness (endomyocarditis) she again fell behind. After this illness (until the age of 14 years) she was educated at home.

The girl was under our observation after the age of 14 years, i.e., from the time she entered the fourth class of a special school. In the course of two years she showed further progress in her development, especially in her emotional-volitional function. Natasha was sensitive to the teacher's evaluation of her and at the same time developed a critical attitude towards her own work. She lost her indifference to her situation. Natasha showed emotions and was very attached to her mother. She was easily hurt, and bitterly resented her failures.

The girl also made considerable progress in learning to read, write, and count. There was also a less obvious additional development of her cognitive activity during those two years.

Clinical Analysis of the Case

The marked maldevelopment of the girl's cognitive functions, due to an intrauterine lesion of the central nervous system, in this case provided the basis for the diagnosis of oligophrenia. The fundamental etiological factor was an intrauterine lesion of the central nervous system, as evidenced by a uterine hemorrhage one month before birth and asphyxia at birth. A severe attack of influenza at the age of three months, and the chronic dysentery at seven months further complicated the girl's development.

Qualitatively, we may postulate hemorrhage in the brain substance associated with the mother's prenatal hemorrhage during late gestation, and the asphyxia.

So far as the distribution of the pathological process is concerned, there is reason to suppose that it was mainly localized in the cortex. Neurological findings (in the form of signs of a differential paresis, innervational disturbances of tone, stereotypy in evaluation of superficial stimuli) also confirmed that the lesion was mainly cortical in character.

In addition the brainstem was to some extent involved. This fundamental pathogenetic factor was associated with a residual hydrocephalus, as indicated by the skull x-rays.

Experimental investigation of the higher nervous activity of this girl clearly showed additional features indicating predominance of the process of inhibition, in addition to the characteristic features of oligophrenia.

The distinctive features of the pathogenesis and pathophysiology explain the qualitative features of the clinical picture. The structure of the defect in this case was determined not only by the maldevelopment of the cognitive functions but also by the sharp diminution of cortical tone, manifested in the clinical picture by the slowness of all her mental reactions and by the inhibition.

Taking into consideration the brainstem disturbances also present in this case it may be assumed that the sharp fall in the tone of the cortical cells was due not only to the hydrocephalus but also to the inadequate stream of impulses to the corte . from the subcortical ganglia. The foregoing facts provide grounds for including this case in this particular variant of oligophrenia.

CASE 4

Yura B., a boy aged 13 years, a pupil in the fifth class at a special school. No abnormal hereditary factors.

History. Yura's mother had four pregnancies. Three children are normal. Yura was born of the second pregnancy, the course of which was normal. He was born in asphyxia. During the first year of life, according to his mother, the boy developed normally. At the age of one year, when he was evacuated during the war, Yura suffered from a severe form of dyspepsia. The illness lasted two years and his condition was serious, with marked signs of general malnutrition (senile, wrinkled skin, prolapse of the rectum). After this illness the boy's general development was severely affected: Yura began to walk during his fourth year, used single words at 4 years and simple sentences at 5 years. Besides the retardation of development, he exhibited lethargy, passivity and drowsiness. The boy showed no interest in anything. He was helpless and had to be fed and dressed. During his preschool years Yura remained constantly lethargic and passive, showed no interest in play nor in other children and mixed little even with neighbors and relatives. Yura was very somnolent. If he was not called in the morning he would sleep until four or five o'clock in the afternoon, and then after being awake for two or three hours would fall asleep again. The boy did not attend kindergarten. A nine years an attempt was made to send Yura to an ordinary school. At school Yura remained lethargic, incapable of spontaneous activity, asocial and unresponsive to the teacher's questions. At school the boy was found to be very retarded, did not discuss school at home, and soon after returning home would fall asleep. Having reached school age, Yura remained passive and very inhibited. He obeyed not only his mother and his elders, but also younger children. Even when 9 years old Yura was incapable of carrying out even the most elementary duties because of his reticence, his extreme inhibition, and his shyness. There were also complaints of frequent headaches and vertigo, nocturnal enuresis, and stammering.

At 9 years of age he was sent to the imbecile class at a special school. At the beginning of his special education the boy remained lethargic, showed little spontaneous activity, and mixed little with other children; he nevertheless gradually became more lively and active, and after one year was transferred to the first class.

Physical State. The skull was deformed and hydrocephalic with well-marked tuberosities. The left occipitoparietal region was flattened. There was a general narrowing of the skeleton, flattening of the chest, winging of the scapulae, the subcutaneous fat was poorly developed, and the muscles weak.

No abnormality of the internal organs. Blood pressure 110/60. His attacks of headache and vertigo persisted to the present time.

State of the Nervous System. Pupils wide, reaction to light adequate. During convergence the right eye was turned laterally. The right nasolabial fold was ill defined. The tongue deviated slightly to the left. Some weakness of the fingers of the right hand was noted.

Slight generalized hypotonia of the muscles. The tendon reflexes were irregularly increased. The knee jerks were increased on the right and the abdominal reflexes also increased on the right. A slight Rossolimo's sign could be produced, although not very clearly, on both sides. Oppenheim's sign was present on the left and Babinski's sign on both sides. Marked vasomotor instability was present: cyanosis of the hands, and slow, sluggish, diffuse and pink dermographism. A slight residual symptomatology was found, more marked on the right.

Ophthalmological Examination. Visual acuity of both eyes 0.4-0.5. Myopia was present. Optic fundus: the optic disk was pale pink and clearly outlined. Slight dilatation of the veins was present. The periphery and region of the macula lutea were normal and perimetry to white light was also normal.

Otorhinolaryngological Examination. Hearing within normal limits.

X-ray Examination of the Skull. Skull turret-shaped. Pattern obliterated, base flattened. Bones of the vault of the skull thinned. Cranial sutures not differentiated. Well marked digital impressions.

Electroencephalography. The alpha-rhythm was well marked in the occipital regions, less so in the parietal regions, and only occasionally could it be seen in the frontal regions. In the anterior regions of the cortex slow waves and rapid fluctuations of potential were predominant (Fig. 38). During the investigation of the reactions of the cortex by the method of rhythmic light, tactile, and sound stimuli, the presence of modification of the cortical rhythm by high-frequency flashes of light was demonstrated. Considerably more modification of the cortical rhythm took place in response to the simultaneous action of several stimuli addressed to different analyzers. Modification also took place in response to a slow rhythm of light flashes.

After a light stimulus prolonged depression of the alpha-rhythm was observed. The cortical neurons were involved in the rhythm of stimulation entering through the optic analyzer only after a long latent period (modification of the cortical rhythm first appeared in response to the tenth light stimulus). In a series of cases rapid and slow waves were observed on the electroencephalogram during the action of light stimuli, and especially during the action of stimuli coming from different analyzers (Fig. 39). These facts may be regarded as indicating the easy transition of the cortical neurons into a state of inhibition.

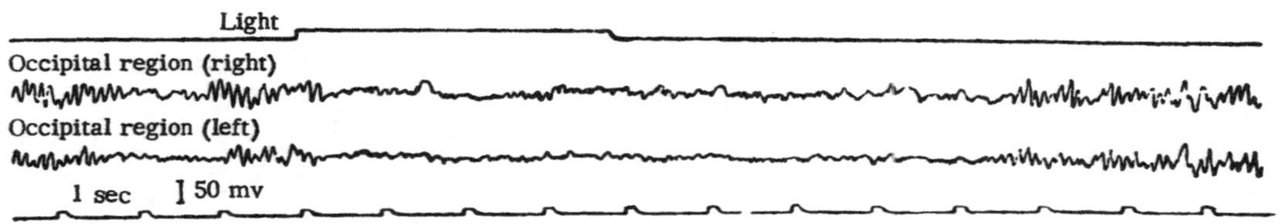

Fig. 38. Yura B., aged 13 years, pupil at a special school (oligophrenia, degree of feeble-mindedness). In response to a single light stimulus, the electroencephalogram showed a depression of the alpha-rhythm in the occipital region, which subsequently lasted 4.5 seconds.

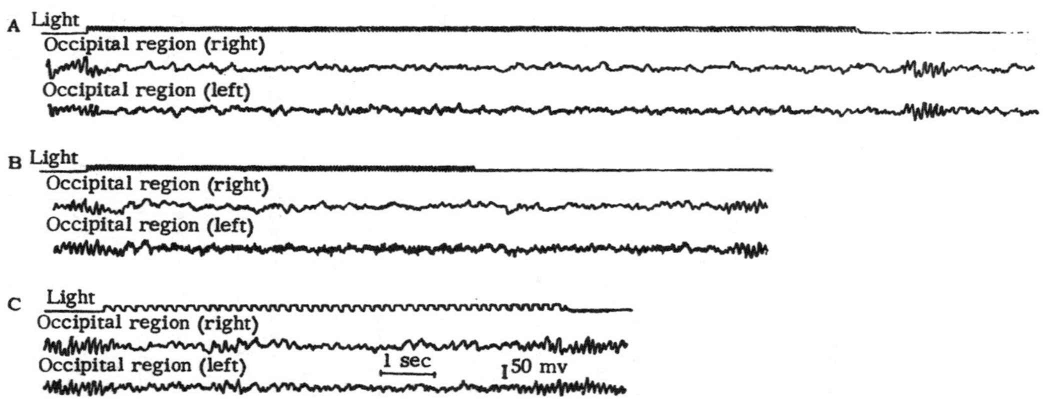

Fig. 39. EEG (of the same subject) during the application of a rhythmic light stimulus. A) A flicker frequency of 21 per second caused in ill-defined modification of the cortical rhythm in the left occipital lead. B) Under the influence of the combined action of light and tactile stimuli the rhythmic reaction became much more marked and longer in duration. C) A flicker frequency of 5 per second caused modification of the cortical rhythm.

Results of the Investigation of the Higher Nervous Activity by the Method of Plethysmography. During the application of an indifferent stimulus an orienting reflex arose only in response to a very strong stimulus, but even in this case a long latent period was observed in comparison with the normal. This fact suggests a decrease in cortical activity and a predominance of the process of inhibition.

After repeated application of the stimulus reactions finally appeared, after 15 to 20 applications, which were pathologically vasodilator in character (normally the reaction is vasoconstrictor in character).

If instructions were introduced, i.e., if the stimulus acquired the meaning of a signal (the child was asked to count the number of stimuli), an adequate and relatively stable vasoconstrictor reaction developed. In this case additional stimulation restored the normal orienting reflex.

The long latent period during the application of indifferent stimuli, and the development of distorted reactions in response to the 15 or 20 applications of the stimulus are suggestive of a lowered excitability of the cortex and of a facile development of limiting inhibition.

Investigation of the Higher Nervous Activity. Yura's reaction to a direct command was extraordinarily unstable. Conditioned reactions to simple light and sound stimuli were produced rapidly. The conditioned reactions were poorly stabilized. When reinforcement was removed a gradual fall in the magnitude of the reaction was observed at the end of the investigation.

A specific feature of the higher nervous activity of this boy was the fact that the primary generalization of new stimuli did not occur at once: in response to the first, or even several applications of the new stimulus, it did not take place, but only developed after repeated applications, increasing in magnitude. Stimuli directed to another analyzer were not generalized with the positive stimulus. At the beginning of a new experiment, during the presentation of the old conditioned stimulus the conditioned reactions were absent, and then they developed and gradually increased in strength.

It was extraordinarily difficult to obtain a verbal projection. The boy replied in monosyllables, sometimes after frequent repetition of the questions, but the projection of the production of simple conditioned reactions and simple differentiation were adequate. In some cases, however, irrelevant connections were mixed up with the projection, which was distorted under the influence of strong, irrelevant stimuli. After modification, the projection showed inertia of the old verbal connections. The development of complex forms of differentiation was difficult. In the verbal projection of the production of the more complex systems of connections, an inert reproduction of the old projection was observed. The inertia of the previously formed verbal connections was revealed particularly clearly when working according to instruction. After modification of the conditioned significance of the stimuli (only verbalized systems of connections were subjected to modification) it was observed that a positive value could become inhibitory quicker than the reverse. For instance, during the attachment of an inhibitory value to a previously positive stimulus only one combination was required, but to attach a positive value to a previously differential stimulus required three combinations.

Extrastimuli had a powerful action. A strong extrastimulus, applied in the middle of the experiment, led to complete inhibition of the conditioned reactions until the end of the experiment.

During the formation of connections by preliminary instruction it was found above all that a connection made in the verbal system did not appear at once in the reactions. Reactions to the first stimuli were usually absent. Regulation of the reaction from the verbal system (by instruction) was unstable when once established. Under these circumstances the connection in the verbal system was retained in most cases. It was sometimes observed that conditioned reactions appeared in accordance with the instruction, but in the projection old verbal stereotypes, as laid down in previous experiments, were repeated.

During investigation by means of preliminary instruction a marked degree of inertia was found during the learning and reproduction of the instruction. During the formation of the more complex connections by means of preliminary instruction a gross motor stereotype developed: the accidentally formed system of motor reactions was extraordinarily inert and was modified with great difficulty.

In addition to the features common to all oligophrenic children (above all the gross inertia, especially at the level of the second signal system), the boy's higher nervous activity was characterized by a series of specific features, indicating pathological imbalance between the nervous processes in the direction of the predominance of inhibition. This is demonstrated by the following facts:

1. At the beginning of each experiment conditioned reactions were absent in response to stimuli to which they had been formed in previous experiments.

2. During the formation of conditioned connections by the method of preliminary instruction conditioned reactions were also absent to the first stimuli applied after the instruction.

3. Primary generalization of stimuli was absent: during the first applications the new stimuli were not generalized with the positive stimulus, but generalization did subsequently take place.

4. Powerful extrastimuli caused complete and prolonged inhibition of conditioned connections which had been formed and consolidated.

5. During modification a positive stimulus more rapidly acquired an inhibitory value than vice versa.

Mental State

Optic Analyzer. Yura correctly identified pictures representing various objects, but he gave his answers slowly and only after additional stimulation. When his general level of inhibition was raised, the boy ceased to recognize objects with which he was well acquainted, but after additional stimulation he easily recognized the same objects which previously he had failed to recognize. Only after additional stimulation did Yura recognize individual objects, crossed-out figures and pictures shown to him upside down.

Spatial Orientation. Yura was capable of orienting himself in space. He understood the concept of right and left. He correctly copied figures from sticks, but performed the task slowly and only after supplementary stimulation. Yura was unable to copy more complicated pictures from matches during his early education, but in later years he could perform more complicated tasks.

Motor and Motor-Speech Analyzers. The boy showed no gross disturbance of postural movements. He carried out the various tests very slowly, sometimes only after additional stimulation, and at times he kept repeating a previous task.

In tests of his dynamic movements Yura experienced difficulties. He had no particularly difficulty in the pronunciation of individual words, and he could rather slowly repeat a difficult sentence. He stammered; sometimes this was hardly noticeable, but if he was fatigued, or faced a more complicated task, especially after physical illness or psychic trauma, his stammer became much more severe. The clarity of his pronunciation of words and sentences was dependent on his general condition. When there was a sharp fall in his general psychic tone, his speech became slurred and indistinct to such an extent that it became difficult to understand. But if he were encouraged and stimulated his pronunciation of words and sentences became clear and comprehensible. Yura's vocabulary was limited and his speech was quiet, inexpressive, slow, and hesitant.

Phonemic Hearing. Yura understood what was said to him. The boy repeated correlated phonemes correctly, even when the scope of the test was extended. There were no gross localized defects, but his general lethargy, passivity, lack of initiative, and sporadic reduction of reactivity became obvious during the performance of some tasks.

Cognitive Function and Behavior. Yura was punctual to class, and very well disciplined, completely obedient, lethargic, shy, taciturn, and reticent. He never asked questions of the teacher or the other children and hardly ever raised his hand, although he often answered questions correctly. Particularly at the beginning he was tense, confused, difficult to engage in any form of activity, and usually half asleep. The boy began any activity extremely slowly, and only after additional stimulation. For instance, in the process of carrying out an task he required constant stimulation, otherwise he would give up. This was clearly shown when Yura's school activities were analyzed.

For example, during a topical lesson the theme "The Family" was discussed. As a preliminary step the teacher told the children in detail, with the help of pictures, what a family consisted of, and what its various members did. The teacher then asked the question: "Who are in the family?" Yura was quiet for a long time and, after a supplementary question, replied "Father." "And who else?" asked the teacher. Yura thought for a long time and then replied "Mother," after which he was silent. Only after constant stimulation by the teacher was Yura able to name his sisters and brothers as well as himself as part of a family. The boy's behavior pattern clearly revealed itself during play, during various school activities and during the tests performed on him.

Sometimes Yura exhibited special states of most severely disturbed activity. These states were most obvious when he did school work. For instance, when extremely inhibited, Yura did not even recognize letters which he had memorized. He would write capital letters in the middle of a word, e.g., "ryBak" [fisherman], although he knew that a capital letter is written at the beginning of a sentence.

When copying from the blackboard he made several foolish mistakes. For example, when he had to copy the following sentence: "Postavit' predlozheniya po poryadku" [put the sentence in its proper order], Yura wrote: "Postavit' pryadku predlozheniya." In this case when copying Yura did not keep the sentence in its proper order.

In another case the boy had to copy a few sentences from a book: "Zagorelsya dom. V dome spala devochka. Poslali sobaku. Sobaka spasla devochku." [The house was on fire. A girl was asleep in the house. A dog was sent. The dog saved the girl.] Yura wrote: "Zagorelsya doma. V dev dome spala devochka. Poslali sobaku. Sobaka spala devochku." These sentences reveal transpositions, omissions of letters and perseverations.

In copying and writing from dictation the boy made several transpositions, failures to finish words and sentences, and omissions of individual letters. When copying from the blackboard he wrote "cherveg" instead of "chetverg" [Thursday], "sanza" instead of "solntse" [sun], "gret" instead of "greet" [it warms] and "ponedel'kik" instead of "ponedel'nik" [Monday]. "Subbota" [Saturday] he wrote "subobta," and "veter" [wind] he wrote "verer." He often duplicated the letters in a word and left words incomplete. Sometimes, however, when less inhibited, Yura would take a perfect dictation.

He had the same characteristic behavior when he learned arithmetic. For example, when he learned his four-times table he forgot his two-times table; when he learned his six-times table he forgot his four-times table, etc.

Yura's state of inhibition influenced his solution of arithmetical problems. He solved a number of these correctly and worked actively, but as he gradually became more lethargic, passive and slow while handling equally difficult problems, he now made mistakes of perseveration, omission of individual elements, and finally stopped working altogether. The teacher then came to his aid and solved a number of problems with the boy. Yura gradually became more alert and active, and solved the next batch of ten problems without a single mistake. This demonstration fully justified the conclusion that his temporary difficulties were caused by an increase in his general level of inhibition.

All these specific features of the boy's neurodynamics were exhibited against a general background of maldevelopment of his cognitive functions. In classifying pictures during his early education the boy's inadequate capacity for abstraction and generalization was very clearly demonstrated. Yura interpreted his instructions literally and arranged the pictures singly. Later he could group together a few situationally related objects. He grouped pictures of a satchel and a book because the book goes in the satchel. He also grouped a table with these, because the satchel and book lie on the table.

At subsequent stages of his education, in this same experiment it was revealed that concrete situational forms of thinking coexisted with memorized categories. In order to classify pictures of various objects Yura employed mechanically learned categories. He grouped pictures representing a fork, a cup, a frying pan, and a saucepan, but in answer to the experimenter's question why he put all these pictures in one group, Yura again reproduced concrete connections in support of each separate picture: "You can take sausage with a fork."; "You can drink milk, tea or water from a cup."; You can wash up in a bowl."; "You can cook in a frying pan." Having grouped together pictures of a cat, fox, crab, goat, and goose, he gave a general definition to them all: "Useful animals," but in his verbal projection he again reproduced concrete connections in support of each separate picture: "The cat catches mice."; "The fox is cunning, it steals hens, geese, and pigeons, and eats them."; "The crab lives in the water. It bites very painfully. Once a crab bit my finger. Crabs taste good and I eat them."; "The goat gives milk which people drink, and it makes leather."; "This is a goose, which has little baby geese and they all give feathers and down and meat."

He grouped together pictures of an apple and a cherry, saying: "They are fruit," but he added to these pictures of flowers, a Christmas tree, a turnip, a carrot, an onion, an oak tree, and blossom. When the experimenter asked the boy why he grouped these pictures together, he again began to reproduce concrete connections in support of each individual picture.

These facts which we have described above show that Yura's cognitive functions had developed to a certain extent. During his years of education Yura had acquired concrete knowledge and had learned to distinguish between groups of objects in accordance with the categories which he had learned. He could not explain, however, why he organized them in this way, and his attempts to explain drifted away into statements of concrete connections in relation to each separate object.

The same inadequacy of his cognitive function appeared when he described similarity and difference. The boy compared the concrete images of a cat and dog by unimportant signs. If the boy was told that the fir tree and birch are similar because they are trees, thereafter he could transfer this information only to closely related, similar objects. After trying to establish the similarity and difference between a cat and a dog, the boy was shown pictures, in some instances of a dog helping a man, and in others looking after its puppies. He was told to put these pictures into two groups. At first Yura did not understand the instructions and attempted to reproduce the inert connections established in the previous experiment, i.e., to compare two dogs represented on different pictures. After this connection had been broken, he correctly arranged the pictures into two groups, but he could not explain why he had done so. Subsequently, the regulatory function of the instruction weakened and he began to recite a list of all details of the picture. The instruction was not now reflected in his verbal projection, and he described the picture without regard to the instruction.

The boy's defective power of thinking was also revealed when bonds of reasoning were established between words and pictures. The simplest connections were formed relatively easily, for example the picture of a mouse, together with the word "cat," gave rise to the connection "The cat catches the mouse." For more complex cases he could not establish any connection at this stage. Yura could not grasp the meaning of a metaphor, for example, when he was asked what an "iron hand" means, he replied, "A man cannot have an iron hand, and so to say that is silly."

The boy also had difficulty understanding passages from stories. He heard the story "The Unsolved Problem." Although Yura listened attentively he could not reach any conclusion about its content. At first he carefully recited the food for each animal in turn, and then came to the conclusion that milk was nicest of all. He confused elements of his own experience with isolated fragments of this story.

Yura had difficulty in understanding the meaning of a series of picture stories. He could not arrange the pictures in order and regarded each one as a complete episode. The maldevelopment of his cognitive functions was also shown in Yura's difficulties in his special education. These were especially marked when the boy was taught how to solve arithmetical problems.

To learn the range of his current development, we attempted to teach Yura how to solve a two-part problem. He was set the following problem: "In one pocket there were five nuts and in the other three nuts more than that. How many nuts were there in both pockets?" Yura correctly repeated the posing of the problem but could not solve it, and instead carried out a simple arithmetical operation. The problem was then presented in concrete terms, and pockets were drawn, but even this procedure did not change Yura's approach, for he added 3 to 5 and obtained 8 which he considered the right answer.

After prolonged explanation of the correct solution, he eventually could understand it, but when he was given a similar problem he was unable to transfer the method to the new set of conditions and again attempted to solve it as a single arithmetical operation.

Against the background of maldevelopment of this boy's cognitive functions the inertia of previously formed connections was clearly apparent, especially at the level of the second signal system. In a clinical conversation the boy was asked to recite the names of the months. He managed to do so only after additional stimulation. The doctor had only to name the first month, and Yura would correctly name all the rest. When after naming the months he was asked to state the days of the week, he persistently continued to enumerate the names of the months, and later instead of the seasons of the year he continued to enumerate the days of the week.

After solving three-component problems. Yura continued to use the old method when transferred to easier two-component problems. The most specific feature of this case was the disturbance of the boy's work capacity, although he expressed a proper attitude towards his work. He showed his low work capacity in the earliest stages of his education, when during a lesson his level of inhibition rose to such an extent that he stopped working. Yura's inhibition level was very variable and unstable and largely dependent on the conditions of the activities.

The presence of a stranger in the class caused an increase in Yura's inhibition level and a fall in his work capacity. This latter was shown by an increase in the number of answers he made in a thoughtless way, the number of guesses, and in the number of mistakes in counting, copying, or solving arithmetical problems. Under familiar conditions he often showed fluctuations in his work capacity, and moreover a very obvious relationship between the boy's work capacity and his general condition of health was established. After an illness (influenza, tonsillitis) his general inhibition level rose sharply, and this led to a considerable diminution of his work capacity.

The relationship between Yura's work capacity and his emotional state was easily shown. Any unpleasant experience caused a significant rise in his general inhibition and a fall in his capacity for work.

Principal Stages of the Child's Development. The disturbance of Yura's development was clearly apparent when still a little child. He was retarded in most complex functions (walking, speech) and was extremely inhibited.

The boy was lethargic, drowsy, and hardly reacted at all to his surroundings. Careful study of the boy and the determination of his basic pathophysiological peculiarities suggested that the paroxysmally developing states of extreme inhibition which were observed in the boy at school age were evidently diffuse in character in earlier stages of his development. These relatively prolonged states of limiting inhibition were quite marked in his preschool years, as proved by the boy's extreme drowsiness. As shown by his history, Yura would sleep until three or four o'clock in the afternoon if he was not roused, and after two or three hours of relative wakefulness, he would then again fall asleep. These observations suggest that the cortical neurons possessed an increased tendency to fall into a state of inhibition.

At the beginning of his school career Yura gradually made some slight progress in his development, so that his parents decided to send him to regular school for his education, but as a result of this there was a sharp decline in his condition. The powerful stimuli which school conditions presented to him led to almost total inhibition. Yura did not answer questions, did not react to his surroundings and, when he came home from school, he immediately fell asleep. The next stage in Yura's development involved his attendance in the imbecile class at the special school where he received an education properly oriented to his abilities.

The restful conditions and the absence of overstrain had a beneficial effect on Yura's development, which soon reached a higher level than that of the other pupils in the imbecile class. During his stay in the imbecile class he became rather more alert and less sleepy. He began to respond to his environment and began to carry out several elementary duties. He developed to such an extent that he was transferred to the first class of the special school.

The greatest development during his education and training took place in the emotional-volitional sphere. In his second school year Yura revealed a responsive attitude towards the teacher's opinion of him and he reacted to unfamiliar situations. He showed a marked interest in his studies and did his school work in a responsible manner.

At the beginning of the first half of the 1955-1956 school year an acute change took place in the boy's behavior. Usually disciplined, obedient, quiet, and attentive, Yura became irritable, tense, and disobedient. His periods of inhibition became more frequent and stronger, and his progress became slower. At this time he had a particularly poor grasp of his tasks, could not keep in mind the details of an assignment, and found it difficult to solve problems previously within his grasp. His stammer got worse. This loss of interest in his studies was utterly incomprehensible.

Yura, who had always done his lessons on time, now only partially prepared them, during lessons he paid little attention to the teacher's explanation, and expressed a desire to quit school and go to work. His mother also noticed a considerable change in the boy's conduct. Yura, who was usually disciplined and attentive, would leave home without permission and remain away for a long time. This change in Yura's behavior was at first incomprehensible and apparent without any motive. Only later was the reason for it discovered. The real reason for the deterioration in the boy's behavior was his reaction to a change in the family circumstances (the father left home). Gradually, however, Yura began to grasp the situation and defined his attitude towards his surroundings. He developed a dislike for his father, but was very attentive to his mother and tried to help her in every way, fetching firewood and water, doing some shopping, looking after his youngest brother, and taking him to and from kindergarten each day. Yura refused to buy clothes which he needed, telling his mother that he would go without. The development of this complex of real emotions was evidence of marked progress in the development of his personality and emotional-volitional functions.

In the course of his schooling Yura showed definite improvement in his analytical and synthetic functions within the limits of individual analyzers. When the boy was given various tasks addressed to a given analyzer, we observed no difficulty in his performance.

There was every reason to believe that the boy's cognitive activity had also developed, as shown specially in the picture classification experiment. It will be remembered that in the first year of education he was incapable of understanding instructions, and that subsequently he was able to group together only identical pictures, but later he was able to make use of memorized categories for classification.

The character of his cognitive activity was primarily determined by the maldevelopment of the generalizing function of speech. This maldevelopment of the capacity for abstraction and generalization, i.e., the fundamental symptom of oligophrenia, was expressed in varying degrees but nevertheless continued at all stages of the child's development. The boy's development was also characterized by a series of specific features, connected very closely with his inhibition. As he matured his general inhibition level fell lower and lower. Yura gradually became more active and alert, states of limiting inhibition arose much less frequently, and were also much shorter in duration.

From the findings described it may be considered that in this particular case the defect was largely compensated. From a slow learner in the imbecile class, Yura became a successful student in the special school. There he became a good worker in the handicrafts department, and there is every reason to suppose that in the future he will be capable of working for his living.

Clinical Analysis of the Case

The marked maldevelopment of the cognitive functions, due to the lesion of the central nervous system in the early stages of postnatal development, provided grounds for the diagnosis of oligophrenia. The principal etiological factors probably were the severe and prolonged malnutrition, after the occurrence of natural asphyxia at birth. The presence of the fundamental symptom of oligophrenia in conjunction with primary preservation of the emotional-volitional function, the absence of disturbances within the limits of the individual analyzers, and the results of neurological investigation suggest that in this case there was a diffuse lesion of the cerebral cortex. The results of craniographic investigations, the dilatation of the veins of the optic fundus, and the attacks of headache of a hypertensive character are evidence that an important role in the pathogenesis of this particular case was played by a residual hydrocephalus.

Experimental investigation of the higher nervous activity revealed, in addition to the common oligophrenic characteristics (especially marked inertia of the nervous processes), a series of specific characteristics of this particular variant of the oligophrenic defect.

At the beginning of each experiment (in the first stage of the investigation) in response to the first positive stimuli Yura showed no reaction in spite of reinforcement. During trials of the established conditioned connections, there was likewise no reaction to several of the initial positive stimuli. Absence of initial generalization of newly introduced stimuli with the positive stimulus was observed. After the development of differentiation, even stimuli close to it were not generalized with the positive stimulus.

External inhibition was especially strong in this case. This relationship between the nervous processes stood out especially clearly during the modification of the established conditioned connections. In the process of modification it was extraordinarily easy to attach an inhibitory value to a formerly positive stimulus, but an inhibitory stimulus was transformed into a positive stimulus more slowly. All these facts suggest a definite predominance of inhibition in the cortex.

The predominance of inhibition was also demonstrated by investigation of the higher nervous activity using the method of plethysmography. A number of facts provide evidence of the lowered excitability of the cortex, the increased liability to fatigue of the cortical neurons and the easy development of limiting inhibition. These facts include: the lengthened latent period during the application of indifferent stimuli, the onset of a reaction only after 15 or 20 applications of the stimulus and the development of distorted reactions in the course of the experiment.

The results of the electroencephalographic investigation also indicated the rapid transition of the cortical neurons into a state of inhibition. These specific changes in the higher nervous activity also lay at the basis of the distinctive clinical picture of this variant of the oligophrenic defect.

As a result of the above analysis, this present case may be classified with that variant of oligophrenia in which the balance between excitation and inhibition is obviously disturbed, and inhibition is the predominant process — which accounts for the characteristic development of the clinical picture in the child whom we have been studying.

ANALYSIS OF ALL THE RESULTS OBTAINED

Special Features of Early Development. Children of this subgroup show disturbed development from earliest childhood. A specific feature of these children is the characteristic dissociation between the very severe developmental disturbance at nursery or even preschool age and the relatively high developmental progress in later periods of the child's education and training.

This dissociation may be more clearly understood if it is remembered that in this variant of the defect general intellectual deficiency is combined with a high level of inhibition. In the earliest stages of development the predominance of inhibition in the cerebral cortex is already very plain to see. As a rule in early childhood these children show no reaction to sounds and to bright objects. They lie in bed most of the time and sleep. They are neither interested nor attracted by toys. Their appetite is severely impaired. At preschool age, even when the children have learned to walk and talk, they still remain lethargic, passive, show no interest in play and are asocial even with neighbors and relatives.

Changed circumstances, especially the introduction of excessively strong stimuli, lead to an even more marked rise in the child's general inhibitory level. In one of our cases a girl, age six, was admitted to the hospital with scarlet fever. This unfamiliar environment caused the development of severe inhibition. The girl did not answer questions, remained immobile for long periods, sometimes refused to eat, and did not react to her surroundings.

In addition to characteristic features common to all oligophrenic children, at preschool age children of this subgroup are generally lethargic, passive and slow in all their mental reactions.

At the beginning of school age these children remain just as extremely inhibited, lethargic and passive, show little concern in their surroundings, and yet are obedient. Children in this subgroup obey not only older persons but also younger children and do not know how to defend themselves. However, in addition to this obedience in these inhibited children, we observed the presence of pseudonegativistic reactions. For instance, against this general background of inhibition, a change in circumstances induces reactions characterized by increased general tension and silence, the appearance of involuntary facial grimaces, and by the cessation of all activity. The difference between this behavior and true negativistic reactions is that this behavior is comparatively easily arrested.

For example, the doctor has only to move the child's finger in a particular task and the child will carry it out by himself, or if the doctor begins to say a word necessary for a particular answer, the child will himself continue the answer.

The children whom we studied had been educated for a year or more in a regular school before they began to attend the special school. The period of their stay in the regular school aggravated their general condition. These children did not learn the elements of reading and writing, even when the child was in the first class of the ordinary school for as long as three years. For example, Zina K. after three years in the first class did not know a single letter or number. While attending the ordinary school the general inhibition, the tendency to fatigue and drowsiness in these children increased. By their behavioral characteristics, the children of this subgroup differed very sharply from their normal siblings. At the regular school many stimuli were too strong for them and this often led to an increase in their negativistic reactions, and to the development of headache, vertigo and anxiety.

X-ray Examination of the Skull. Of the 18 children studied belonging to this subgroup, 16 showed an increase in the head circumference (from 54 to 57 cm), characteristic of hydrocephalus. In x-ray examination of the head, which is of great importance in the diagnosis of hydrocephalus, attention is paid to changes in the size and shape of the skull and of its vertex and base. In anteroposterior films the skull is usually spherical in shape. Associated with changes in the configuration of the vault of the skull changes are observed in the base, i.e., the cranial fossae are flattened. It is only in hydrocephalus developing in the early stages of the child's life that changes of this type are always found in the vault and base of the skull. In some cases we observed in children with this variant of oligophrenia, besides thinning of the bones, an extremely poor and ill-defined relief of the inner table, indicating the presence of an open form of hydrocephalus, existing from an early age.

In all the children of this subgroup the so-called digital impressions were found on the internal surface of the cranial bones over the cerebral hemispheres. The work of Kopylov (1935) showed that the digital impressions pass through a stage of growth and then undergo regression, and that they are dependent on the presence of prolonged increased intracranial pressure.

The conditions in which these characteristic impressions arise are essentially such that as a result of the creation of a barrier between the ventricular system and the subarachnoid spaces, the volume of cerebrospinal fluid surrounding the brain surface decreases. This creates an inequality of pressure on the bone from the gyri of the brain and the fissures, as a result of which localized thinning of the bones occurs, and the markings take their shape from the underlying gyri.

Kopylov's explanation implies that digital impressions are found only in closed forms of hydrocephalus. Arendt (1948) reported digital impressions also in open forms of hydrocephalus. Arendt states that in open forms of hydrocephalus ill-defined digital impressions are observed. The presence of ill-defined digital impressions in our cases is evidence that we were dealing with open hydrocephalus.

The disturbance of the circulation of the blood and cerebrospinal fluid is revealed by the presence of a general cerebral symptomatology, such as episodic headache and vertigo. We observed these headaches, which change their character in the course of time, and are well marked in early stages of the development of these oligophrenic children. The headaches were often accompanied by nausea and, in isolated cases, by vomiting. At school age the episodic headaches developed much less frequently. Unfavorable conditions (the time spent by the child at the regular school, physical illness, psychic trauma) led to a state of decompensation, which was shown by recurrence of the headaches.

Neurological Investigation. The neurological symptomatology in children of this subgroup is characterized by a series of signs bearing a diffuse, residual, and mainly cortical character. The specific feature of the residual neurological signs is the briskness of the tendon reflexes, which are often of unequal amplitude. A number of pathological reflexes are seen (Rossolimo's, Oppenheim's and Babinski's signs), which are vague and inconstant in character.

Considerable vasomotor disturbances only occur in children of this subgroup, characterized by cyanosis of the limbs, and by erythemic and cyanotic changes in the fingers and toes. Investigation of the optic fundus showed a significant dilation of the veins in most of these children.

Our clinical findings thus point to the complex pathogenesis of this variant of oligophrenia, which is characterized by the combination of a general diffuse lesion mainly affecting the cerebral cortex with disturbances of the circulation of the blood and cerebrospinal fluid.

Investigation of the Electrical Activity of the Brain. Electroencephalographic investigations in children of this subgroup revealed specific features as well as general features common to all oligophrenic children. These specific features take the form of depression of the electrical activity of the brain, and in the predominance of low-voltage slow waves in the electroencephalogram. These may be interpreted as meaning a predominance of inhibitory processes in the cortex (Fig. 40).

During the investigation of the cortical reactions by the method of rhythmic light, tactile and sound stimuli, prolonged depression of the alpha-rhythm after light stimulation was established (Fig. 41).

The appearance of fast and slow waves on the electroencephalo-

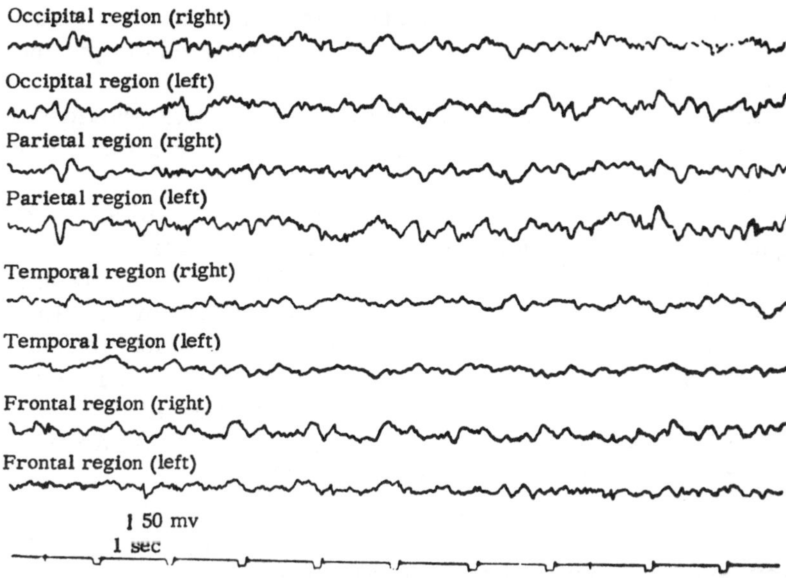

Fig. 40. Valerii S., aged 12 years, a male student at a special school (oligophrenia, feeble-minded degree). EEG taken in a state of relative rest; alpha-rhythm absent. Slow pathological waves predominate and are more marked in the posterior regions of the left hemisphere.

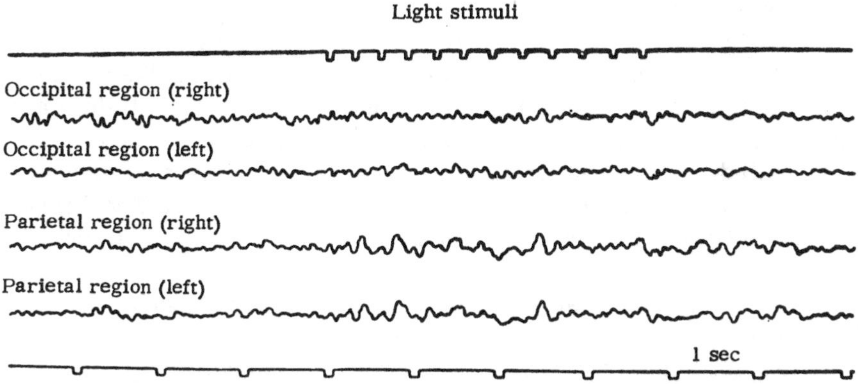

Fig. 41. Investigation of the EEG (of the same object) during application of a rhythmic light stimulus. The rhythmic light stimulation induces an increase of slow waves.

gram during the action of stimuli directed to different analyzers is also an indication that the cortical neurons are easily put into a state of inhibition.

Comparison of the clinical and experimental data provides a firm basis for the diagnosis of this particular variant of oligophrenic defect.

Special Features of the Higher Nervous Activity. The results of the investigation of the higher nervous activity by the method of plethysmography, which was undertaken in these children by O. S. Vinogradova, clearly showed the presence of a state of inhibition of the cerebral cortex. During the recording of the vascular reactions in the normal child of school age (10-14 years) it is found that any stimulus which is new to the child and unfamiliar, will cause a marked vasoconstrictor reaction in that child, which is a component of the orienting reflex (Fig. 42). Vascular reactions even to relatively weak stimuli are readily produced in normal children, are reasonably stable, and are gradually extinguished only after repeated application of the stimulus.

Plethysmographic investigation of children with this type of defect revealed specifically the predominance of cortical inhibition. This statement is proven by the presence in certain cases of marked waves of the third order, and by the respiratory and cardiac arrhythmia. Weakness or absence of the vascular reactions to indifferent stimuli were observed, together with marked delay in the appearance of the reactions, longer latent periods, an inert course of both the conditioned and the unconditioned reactions, and the presence of distorted vasodilator reactions (Fig. 43).

These findings clearly indicate the predominance of a state of inhibition of the cerebral cortex.

Investigation of the higher nervous activity showed most clearly the distinctive feature of this variant of the defect. We used the motor method with speech reinforcement. In each case clinical and experimental findings were compared. This experiment particularly revealed the inertia of the fundamental nervous processes as well as other common oligophrenic characteristics. The higher nervous activity of these children also showed a number of specific features.

Primary generalization of new stimuli does not occur at once. No reaction is present to the first or even to several of the initial applications, and a reaction appears only after repeated applications, and it usually increases gradually in magnitude. Stimuli not

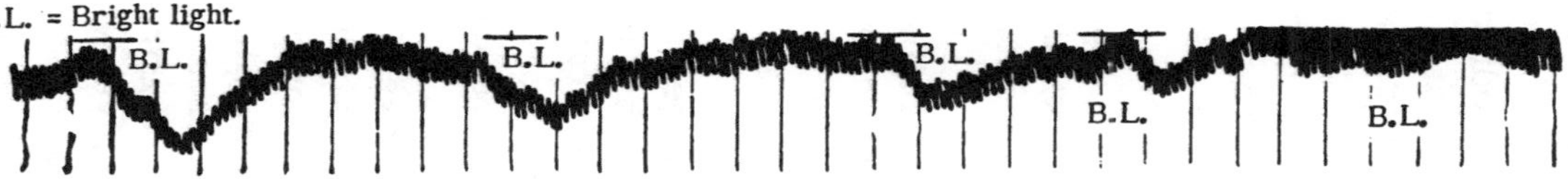

Fig. 42. Vascular reactions to a light stimulus in a normal child of 12 years old. The reactions are clearly expressed and are gradually extinguished in the course of repeated applications of the stimulus.

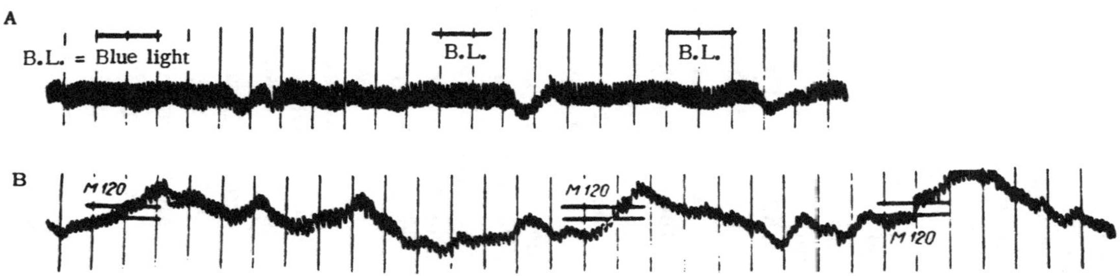

Fig. 43. A) Sasha Kh., aged 12 years, a boy at a special school. Reactive curve with primitive reactions arising after application of a stimulus. B) Yura B., aged 14 years, a male pupil at a special school. Distorted vasodilator reactions to a sound stimulus (a metronome).

addressed to the same analyzer as the positive stimulus are usually not generalized with the latter.

At the beginning of a new experiment, during the presentation of the old conditioned stimulus the conditioned reactions to this stimulus are absent, and they only gradually begin to appear thereafter. A verbal projection can be obtained in these children only after the frequent repetition of the question, although the projection of the formation of simple conditioned reactions and of simple forms of differentiation is adequate. During the modification of the conditioned value of the stimuli it was observed that a positive stimulus may be converted into a inhibitory value more rapidly than an inhibitory signal to a positive stimulus. Only one combination was required to produce an inhibitory value from a positive stimulus, but two or three or more combinations were necessary to transform a previously differential stimulus into a positive one.

Extrastimuli have a powerful and specific action. A strong extrastimulus, applied in the middle of the experiment, leads to complete inhibition of the conditioned reactions to several conditioned stimuli. In individual cases the reactions were inhibited until the end of the experiment.

During the formation of connections by preliminary instruction it was found that the instruction does not produce a response at once and that reactions are usually absent to the first stimuli. Thus a connection established in the verbal system is not manifested at once in the reactions. The regulation of the reaction by the verbal system remains unstable. The experimental findings all point convincingly to the fact that in oligophrenic children of this subgroup the higher nervous activity is characterized by both a marked inertia of the fundamental nervous processes and a series of specific features, indicating a severe imbalance of the nervous modalities, with predominance of inhibition.

Investigation of Individual Cortical Functions. Investigation of the level of development of analysis and integration within the limits of the various analyzers showed the absence of any gross localized defects of individual cortical functions. Meanwhile dynamic investigations revealed certain characteristic features.

Pictures depicting various objects were correctly recognized by these children, but their answers were given very slowly. After the pictures were presented there were at first no reactions, and the instructions had to be repeated two or three times before the children responded. In the first stage of their education these children recognized the picture of an object only when presented in the correct position. They did not recognize pictures shown upside down, dotted-line drawings, geometrical figures, or crossed-out figures.

In the second year of their education, these children recognized pictures shown upside down and crossed-out figures, but they did not recognize dotted-line drawings. In the fourth year of their education this investigation of analysis and integration in the visual analyzer showed that this group of oligophrenic children experienced no difficulties.

These experiments demonstrated very clearly the neurodynamic features of these children. As the degree of inhibition increased their reactions disappeared, and the child either failed to name the picture at all or recognized only its individual parts, i.e., a very indefinite symptom of pseudo-optic agnosia developed. After one or two minutes, with additional stimulation, the children again correctly recognized pictures shown to them. In no case, however, did we detect impulsive answers.

The experimental investigations very clearly demonstrated the predominance of the state of inhibition in the cortex, as manifested by the development of this particular reaction, viz., the naming of pictures only after additional stimulation. This investigation also clearly revealed the inertia of the mental processes. For example, the girl was shown the picture of a frog. She looked at it for a long time and then gave the correct answer, but the next five pictures shown to her immediately after, a turkey, a pencil, a ruler, a trolley-car and a table, were also described by the word "frog." When she finally named the picture of the turkey correctly, the next series of pictures of a bear, a goat, an onion, and a cock were all called "turkey." When presented to her a second time, all these pictures were usually correctly recognized and named.

The investigation of analysis and integration within the limits of the optic analyzer in children with predominance of inhibition thus showed a series of special features which differed markedly from those which were described during the investigation of the children in whom excitation predominated. In these cases we observed no tendency to overstep the limits of the task and no impulsive answers. On the contrary, these children produced their answers very slowly and only after additional stimulation.

In some of the children whom we studied we investigated analysis and integration in the optic analyzer after injection of caffein. After receiving an injection of caffein the children became more active and gave correct answers. At the same time certain special features, hitherto unobserved, became apparent in these children under these conditions: their answers showed the arousal of a cluster of associations which they could not inhibit. For example, when a picture was shown representing a raspberry, the child examined it for a long time and said: "Plum, strawberry, pear, berries," and only then was the correct answer given. It may be assumed that in these cases a slight decrease in the degree of inhibition discloses the presence of a weakness of excitation with a tendency to irradiation.

We also found no gross disturbances during the investigation of spatial orientation in the children of this subgroup. They grasp the notion of right and left. They correctly copy stick figures. In the initial stages of their education these children can only cope with the simplest tasks, but subsequently they learn to do more complicated tasks by themsleves. However, to do this they require additional stimulation. Without such stimulation their activity sometimes ceases. They may stop work even in the presence of verbal stimulation. On such occasions other stimulating factors have to be introduced, for example by initiating the movement of the child's hand, so that the child is activated and begins to carry out the task. These children obviously have great difficulty getting started on a task, and once started they tire very quickly.

We found no appreciable disturbances in the auditory and motor-speech analyzers in the children of this subgroup. These children understood what was said to them. They correctly repeated phonemes even when the range of the task was slightly extended. They could pronounce a difficult sentence slowly but accurately. The clarity with which these children pronounced words and sentences was dependent upon their general condition. With an increase in inhibition their speech became slurred and incomprehensible, but with additional stimulation such a child would begin to pronounce words and sentences distinctly and clearly. We may observe that their speech on the whole was limited in vocabulary, was quiet, inexpressive, slow, and indecisive.

No gross disturbances were noted in their motor analyzer. With external stimulation these children could perform various postural and dynamic movements. The separate components of their motor functions were very clearly demarcated, however. The postures and movements of these children were poor in quality and unvaried, and the tempo of movement was slow. If the child carried out a task incorporating some action with small objects, the tempo gradually slowed and the movements weakened, diminished in scope, and eventually ceased altogether. The facial expressions were undifferentiated, dull in quality and somewhat frozen.

Investigation of this group of oligophrenic children thus shows the absence of gross disturbances within the limits of any analyzer, but at the same time reveals the specific neurodynamic features described above, which are characteristic of this particular variant of the defect.

Peculiarities of Cognitive Activity. Like other oligophrenic children, the children of this subgroup show the presence of the fundamental symptom of oligophrenia, the maldevelopment of the capacity for abstraction and generalization. At the same time the development of these children's cognitive functions shows a series of specific features. They all showed very severe maldevelopment of the cognitive function early in their training at the special school. For example, when instructed to classify pictures, they comprehended only the word "arrange," and even with help were unable to accomplish the task of classification. These children could not order the simplest series of story pictures nor establish a relationship between words and pictures. In view of these characteristics, it is not without reason that they were graded as imbeciles.

In later stages, as their general inhibition diminished, these children showed good progress in their development. The distinctive developmental pattern of their cognitive activity is explained by the combination of decreased cognitive activity with a general state of inhibition.

Certain characteristic traits appeared during all the testing procedures, and disturbed the normal course of the experiment. In the picture classification experiment they listen to the instructions given to them, apparently attentively, but they do not start to tackle the job. Only after repeated additional stimulation does the child start work, but he does everything very slowly, uncertainly, and clumsily, and gradually stops altogether. After additional stimulation he undertakes the task, showing doubly concrete forms of thinking.

In contrast to the excitable oligophrenics, in whom an abundance of ideas appear when classifying pictures, each of which distracts them from solving the problem, in the inhibited children we observed no tendency to overstep the limits of the task. During the investigation of the cognitive activity of children with this particular variant of the defect, against the background of their general lethargy and inhibition special states arise sporadically, in which all their activity ceases. Thus the characteristic sign of the oligophrenic children of this subgroup, besides the disability which they have in common, is their difficulty in initiation of an assigned task, and their liability to rapid fatigue, which leads to the cessation of any form of activity.

Special Features of the Emotional-Volitional Functions. The characteristic pathogenetic feature of this variant is the predominantly diffuse cortical lesion with no evidence of involvement of the subcortical structures. This characteristic distribution of the pathological process explains the absence of primary gross disturbances in the emotional-volitional function in this subgroup of oligophrenic children.

The development of their emotional-volitional life follows a characteristic course. In the early stages of their development their lethargy and passivity, and the lack of reaction to their surroundings suggest a considerable diminution of their emotional tone, and in individual cases they may even suggest emotional dullness. The study of the dynamics of the development of these children shows that in the course of their education and training, as the general level of their inhibition diminishes, the signs of development of their emotional-volitional function become more and more obvious. In the second year of their education the children of this subgroup were much more obviously concerned about the teacher's opinion of them than were other oligophrenic children. A further indication of the development of their emotional-volitional function can be found in the appearance of self-criticism of their own work.

A specific feature of this variant of the defect is the monotonous character of the reaction of these children to unfavorable external conditions. They do not express their dissatisfaction by vocal reactions or by increased excitability, but they react by a further increase in their inhibition, by tenseness, reticence, and negativism. Such children very clearly show the correlation between their increased activity and the development of their emotional-volitional function.

During the third school year the children behaved in a manner indicative of an appreciable fall in inhibition level, which favored the development of all aspects of their personality, and which was revealed specially clearly in the development of their emotional-volitional functions. In the course of the development there emerged a sense of duty and responsibility toward school work, an interest in learning, a widening interest in reading and the cinema, increased participation in group activities, etc.

It was in subsequent stages (fourth and fifth years of education) in children of this subgroup of oligophrenia, that in isolated cases we observed well-marked reactive states, based on complex emotional experiences. These reactive states appeared to have two phases. The first phase took the form of an augmentation or exacerbation of the fundamental characteristics of these children. Under the influence of psychotherapy the reactive state passed into a new phase, brought about by the recognition of the situation, which led to the development of a discriminatory attitude toward their surroundings. The appearance of this complex group of emotional experiences and the ability of these children to recognize a situation indicate a considerable development of their personality as a whole and of their emotional-volitional functions in particular.

This fact may be understood from the special pathophysiological mechanism found in this particular subgroup. The whole clinical analysis demonstrates the predominance of a state of inhibition of the cerebral cortex, which in turn leads to a slowness of reaction. Conditions are thereby created for much greater fixation on their experiences, and this, in the absence of primary disturbances in the emotional-volitional function, leads to a much higher level of development of both the emotional-volitional function and of the personality make-up as a whole.

Besides the features indicating an adequate level of development of the emotional-volitional function, however, these children also showed a number of signs indicating the distinctive nature of their emotional-volitional function as it relates to the maldevelopment of their cognitive function. It is because of the inadequacy of the cognitive function of this subgroup that they often cannot work out a complicated or conflicting situation. The same child may show an adequate emotional attitude to his surroundings and an appropriate attitude towards the situation but may still behave incorrectly because of his inadequate grasp of the situation.

A prolonged clinical study of children of this group showed a series of specific behavioral features. In the most marked cases their behavior lapsed into extreme lethargy, passivity, and inhibition. If such children were not goaded into activity or encouraged, if they were not asked questions, they would persist in the same attitude – immobile, indifferent, and inactive.

In the initial stage of our observation the children did not become animated and were not disinhibited even at play. In a group they were well disciplined and almost excessively obedient. Phrases such as "I don't want" or "I won't," or demands on others for any reason were quite uncharacteristic. They never asked questions of the teacher nor tried to answer although if asked a direct question they would often answer correctly. If such a child is called to the blackboard, especially if the teacher paid too little attention to his individual peculiarities, he would become more inhibited, negativistic, and incapacitated. The presence of a stranger in the class would usually lead him to become much more tense, reticent, and taciturn, and to react with characteristic negativism.

Characteristics of the Motor Activity. During investigation of the motor activity of these children, no marked disturbances of the motor analyzer were found. Their motor activity is characterized by lethargy, uncertainty, and indefiniteness in all movements. The children initiate their movements badly and often aim them poorly. The posture and motility of these children are poorly integrated and unvaried. Their customary posture is slightly stooped. Their facial expressions are undifferentiated, dull, and frozen. Their gestures are constricted and indecisive. The tempo of their movements is slow and tends to become even slower. If one of these children is asked to repeat some activity involving small objects, the tempo of his movements will gradually become slower, they will become constricted and weak, diminish in scope, and eventually stop completely. The finer movements of these children are inadequately coordinated though their gross movements (for example, throwing a ball or reaching high in the air) are better coordinated. The latter type of activity helps to liven up these children perceptibly and draws them out of their semi-lethargic state. However dynamic movements such as running, jumping and marching, are undertaken with reluctance; these children often lose their motivation and mechanically follow the children ahead of them.

Certain Specific Features of the Children of This Subgroup Appearing During Education. When learning to read these children experienced no particular difficulties aside from the usual ones characteristic of oligophrenic children. They have much more difficulty with writing. The visual organization of writing presents no special difficulty to this group. We also observed no writing difficulties in this group that could be attributable to disturbances of phonematic hearing. These children learned to write after a long instruction period involving a proper educational approach of encouragement and stimulation. When taking dictation or when copying without any additional organizing help from the teacher, they made mistakes of contamination, perseveration, and omission of individual letters, syllables, or words. With organizing help from the teacher to stimulate and encourage them the quality of their work improved and there was a perceptible decrease in the number of mistakes.

In less severe forms, or at later stages of their education they had periodic lapses with increased mistakes in writing. The child would copy correctly from a book or take dictation, but characteristic mistakes reappeared with an increase in inhibition due to changes in the circumstances or changes in the child's condition. Over an extended period, we observed a relationship between an increase in the number of mistakes and the child's general condition. In individual tasks, with stimulation from the teacher, such a child could write down dictation or copy from a book without any mistake. With a change in his condition the number of mistakes increased considerably.

These children experienced similar difficulties when solving arithmetical problems. When inhibited, in attempting to solve arithmetical problems by themselves, these children could not even use their elementary skill in counting. If a child were asked to solve a series of problems in addition up to ten by means of visual aids, he would present some random number as an answer, or he would persistently repeat the same number as the answer to all the problems, replacing the solution of the particular problem with some stereotyped repetition of any number that happened to be fixed in his mind.

If problems of similar difficulty were given to the child but with organizing help to encourage him, his performance would improve although he would occasionally make mistakes.

Certain pharmacological agents also act in this direction. Problems of similar difficulty are solved without mistakes by such children after receiving an injection of caffeine.

In later stages of these children's schooling the disturbance of their capacity for work appears only sporadically and is clearly induced by an increase in their degree of inhibition. For instance, at the beginning of an assignment a child may work actively and with adequate intensity, but gradually his slowness, lethargy and passivity increase. This is shown by the appearance of errors of perseveration during the solution of arithmetic problems. Also, individual elements are left out, and eventually activity ceases. If the child is encouraged and stimulated, however, he will gradually begin to do a better job and will often solve subsequent problems perfectly.

Because the specific neurodynamic features of oligophrenics are combined with marked maldevelopment of their cognitive activity, they have difficulty sloving arithmetical problems; they cannot independently establish the necessary bonds of reasoning between problem conditions, nomenclature of the examples, and numerical data.

The Principal Ways of Compensation of the Disability in Children of this Subgroup. A dynamic study of the children of this subgroup clearly revealed a complex clinical picture combining the fundamental symptom of oligophrenia with a series of additional nonspecific symptoms (inhibition, psychomotor retardation). The qualitative nature of the structure of the disability determines the character of the corrective training required by these children.

In working with these children it is most important to employ methods which will increase the child's activity. When these children carry out their various tasks they need encouragement and stimulation. Sometimes the teacher must begin the task with the pupil.

In certain cases, especially in the initial stages of education, it is desirable to instruct these children step by step, and to reinforce each separate element verbally. It is sometimes helpful for the child to verbally describe the solution as he goes through it. This conversational approach increases the child's activity and thereby improves his performance. Since the children of this subgroup find their school work very difficult, not only do they need individual attention during general class work, but also, as our experience shows, they need supplementary individual tuition.

These mentally inhibited and slow children are unable to keep up with the class's general rate of progress. To prevent this, the teacher must, as a preliminary measure, discuss the class work during individual lessons, or the child must be taught these subjects at home. It is very important that the teacher take into consideration the child's special characteristics when working with him, and recognize the inept answers during an intense state of inhibition, or the presence of paroxysmal phases of cessation of activity. Although this subgroup presents behavioral problems it is still necessary to take account of these special features. It must be remembered that these children are characterized by pseudonegativistic reactions. The teacher who knows the distinctive features of these children can easily mitigate or relieve these states. For example, it is sufficient to begin to carry out a particular action for the child and he will readily begin to do the task himself. These children are silent and reserved, difficult to approach and easily confused. These features must also be taken into consideration during their corrective training. These children must be helped to fit into groups of other children, they must be given various errands to do, and the teacher must praise their achievements before the group.

As shown above, the emotional-volitional function attains a relatively high level of development in these oligophrenic children. Characteristically their emotional experiences are more complex in structure, they are touchy and easily hurt, and they often take their failures badly. All these features must be taken into consideration by the teacher working with these children, and may sometimes require special psychotherapeutic measures.

When educational measures are accompanied by medical treatment directed towards the stimulation of development and to the improvement of the flow of cerebrospinal fluid, the development of these children is greatly facilitated.

After our observations on the same children for six years we could see how an increase in their activity led to considerable progress in their development, as was most clearly shown in relation to their emotional-volitional function. The development of analysis and integration within the limits of individual analyzers, and the development of their cognitive functions were no less well marked. In the first stages their capacity for abstraction and generalization was so low that of the 18 children under our observation, ten began their education in the imbecile class. Subsequently they were transferred to the ordinary classes, and later still they became quite successful pupils.

Properly organized corrective training work stimulates the development of these children and their adaptation to working life can be confidently anticipated.

CHAPTER 6

OLIGOPHRENIC CHILDREN IN WHOM DISTURBANCE OF THE CORTICAL NEURODYNAMICS IS CHARACTERIZED BY MARKED WEAKNESS OF THE FUNDAMENTAL NERVOUS PROCESSES

In the third subgroup of oligophrenia we include those forms in which the characteristic clinical picture is associated with very great weakness of the fundamental nervous processes. Our analysis of the clinical findings is based on the study of ten cases, only two of which will be described in detail.

CASE 1

Valerii S., a boy aged 14 years, a pupil in the fifth year at a special school. No abnormal hereditary features.

History. This boy was born of his mother's second pregnancy, which took place during difficult wartime conditions. In the seventh month of pregnancy his mother sustained an abdominal injury. Labor took place at term; the boy was born in profound asphyxia. He was bottle fed. Disturbances of development were observed from his very earliest childhood. He began to cut his teeth at eight months and began to walk at two years. He did not speak his first words until he was two. From an early age those around the boy noticed his general lethargy, the obviously defective development of his motor activity, the emptiness of his facial expression, and his lack of interest in toys, games, and stories. In kindergarten Valerii was at times extremely lethargic and passive and sometimes undisciplined and excitable.

The boy began his formal education in the first class of a special school. From the beginning the teacher was struck by Valerii's considerable motor difficulty. He showed inadequate awareness of his environment, and for a long time he could not find his seat in class. He did not know the way home. Furthermore, when writing he did not follow the lines in his exercise book, and his writing was poor, even when tracing. His attention was readily distracted, and he was unable to concentrate upon anything. His memory was poor. He became easily fatigued. In his first six months Valerii was backward in every subject. For this reason he was investigated by the medicopedagogic department of the Institute of Defectology. This investigation showed that, against a background of general lethargy and apathy, he had a well marked disturbance of spatial orientation. He confused his right and left hands, the right and left sides of his body, and could not tell on which side of him objects lay. When he attempted to arrange matches into figures he was unable to copy any example given to him, especially if the lines pointed in different directions. He could not form simple figures when told to do so. Disturbance of spatial orientation was shown in the difficulties experienced by the boy when arranging sticks. These distinctive features as described above were combined with a maldevelopment of cognitive functions. In the second six months the boy was helped, as a result of which he began to show a better understanding of what he was studying. He quickly learned to arrange individual words correctly from cut-out letters. He also learned to solve mentally, without visual aids, easy problems in addition and subtraction of numbers up to ten. Valerii began to learn poetry by heart. He ran errands for the teacher, and developed a sense of responsibility towards tasks entrusted to him. He began to be much more capable of orienting himself in space; he easily found his classroom and his own desk and learned to find his way home from school and back again. At this stage he was transferred to the second class of the special school. In the summer of 1951 Valerii sustained a head injury and was admitted to a hospital. After his discharge from the hospital the boy again began to attend school. His teacher noticed a marked set-back in his condition. Particularly noteworthy were the boy's motor restlessness and inattentiveness. He could not concentrate on anything. The boy repeated the same class for a second year. It was at that time that we began to study him.

Physical State. Valerii's physical development was normal for his age. Slight muffling of the heart sounds was noted, and his pulse was 78 beats per minute, regular. The blood pressure was 96/55.

State of the Nervous System. The pupillary reactions were brisk. The range of eye movements was adequate. He could not converge. He found it difficult to close one eye at a time, especially the left. The right nasolabial fold was ill-defined; the tongue deviated to the right; the uvula was in midline. His movements were clumsy: he could barely hop on one leg, the change-over from one movement to another was difficult and carried out at a slow tempo, especially when he had to combine the hops with coordinated movements of the right and left hands. No obvious signs of paresis were present. Hypotonia and denervatory disturbances of tone were observed. Imitative synkineses were observed during movements of the fingers, especially in the left hand in response to the right. The tendon reflexes were brisk. The plantar reflexes were sluggish. No pathological signs were present. Neurological investigation indicated an inadequacy in the motor sphere with the left cerebral hemisphere more severely affected.

Ophthalmological Examination. Visual acuity of both eyes 1.0. No nystagmus, media transparent. Optic fundus: optic disk whitish-pink, clearly outlined; veins slightly dilated; periphery of the region of the macula lutea normal.

Otorhinolaryngological Examination. Hearing within normal limits.

X-ray Examination of the Skull. Skull spherical in shape. Base of the skull slightly flattened. Cranial sutures ill defined. Well marked digital impressions present.

Electroencephalography. The alpha-rhythm was absent from the EEG. In all regions of the cortex slow pathological waves were predominant, more marked in the parieto-occipital region, and especially in the left hemisphere. In the frontal regions beta-waves were present in association with delta waves of low amplitude. The electroencephalogram showed marked abnormalities. Against the background of a diffuse pathological process a focus of pathological activity was found in the posterior regions of the left hemisphere (Fig. 44).

Investigation of the Higher Nervous Activity. A characteristic feature of the higher nervous activity of this child was the presence of considerable fluctuation in his neurodynamics, changing from one experiment to the next, or even in the course of the same experiment: an easily formed positive temporary connection was inhibited in the course of the experiment, a rapidly produced differentiation was disinhibited and, in spite of continuous reinforcement, it was only slowly restored, while an established motor conditioned reaction was absent in the next experiment. These fluctuations were evidently associated with phasic states (of partial inhibition) which were observed in the experiments. These phasic states were expressed as the presence of a motor reaction to a differential stimulus in the absence of a reaction to a positive stimulus (this was observed, moreover, when the connections in the verbal system were maintained), and also, probably, as distorted reactions to a

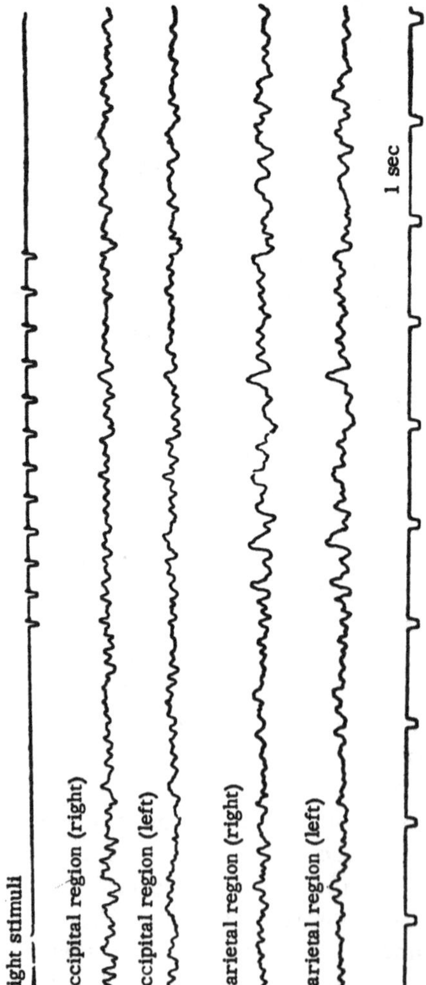

Fig. 44. Valerii S., aged 14 years, pupil at a special school. It is clear from the EEG that the alpha-rhythm is absent. Slow pathological waves are predominant in all regions of the cortex, and are more marked in the parieto-occipital region of the left hemisphere.

positive stimulus (he lifts up the push-button instead of depressing it). Wave-like fluctuations in the level of excitation were noted, as expressed by differences in the magnitude of the reactions and by their extreme instability. These fluctuations were found both during the same experiment and from one experiment to another.

The process of excitation showed a tendency towards irradiation, which was manifested both by differences in the duration and the strength of the motor reactions, and by the presence of prolonged and frequent press responses and large number of intersignal reactions, which were found in the experiments with reactions to a direct spoken command. In the course of the experiment the powerful inhibitory action of certain extrastimuli was revealed (the faint noise of an opening door caused complete inhibition of the conditioned motor reaction). Other extrastimuli (for example, a bell) had a weaker action, merely increasing the latent period and decreasing the strength of the reaction. Disinhibition of differentiation was observed under the influence of extrastimuli. Simple differentiation of light stimuli by their color was rapidly established (after one combination) but was not sufficiently stable: in a series of experiments it was disinhibited and, in spite of the presence of reinforcement, was not at once restored.

Irradiation of inhibition took place: restoration of the disinhibited differentiation led to inhibition of the reaction to the next positive stimuli.

In the verbal projection, in the first experiments there was a reverse image of the connection between the stimulus and the motor reaction ("When I pressed, the light came on.") Other disturbances were noted in the projection. Sometimes, for instance, the subject reported stimuli which did not, in fact, exist. ("It rang," when the bell did not ring, and, "The blue light came on, but not the green," when in fact the reverse was the case.)

Mental State

Visual Analyzer. Valerii quickly recognized and named objects placed in front of him as well as crossed-out pictures drawn on cards, dotted-line drawings, and geometrical figures. Frequently, however, he drifted away from his task into an excitable state or lapsed into a state of lethargy with no reaction.

Spatial Orientation. During the investigation it was found that Valerii had overcome to a large extent those severe disturbances of spatial orientation that were formerly typical for him. Now, for example, he could correctly point out his right and left hands (and those of his neighbor); he could state which objects were on his right and left sides, and he could correctly copy an example of a match figure. Difficulties arose only when the task was made more complicated, and even then he usually surmounted them himself. In the course of performing these tasks, however, Valerii often produced incorrect solutions, the character of which depended on his condition. When in a state of increased excitability he drifted away from his task and completed only a part of it. When in a state of inhibition he usually would not even begin his task, and only after additional stimulation would he make a move in that direction.

Motor and Motor-Speech Analyzers. When the boy carried out various tests of postural movements or of dynamic movements, it was noted that he understood the task and was capable of accomplishing it properly, but that when he did so he revealed the same distinctive features. He drifted away from the task as his excitability increased, and needed additional stimulation when his degree of inhibition increased.

The articulatory aspect of the boy's speech showed no significant disturbance, and he could easily repeat sentences that were difficult to pronounce. The tempo of his speech varied depending on his condition. When the boy was in an excitable state the tempo of his speech increased to such a degree that his speech became slurred, but when he was in a state of inhibition, on the other hand, the tempo of his speech was slowed and it became very subdued.

Phonemic Hearing. The boy readily understood what was said to him, distinguished correlated phonemes and correctly reproduced a rhythm, but he easily drifted away from a task of wider scope, revealing perseverations from previous tasks. When in a lethargic state all these tasks were undertaken only after additional stimulation. These investigations demonstrate that the boy had no gross localized disturbances within the limits of any analyzer, and at the same time they revealed disturbances of purposeful activity.

Cognitive Function and Behavior. Observations on the boy revealed the following features of his behavior. He adjusted poorly to general work of the class, his gaze wandered, he bit his fingernails, kept fingering his pencil, opened and shut his desk, moved his things about, pushed other children when sitting in class, chattered with his neighbors, and got up from his seat and walked about the classroom.

Sometimes the state of excitation gave way to lethargy and apathy. Whether in a state of excitation, or of lethargy and apathy he was incapable of work, and drifted away from a task or performed it piece-meal. At the blackboard he also behaved in a disorganized manner.

Other investigations also revealed a sharp fall in his capacity for work. For example, if Valerii was asked to count the number of dots inside a small circle he would at first understand the task correctly, but soon the idea of number would become separated from the operation of counting which would lapse into the stereotyped recital of some automatic numerical series. When counting a random distribution of dots he would count the same ones over and over again, or count the empty spaces between the dots. In all these tests it was found that the operation of counting lost its purposeful character and degenerated into the automatic recitation of a familiar series of numbers. The same was found in an experiment on discrimination of acoustic rhythms. Here again the boy very quickly replaced the required discrimination between the rhythms by the reproduction of a series of numbers learned by heart.

Attempts to organize his activity by means of spoken instructions more clearly demonstrated his forgetfulness of a task and its replacement by a reproduction of some consolidated, stereotyped activity.

He was able to reproduce a given rhythm from a visual example, but if he had to do this upon verbal instruction, the situation was quite different. Speech did not have the required regulatory effect, and his tapping movements lost their rhythmic character and were converted into a monotonous, hurried and stereotyped series. This disturbance of purposeful activity was demonstrated very clearly in his school work. He even wandered from simple counting operations, for instance, and gave stereotyped answers. His reading also demonstrated his impulsiveness, lack of organization, and impatience. The boy often lost his place on the page and could not move on to the next line even using his finger. While reading he would join the beginning of one word to the end of the next, distort words, and omit the end of a word. For example, instead of the word "vlez" [climb in] he read "vylez" [climb out], instead of the word "stara" [old, f.] he read "staryi" [old, m.]. He would add various words which were not in the text.

When in a state of inhibition, the boy's activity changed sharply in the opposite direction. He became extremely slow and required constant stimulation, and at times his degree of inhibition grew to such an extent that Valerii gave the impression of being in a stunned condition.

These sharp changes in cortical tone were clearly revealed in his writing. In spite of the fact that the boy was familiar with the analysis of sounds and letters, and had overcome his opticospatial disturbances, his writing remained extremely pathological. The boy's characteristic mistakes were as follows: fusion of a complete sentence into one word with omission and transposition of individual elements, leading to complete loss of meaning of a dictated sentence; omission of letters; transposition of letters within a word and of words within a sentence; and the addition of superfluous letters.

He made mistakes both when copying and when writing from dictation. One of Valerii's characteristics was the extreme inconstancy of his mistakes. After writing a difficult sentence correctly, he would make a series of mistakes in an easier sentence. The number of mistakes in the boy's writing was dependent on the condition in which he found himself. For instance, during individual work with the boy, the teacher could reduce the number of mistakes considerably simply by standing near him to organize his work, slow his tempo, or stimulate him if he was inhibited (Fig. 45).

The boy wrote the first sentence without the aid of the teacher and made a number of mistakes (fusion of several words, omissions, transpositions). He wrote the second sentence with the teacher's assistance. The help given by the teacher in this case consisted of slowing the tempo of the boy's work and directing his activity into more complete analysis of sounds and letters. Sometimes a single remark ("Think, don't be in such a hurry!") was enough to ensure correct performance of the task.

During the investigation of Valerii's cognitive functions, he showed the characteristic oligophrenic maldevelopment of the capacity for abstraction and generalization. This was demonstrated by doubly concrete forms of classification. For example, he grouped the picture representing a tree together with the picture of a deer, because "The deer is in the woods and walks by the trees."

He grouped together pictures of a cabbage, a pencil, and a knife, his explanation being that, "a knife is used to cut a cabbage and to sharpen a pencil." He grouped the pictures of a cat and dog separately from pictures of a goat and a pig, only for the reason that "the cat and dog live at home but the goat and pig live in the yard." He grouped the picture of a table together with pictures of vegetables and pots and pans because "plates, glasses, cups, and carrots can be put on a table."

In the course of his school lessons he grasped a series of concepts ("vegetables, animals, pots, and pans"). These concepts were learned by heart, however, and he could not form independent ideas.

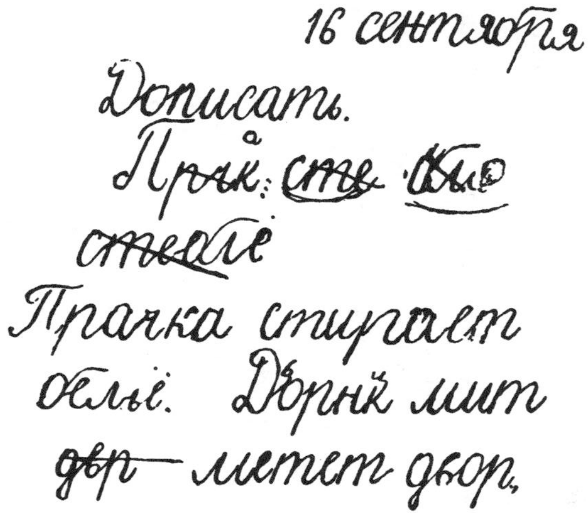

Actually written	Should have written	English equivalent
16 Sentyabrya	correct	16 September
Dopisat'	correct	To write
Prchk ste ble steble	(see below)	(see below)
Prachka stiraet bel'e	correct	The washwoman washes the clothes
Dornk mit dor metet dvor	Dvornik metet dvor	The janitor sweeps the courtyard

Fig. 45. Valerii S., aged 14 years, pupil at a special school (oligophrenia, feeble-minded degree). Severe disturbances in writing in the form of omission of letters, incomplete words and contamination.

His low capacity for abstraction and generalization also showed itself in his inability to understand the meaning of an arithmetical problem or a grammatical rule. A unique feature of the cognitive activity of this boy was his constant tendency to drift away from the task, to overstep its limits, and to develop a series of irrelevant associations or random connections, a tendency toward perseveration, and at times a complete inhibition and total absence of reaction. No sooner had he been given a set of pictures to classify but he developed irrelevant associations. He would say, "Oh, this is a grey cap, it is worn on the head, and here are galoshes, they are worn on the feet when it is very muddy and it is raining."; "Here is a goat, it chews grass and it will butt."

His tendency to form only a concrete connection was revealed in the aided memorization experiment, in which the boy had to use a picture as a means of remembering a given word and to establish a bond of meaning between the word and the picture. In this experiment he also developed a series of irrelevant associations, which prevented him from fulfilling his task. For example, when the boy was given a picture of a galosh and was asked to remember the word "rain," he said, "Where the rain falls it makes a puddle, and shoes mustn't go in the water without galoshes but galoshes don't let the water in."

Principal Stages of the Child's Development. Against the background of his general maldevelopment, even at an early stage, the boy's lethargy, drowsiness, and passivity were apparent. At preschool age his condition changed and he became restless, fussy, and timid in his motor activity. At school age, against the background of maldevelopment of his cognitive function, the structure of his disability showed some degree of motor inadequacy, a disturbance of visual-spatial integration and a decrease in his capacity for work.

The next stage in the boy's development began with his attendance in the first class at the special school, where at the end of the year considerable compensation of his disability was observed.

The closed head injury which he sustained led to a decompensation of his condition. It may be assumed that the concussion from which he suffered caused an increase in the manifestations of hydrocephalus, and that, for this reason, the clinical picture revealed a sharp decrease in his capacity for work, as a result of the shifts in the boy's state from excitability to lethargy and vice versa.

At later stages in his education his condition improved somewhat, and his capacity for work was restored to some extent, but the boy remained extremely unstable insofar as his achievements were concerned. Unfavorable additional pathogenetic factors (influenza, overfatigue) usually led to decompensation of his condition.

Clinical Analysis of the Case

The etiological factor in this case must be regarded as a traumatic injury to the fetus, complicated by subsequent postnatal trauma. There is every reason to assume that the pathogenesis in this case was complex, combining a diffuse lesion of the cerebral cortex and a residual and well-marked hydrocephalus. These pathogenetic features were responsible for the unusual type of higher nervous activity, dominated by a combination of inertia with a sharp decrease in the strength of the fundamental nervous processes. The cortical neurodynamics in this boy were highly variable and changed from one experiment to another, or even during the course of the same experiment.

These pathological features were responsible for the distinctive pattern of the clinical picture. This was unusual because in this boy there was at times an obvious predominance of excitation, but at other times inhibition was clearly demonstrated. These paroxysmally developing states of excitation and inhibition sometimes became so strong that the patient gave the impression of a person who had been stunned. It is obvious that the phasic states observed during investigation of the higher nervous activity are of essential importance in the clinical picture.

CASE 2

Aleksandr Z., a boy aged 10 years. At the end of November 1955 he was referred to the diagnostic clinic of the medicopedagogic service of the Institute of Defectology. There were no abnormal hereditary factors.

History. Sasha (Aleksandr) was born from the first pregnancy, during which his mother's general condition was poor. (Her hemoglobin fell to a very low level and her cardiac function was impaired.) Labor was difficult and protracted and the boy was born in deep asphyxia. From the first days of his life he was weak and he nursed poorly. His early development showed considerable delay, especially with regard to his speech. He did not speak his first words until he was five years of age. In infancy he suffered from bronchitis and pneumonia. At preschool age the boy remained lethargic and passive, took no part in games and did not mix with other children. At the beginning of school age Sasha had become somewhat stronger physically and began to show interest in toys, though he preferred to play alone. The boy's motor insufficiency was apparent from a very early age, and became especially pronounced when he reached school age, when Sasha was unable to look after himself as a boy of that age should. At eight years of age Sasha was sent to regular school where he made little progress. He returned from school exhausted and usually went straight to sleep. When attending school the boy's temperature periodically rose (with no obvious external cause), his general physical condition deteriorated sharply, and he developed severe and sudden attacks of headache, sometimes accompanied by vomiting.

Physical State. Deformed, hydrocephalic skull (circumference 53 cm). Narrow, flattened chest, with winging of the scapulae. No abnormality of the internal organs.

State of the Nervous System. The right nasolabial fold was very ill-defined. The tongue deviated slightly to the right. All tendon reflexes were inhibited. Even when the boy's attention was distracted, the reflexes were elicited with difficulty. Pathological reflexes were absent, but after the least physical exertion a tonic Babinski's sign appeared spontaneously on the right side. Investigation revealed apraxia of the tongue; the boy could not perform even elementary movements of the tongue to the side, upward, or downward, and he found it difficult to make alternate sounds with his mouth open a little and then opened wide.

Ophthalmological Examination. Visual acuity of the right eye 0.3, left 0.4. The gaze was steady and the media transparent. Optic fundus: optic disk whitish-pink in color, outline clear, veins tortuous and dilated, periphery of the region of the macula lutea normal, perimetry to white light normal.

Otorhinolaryngological Examination. Hearing within normal limits.

X-ray Examination of the Skull. Skull increased in size, spherical in shape and with a flattened base. The cranial sutures were ill defined. Well marked digital impressions present. Intensified shadows of the diploic veins and the emissary vessels.

Electroencephalography. The alpha-rhythm was recorded on the EEG in conjunction with slow waves. The application of frequent rhythmic light stimuli did not produce modification of the cortical rhythm (Fig. 46).

Investigation of the Higher Nervous Activity. The motor reactions in response to a command preserved their tonic character for a long time. Superfluous movements of perseveratory type were observed

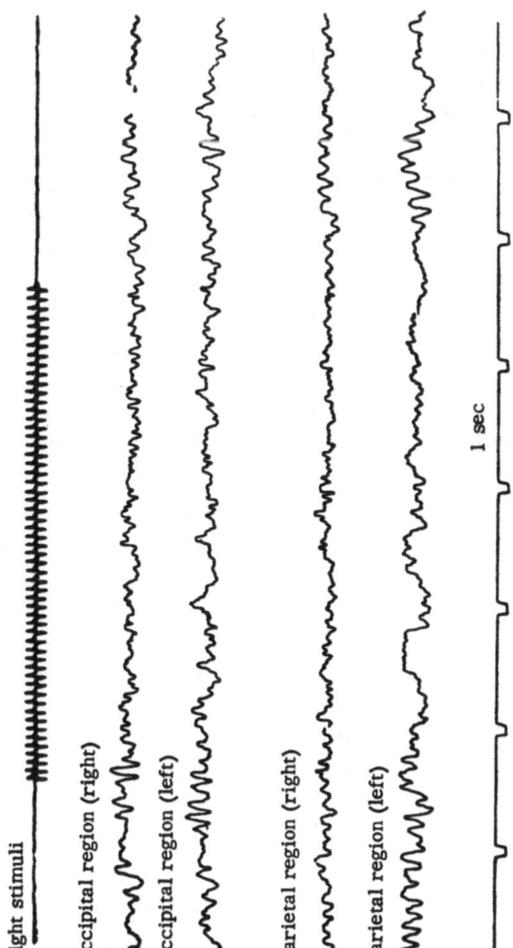

Fig. 46. Aleksandr Z., aged 10 years, pupil at a special school (oligophrenia, feeble-minded degree). The alpha-rhythm is recorded on the EEG in conjunction with slow waves. Application of frequent rhythmic light stimuli did not cause modification of the cortical rhythm.

after a rhythmic succession of several commands. Intersignal reactions were present. Wide generalization of the stimuli beyond the limits of a single analyzer was observed.

The verbal projection was marked by irrelevant associations. After the introduction of verbal equivalents of direct stimuli, echolalic reactions were observed. The motor reaction to a word given out of place was absent, and appeared only after one combination with reinforcement. In all the experiments (until the end of the investigation) the boy showed a tendency to give response reactions in the form of repeated press responses. This was especially obvious at the end of an experiment during the course of which difficulty had been experienced. Differentiation (to a stimulus of another color) arose after one combination.

Extrastimuli (of average strength) led to a single lapse of the conditioned reactions, and sometimes also to a lengthening of the latent period to subsequent conditioned stimuli, and also to a single disinhibition of differentiation.

Transformation of a negative reaction into a positive one took place after one combination, and from positive to negative after only three. Differentiation by intensity first developed after four combinations and did not become complete even after attempts to consolidate it in subsequent experiments. The production of differentiation led to manifestations of a diffuse inhibition (the boy began to yawn, his head drooped, and he began to doze).

The boy gave very poor verbal projections of preceding experiments, which indicates the inadequate stability of the trace impressions. Meanwhile verbal stereotypes, established in older experiments, figured in the projections. Differentiation by duration developed first after four combinations, and then only occasionally. During the subsequent presentation of stimuli in this and in subsequent experiments, instances of differentiation were observed less frequently than at first. Differentiation by duration was not obtained for a long time, and in response to another stimulus (a sound) it appeared only episodically.

During the production of complex forms of differentiation, fluctuating waves of irradiation of excitation were observed (repeated pressures, intersignal reactions, tonic reactions, shortened latent periods) and of inhibition (drowsiness, omission of conditioned reactions). The production of complex forms of differentiation by means of verbal instruction was also difficult; differentiation by intensity and by duration could not be produced. So far as his general behavior during the experiments is concerned, he was passive and showed no interest. (At the same time, he was very easily distracted by irrelevant stimuli.)

In addition to the presence of features common to all oligophrenic children (inertia of the nervous processes and, in particular, inertia of the verbal connections, wide generalization of the nervous processes, weakness of active inhibition) this boy was characterized by the presence of signs of predominance of the process of excitation: 1) the especially wide generalization of stimuli; 2) the large number of intersignal reactions; 3) the frequent pressures on the push-button during the conditioned reactions; 4) the special difficulties (the practical impossibility) of production of complex forms of differentiation; 5) the more rapid transformation of inhibitory stimuli into positive than vice versa.

The development of sleep inhibition was observed during the production of complex forms of differentiation, and waves of irradiation of inhibition and excitation could alternate with each other. A special characteristic of this boy was his passivity (in contrast to other excitable children) and his increased tendency to fatigue.

Mental State

Visual Analyzer. Sasha recognized pictures representing individual objects and named them correctly. Sometimes the presentation of an object to the boy aroused a series of associations which he could not inhibit. For example, when he was shown a drawing of an ewe, Sasha said, "Goat, ram, horse, cow." Only then did he give the right answer. Sasha had no difficulty in recognizing pictures of objects shown to him upside down, crossed-out figures, and outline drawings. When in a state of inhibition he sometimes ceased to recognize familiar objects.

Spatial Orientation. Sasha could orientate himself in space. He was aware of the difference between right and left. With a little help from the experimenter he could correctly copy shapes shown to him with matches, even when the forms were fairly complicated.

Motor and Motor-Speech Analyzers. During the investigation of the motor analyzer, various inconstant symptoms were discovered; in some tests a marked apraxia in the carriage of the upper limbs was observed, together with obvious disturbances of dynamic movements, whereas in others, no disturbances of the motor analyzer were found.

The boy sometimes found difficulty in the pronunciation of difficult words. For instance, instead of saying "verblyud" [camel] he said "irblyud," instead of "sentyabr'" [September], "senbabr'" or "sembar'," instead of "prostokvasha" [sour milk], "patokvasha," "prostkvokvasha," "prostokarakvasha," or "proskvasha." In the pronunciation of words the boy sometimes had difficulty in switching from one articulation to another. If his attention was directed and organized, however, Sasha could easily and correctly repeat even difficult words and sentences.

Phonemic Hearing. Sasha understood what was said to him, although at the same time he had some impairment of hearing, and could not distinguish precisely between correlated phonemes. Disturbances localized to the individual analyzers were unstable in character.

Cognitive Function and Behavior. During his lessons at school the boy was usually lethargic, passive, and lacking in initiative. Sasha showed little reaction to his surroundings at first, and would then react only gradually. During recess Sasha was slightly more excited than during lessons. His school interests were inadequate, although he never refused to do tasks assigned to him. If he could not perform a task by himself he would soon stop trying and he would not turn to the teacher for help. Sasha was competent at certain tasks, for example, coloring through a stencil, and he could do these independently without any need for special stimulation.

Sasha's extremely low work capacity stood out clearly whatever his task. Nothing held his interest for long; his attention soon drifted from a task, and he would begin to introduce a series of irrelevant associations. For example, in the course of a conversation at the clinic, when he was asked with whom he lived, the boy replied, "Grandma Polya cooks the soup; we have a sheep dog, a television set, a pretty box; there was a Christmas tree; I sang 'The Birch Tree in the Field' and uncle gave it to me; the Christmas tree was a very big one; we will paste it on." After a short pause, Sasha continued: "We bought a 'gaberot' (he meant 'garderob' [wardrobe]), a big cupboard, a glass fish, a squirrel, a little rabbit, and a little bird."

The same tendency to drift from a task and the severe impairment of purposeful activity were clearly revealed in the initial stages of teaching the boy the rudiments of reading, writing, and arithmetic. When a series of syllables with familiar letters were dictated to him, and he was told to write them down, the teacher had only to go away from him and the boy's activity would go to pieces; he would stop writing and in various parts of the page he would begin to draw lines, sketches, copy figures or numbers (the date), then turn the paper over and continue to write bits of letters haphazardly on the other side. Even if he were asked to perform the simple and short task of writing a line of capital "B"s [Ve] he would write the first one or two letters quite well, after which the shape of the letter would change and it would begin to resemble the other letter "Б" [Be], and later still his letters would incorporate the elements of both letters, etc. (Fig. 47).

A similar pattern was observed when the boy was asked to trace the letter "y." He wrote the letter several times correctly, and then he began to distort it, omitting certain elements (Fig. 48). Even if his task was restricted to writing only a single element of the letter, Sasha could not cope with it.

When he went on to writing individual words from dictation, after a preliminary analysis of each word the boy revealed certain

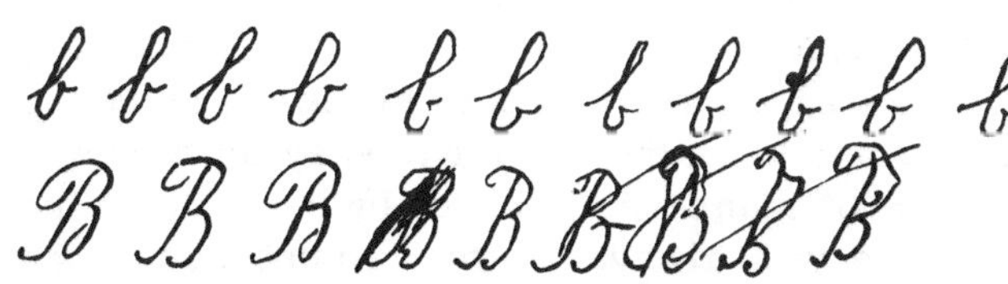

Fig. 47. Aleksandr Z., aged 10 years, pupil at a special school (oligophrenia). When writing a series of single letters its form is changed and it begins to look like another letter.

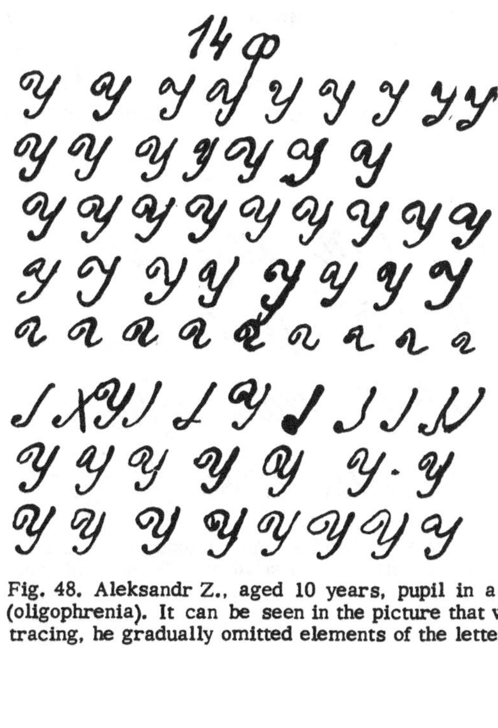

Fig. 48. Aleksandr Z., aged 10 years, pupil in a special school (oligophrenia). It can be seen in the picture that when writing by tracing, he gradually omitted elements of the letters.

specific difficulties: he transposed the letters in the word (instead of the word "luk" [onion] he wrote "lku"). Unfinished words and the perseverative reproduction of the same letter were observed in his writing (Fig. 49).

With the assistance of the teacher he could write a series of words without a mistake. His reduced capacity for work and his inability to concentrate were especially noticeable when the boy was taught to count. The boy could count up to ten, but he could not count backwards even from five. With the organizing help of the teacher Sasha could perform the elementary arithmetical operations (addition and subtraction) with numbers up to five, but when working by himself even at this level he would either make many mistakes, give impulsive and thoughtless answers, or make no effort whatsoever to solve the problem.

Subsequently, when he was asked to take away a certain number of sticks and make a record of the arithmetical operation, he was able to arrive at the answer to easy problems in addition and subtraction of numbers up to ten by counting on his fingers. His performance was always uneven; sometimes he got the right answer, sometimes not. Sasha knew the shapes of all the numbers, but he could not arrange them in the proper order.

If Sasha was asked to fit variously shaped pegs into their corresponding holes, he was quite unable to do so by himself and he made several inept tries. The same thing happened when he put together the pieces of a cut-up picture. However, help from the teacher in directing his attention improved the quality of his work.

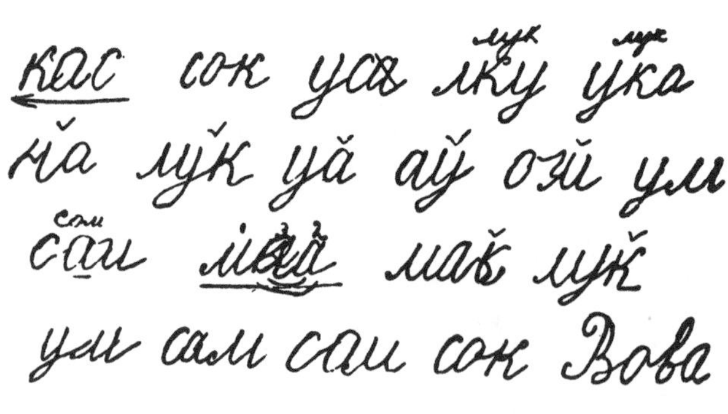

Fig. 49. The same subject's writing. The various words clearly show transpositions of letters in the word, unfinished words and the perseverative reproduction of the same letter.

The boy's capacity for work varied with his surroundings. He worked better alone than in a group. When with other children his productivity was considerably lowered. The boy's capacity for work also depended on his condition. Sometimes he was active and purposeful; at other times he was passive and indifferent. During experimental investigation, just as in his lessons, the boy rapidly became fatigued. He was extremely passive and quite indifferent to his studies, inactive, scattered, forgetful, and aimless. When he left the workroom he never tidied up; he forgot his book-bag and returned for it only when told to do so by his mother. No sooner did Sasha leave the classroom for recess, than he became perceptibly livelier. After four months of group training Sasha became more active, developed an interest in his work, and began to turn to the teacher for help when he had difficulty with his lessons. Sometimes, when he had finished his assigned task, he would ask the teacher what he had to do next. This demonstrated the increase in his activity. He mixed more freely with the other children; he played with them at recess and chatted with them, which he had not done when he first joined the group.

He still remained lethargic and passive, however, and often could not make the necessary effort when performing various school tasks. All these distinctive characteristics, however, stood out against a background of maldevelopment of cognitive function. In the experiment in which he had to discard a fourth superfluous picture, if leading questions were asked the boy could identify the unwanted picture, but he could not give a proper motive for his action.

When asked why he had rejected a particular picture, Sasha often gave silly explanations. Sasha tended to stick to inert verbal stereotypes. When this experiment was repeated two days later, Sasha was able to identify the pictures concerned when helped by leading questions, but in explaining why he had chosen one particular picture he reproduced an old inert connection, established in the first experiment, when he had distributed the pictures purely according to size ("big," "little"). Sometimes the boy tried to compare pictures by size. If the experimenter told the boy that his answer was wrong, he would try to modify his answer but still remained within the bounds of the old inert connection ("a little bigger" and "a little smaller").

A series of wild animal pictures was used next. Sasha had to pick out similar pictures. Sasha was then shown pictures representing objects differing altogether from wild animals (a bicyclé, a steamship, a trolley car, etc.). With each picture the experimenter asked, "Is this a wild animal?" and Sasha correctly replied, "It is not a wild animal." After two or three reinforcements Sasha grouped the pictures correctly. This connection, reinforced by his own conversation, helped Sasha to correctly distinguish the pictures of the wild animals from the other pictures. Later, Sasha was given three pictures representing vegetables, one of a fox, as the extraneous picture. The boy carried out this task with the aid of the reinforced inert connection: "It is not a wild animal," which he repeated three times and discarded all three pictures of vegetables. When the experimenter said that the answer was unsatisfactory, the boy changed his answer "It is not a wild animal" to "It is not a fox."

The experimenter's helpful question, "Which of these are vegetables?" elicited a response which revealed how completely unsure Sasha was, for he failed to recognize that the task was one of generalization. At a later stage in the investigation the two concepts of "vegetable" and "wild animal" were established in the boy. However, when he was given a similar problem but with a different series of pictures, the boy was again helpless: he could not make the transition, but distinguished the pictures on the basis of the former inert connection ("little," "big"). The experimenter's remark that the answer was wrong led the boy to reproduce all the connections that he had formed earlier in the experiment, but which bore no relation to the task nor to the objects to be identified. From this experiment it may be concluded, not only that the boy's cognitive function was on a very low level, but also that his potential area of immediate development was small.

The maldevelopment of his cognitive function was also demonstrated in an experiment in which the boy had to bring together a series of pictures related by a common theme. With assistance, the boy succeeded in properly arranging only a simple series of three pictures. He was quite incapable of dealing with a more complicated series, but looked upon each picture as an isolated entity. When Sasha was asked to tell the composite story shown by the four pictures arranged in the proper order, the boy could not do so, but instead began to describe each picture separately, without recognizing the general theme running through the series.

In this case we shall not offer an analysis of the fundamental stages of the boy's development, since our observations on him were limited to a period of only six months.

Clinical Analysis of the Case

The principal etiological factor in this case must be regarded as natural trauma, the evidence in favor of this being: the protracted labor, the asphyxia, and the disturbance of development from the first days of life.

It may be postulated that the pathogenetic factors are: a diffuse lesion of the cerebral cortex and a residual hydrocephalus. The distinctive pathogenetic features are responsible for the pattern of the higher nervous activity.

The higher nervous activity in this case is characterized by a combination of inertia of the fundamental nervous processes with a periodically developing predominance sometimes of inhibition over excitation, and at other times of excitation over inhibition. In turn, these pathophysiological features are responsible for the complexity of the clinical picture, in which a sharp decrease in the capacity for work and considerable variations in the general tone—from lethargy and passivity to a state of increased excitability—stand out against the background of a considerable maldevelopment of cognitive functions. At times the boy is disinhibited, impulsive, and restless in his motor activity, and at other times he becomes lethargic, passive, and lacking in spontaneous activity. When his degree of general inhibition increased, in these lethargic states he was apparently half asleep; at such times Sasha's actions were unmotivated: for example, he would suddenly begin to write on the wall and not in his work book, or he would write odd sorts of lines instead of letters. His mental state showed paroxysmal symptoms of oral apraxia, difficulty in switching from one articulation to another, and difficulty in the pronunciation of individual words. If the oral apraxia in this particular case had been prolonged, the development of spontaneous speech would have been impossible. Since spontaneous speech did in fact develop, and since the articulatory vocal apparatus was adequate, it may be assumed that in this case the apraxia was pseudo-oral in type, i.e., movements of the articulatory apparatus were possible, but the child could not activate them upon demand because of the marked lowering of his cortical tone.

In this particular case, during the course of investigation, we also discovered evidence of pseudo-optic agnosia and paroxysmally developing manifestations of disturbance of postural and dynamic movements. Taken as a whole, these symptoms (pseudo-oral apraxia, pseudo-optic agnosia, paroxysmal disturbances of dynamic and postural movements) are evidence of the gross disturbance of the cortical neurodynamics. From the foregoing remarks it is clear that this case may be included in that subgroup of oligophrenia which is characterized by a distinctive pattern of the cortical neurodynamics in which there is weakness of both nervous processes, i.e., excitation and inhibition, without evident predominance of either.

ANALYSIS OF ALL THE RESULTS OBTAINED

Special Features of Early Development. In the early stages of their development these children revealed the characteristic features common to all oligophrenic children. Besides these general features, however, there were also other prominent and specific features, namely transient and shifting phases of lethargy, passivity, and drowsiness on the one hand and states of increased excitability on the other.

These recurrent phases are responsible for the peculiar changes in the behavior noted in these children from early childhood. Before they started special school, some of these children attended regular school, where they showed various specific peculiarities and difficulties in reading, writing, and arithmetic. The demands of the regular school, which exceeded their capacity, provoked and exacerbated these periodic fluctuations in their condition (their headaches became more frequent and there was a much greater susceptibility to fatigue).

X-ray Examination of the Skull. Qualitative analysis of the findings described above shows that the unique pathogenetic feature of this subgroup is the combination of a diffuse lesion of the cerebral cortex with a residual hydrocephalus. In all cases we observed attacks of headache of a hypertensive character. X-ray examination of the skull also gave a clearer picture of the residual hydrocephalus.

Neurological Investigation. Upon neurological examination of this subgroup of children, a very varied symptomatology emerged. For instance, in addition to the general residual diffuse symptomatology, at the time of the first examination there was a noticeable preponderance of right-sided signs, but at the next examination these signs were more marked on the left; a similar state of affairs was found with the abnormal reflexes, which in the same child might be absent or become strongly positive.

Investigation of the Electrical Activity of the Brain. In some of the children we examined we found changes in the electrical activity of the brain, testifying to the gross neurodynamic disturbances. These changes took the form of a distinctive reaction to various afferent stimuli, which exceeded the upper limit of working capacity of the cortical cells, and led to a parabiotic state of the cortex, expressed in the form of slow waves of high amplitude. It must be pointed out that the character of this parabiotic reaction in one of the children whom we investigated was much more pronounced than in any other case of oligophrenia under our observation. The gross neurodynamic disturbances were also demonstrated by the presence of modification of the cortical activity by low-frequency light stimulation in the children of this subgroup.

This modification of cortical rhythm in response to low-frequency flicker indicates a very gross neurodynamic disturbance and is observed in normal individuals during the development of cortical sleep inhibition.

Special Features of the Higher Nervous Activity. In addition to the characteristic features of higher nervous activity common to all three subgroups, in the children of this particular subgroup a number of specific features affecting the neurodynamics were observed.

The most prominent of these features was the instability of the neurodynamic indices: conditioned connections which were easily formed in one experiment were absent and re-established only with difficulty in the next, intersignal reactions which were not observed in one test situation were present in large numbers in the same child on another occasion, and so on.

A unique aspect of the higher nervous activity of these children was that in the course of investigation they revealed both the characteristic features of the children with the inhibitory variant as well as some characteristic features of the children in whom the process of excitation is predominant. On different occasions the condition of these children showed marked variations in phase. These differences were observed mainly when the children, for some reason or other, had been in a state of excitation before they were examined.

Analysis of all these findings shows that the specific features of the higher nervous activity of the children of this subgroup are associated with a marked decrease in the strength of the fundamental nervous processes. It is these distinctive features of the higher nervous activity which are responsible for the unique clinical pattern.

Investigation of the Individual Cortical Function. The variability and inconstancy of the various manifestations were demonstrated with particular clarity during the investigation of the levels of analysis and integration within the limits of the individual analyzers. For example, though the capacity for visual analysis and integration was found intact, and the children were ordinarily able to recognize correctly real objects shown to them, dotted-line drawings of objects, geometrical figures, or crossed-out pictures, at times they could not recognize them, presenting a picture resembling optic agnosia. This "optic agnosia" disappeared, however, when the child was stimulated and organized. When their degree of inhibition increased, the children ceased to react to pictures of objects which were shown to them. In a state of excitation the same subjects gave unreliable, impulsive answers or recited a list of objects closely resembling those shown, due to the development of a cluster of associations as the children examined the pictures. The same phenomenon was observed during the investigation of spatial integration. It was only in the children of this subgroup that manifestations of oral apraxia developed paroxysmally during investigation of the motor-speech analyzer. During the investigation of auditory analysis and integration in these children, what were apparently manifestations of acoustic agnosia developed periodically.

The inconstancy of all the phenomena described above, the fact that their appearance was dependent on the child's condition, and the absence of erroneous answers of this type when the children were organized and stimulated as they performed their tasks all suggested that they were symptoms of pseudo-optic agnosia, pseudo-acoustic agnosia, pseudo-oral apraxia, and so on. The periodic development of all these manifestations was due to phasic changes in the condition of the cerebral cortex.

Peculiarities of Cognitive Function. Like other oligophrenic children, when performing various tasks these children showed maldevelopment of the generalizing function of speech, typically revealed in their doubly concrete forms of classification and in the vagueness of their generic concepts. Their specific characteristics were revealed, however, in the special abnormalities of the dynamics of their intellectual processes. During their paroxysmally developing states of excitation, the children did not listen to any complete instruction given to them, or assimilated only some fragment of it. When they carried out their tasks they became distracted and drifted away from the assigned problem. With an increase in their degree of general inhibition these children became lethargic and passive, often did not even begin to carry out their tasks and required additional stimulation. Intellectual disturbances characteristic both of oligophrenic children in whom excitation predominates over inhibition and of those groups of oligophrenic children in whom inhibition predominates over excitation developed paroxysmally in one and the same subject.

Characteristics of the Emotional-Volitional Function. The specific feature of the whole psychopathological picture of the children of this subgroup was the extreme variability of their condition. In the selfsame child we could observe various states of lethargy ranging from a slight decrease of tone when, with some external stimulation, the child could tackle a problem presented to him, and when, moreover, no disturbances of analysis and integration were apparent in the various analyzers, to a state of profound inhibition when the child could not deal with a problem presented to him, and when he would often answer familiar questions quite within his capacity by saying that he did not know. If he could be guided a little toward the solution of his problem, disturbances of analysis and integration within the limits of an individual analyzer were easily found. With a further increase in their inhibition these children passed into a dazed state in which unmotivated and unconscious forms of absurd behavior developed. A distinguishing feature of all these various phases was the fact that external stimulation could draw the child out of that state. These manifestations of their condition were very reminiscent of those found in oligophrenic children in whom inhibition was predominant. This unique characteristic of this group of children is determined by the fact that a state of extreme lethargy and inhibition may be succeeded by general excitation, as revealed both by their behavior and by the distinctive features of their intellectual activity. In these states of excitation the children were extremely disinhibited, readily distracted, with speech and actions responsive to incidental stimuli; they rapidly drifted away from a task, displaying all the characteristic features of oligophrenic children in whom the process of excitation is predominant. All these cortical neurodynamic features were combined with a maldevelopment of cognitive activity.

Characteristics of Motor Activity. Investigation of the motor activity in these children revealed typical changes. One of the distinguishing features in the motor sphere was the fact that it was dependent upon general changes in cortical tone. While in a state of lethargy or inhibition their movements became inhibited, their tempo markedly retarded and their facial expression became flat, inexpressive, and fixed. As their excitation increased their facial expressions became livelier, the tempo of their movements quickened, many superfluous movements appeared, and at times they showed general motor restlessness.

Specific Characteristics of the Children of this Subgroup Emerging in the Course of Their Education. These children experienced great difficulty in learning elementary reading and writing. They quickly forgot the letters they learned, frequently became confused, and found it very hard to master reading by syllables. Particular difficulty was encountered by these children in learning to write. In the initial stages of their education their difficulty in writing was mainly due to the fact that they could not persist at the most elementary tasks for long. Gradually, however, they mastered the operations of writing, and it was then easily demonstrated that their difficulties in writing were due neither to weakness of auditory analysis and integration nor to disturbances of spatial orientation. These two elements, however, by no means exhaust the factors involved in the complex writing process. Arrangement of the individual word elements and of the words in the sentence is a matter of fundamental importance. The children of this subgroup had trouble arranging individual elements of sound-letter complexes, which led to a variety of mistakes such as omission of individual letters, syllables, and words, as well as transpositions and premature insertions. As a result of these features their words lost their clarity (Fig. 50).

Gross writing defects, such as we noted in the children of this subgroup, were not observed in any other forms of oligophrenia.

These children experienced still greater difficulty in learning arithmetical operations. In the initial stages of their education they had the difficulties common to all oligophrenic children, namely, mastering the number concept and the correlations between numbers and objects. Certain specific difficulties were also displayed, however: loss of component elements of arithmetical problems posed for them, and difficulty in remembering the concrete features of the task. Since we had a comparatively limited time to observe these children, we are unable at this time to recommend the main lines of corrective training to be adopted. This will be a matter for future investigation.

DIFFERENTIATION BETWEEN OLIGOPHRENIC CHILDREN WITH GROSS DISTURBANCES OF CORTICAL NEURODYNAMICS AND CHILDREN WITH SIMILAR CONDITIONS

Whereas the oligophrenic children of our first subgroup are usually confused with children who have a temporary arrest of

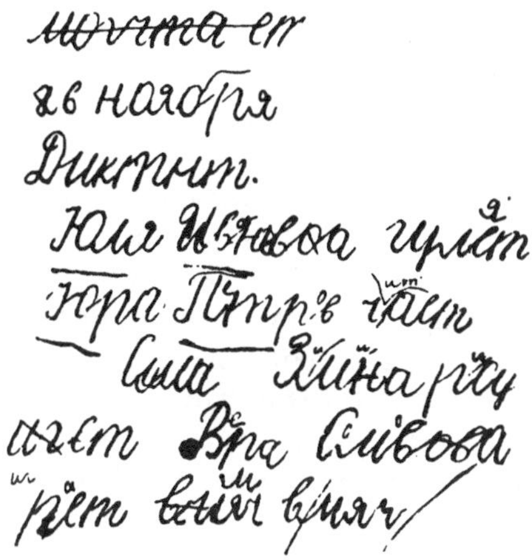

Fig. 50. Subject S., aged 11, pupil at a special school. The figure clearly shows various mistakes: omission of letters, syllables and words, transpositions, and fusion of several words into one.

development, those with gross neurodynamic disturbances are more often confused with cerebroasthenic states in childhood.

Cerebral asthenia is one of the commonest forms of reaction of the nervous system to various noxious agents. Clinically, several forms of asthenia are usually distinguished.

Somatogenic asthenia arises in association with general physical weakness in the child. Such children often become unsuccessful pupils because of their increased liability to fatigue and exhaustion. Somatic asthenia is much more easily distinguished from oligophrenia because in these children the capacity for intellectual development is completely preserved, and the introduction of certain therapeutic measures leads to fairly good compensation.

The differential diagnosis is much more complicated and difficult in relation to those forms of cerebral asthenia which arise as a result of traumatic or inflammatory lesions of the central nervous system.

In contrast to oligopbrenia, these cerebral asthenias are based upon functional, dynamic disturbances alone. These functional, dynamic disturbances arise as a result of the distinctive pathogenesis of these cases. The fundamental pathogenetic feature in these states is the presence of a residual hydrocephalus with no gross morphological changes in the brain substance. The disturbance of higher nervous activity in these states is characterized by a considerable weakness of the fundamental nervous processes and by the rapid passage of the nerve cell into a state of limiting inhibition.

In these states the weakness of the processes of active cortical inhibition is clearly exhibited, leading inevitably to irradiation of the fundamental nervous processes, which in turn is responsible for the instability of the traces of connections previously formed. These distinctive pathophysiological conditions cause the child to develop a series of symptoms; signs of disorganization of behavior and impairment of the capacity for work. These in turn lead to educational difficulties in the regular school.

Fundamental symptoms in the clinical picture of these asthenic states are weakness of excitation combined with headache, vertigo, and attacks of syncope. These children are highly sensitive to loud noises, odors, or temperature changes. They often have sleep disturbances, poor appetite, and a general tendency to increased fatigue. Depending on their behavioral characteristics, these children may be considered as excitable or inhibited.

In the former case excitation predominates over inhibition; their behavior is characterized by increased excitability and general motor restlessness. During school hours their increased liability to fatigue, their extreme forgetfulness, and their greatly diminished capacity for work are all very conspicuous. During a lesson such a child will begin to occupy himself with other things, he will play with something on his desk, bother his neighbors, and chatter. In the absence of any marked disturbances in the individual analyzers, they may give incorrect as well as correct answers. In the course of their education at school such children have a poor memory for letters, read by guessing, and make a number of mistakes in their writing; they do not finish words; they duplicate words and syllables; they transpose letters and syllables within a word and words within a sentence. Their diminished work capacity is shown even more when they try to learn arithmetic, especially mental arithmetic. Such children cannot retain simple problems or concrete features of a problem, and in attempting to solve a problem they omit component elements.

Another distinctive characteristic of these children is the extreme instability of their symptoms. The character of their performance of a particular task is dependent on the child's general condition. With increasing fatigue they cannot do even simple tasks, normally quite within their reach. After sleep or rest these children can accomplish more complicated tasks. Their productivity also varies with conditions surrounding their activity. During individual study, and with the right approach by the teacher, their productivity improves markedly. Their productivity declines if the teacher does not use the correct individual approach to these children.

The fluctuations in their capacity for work lead to a lack of consistency in their answers. For instance, besides giving incorrect answers they may also give perfect answers. The diminution of work capacity in these asthenic children is displayed against a background of a well-preserved personality. The children recognize their difficulties in learning and are greatly upset by their failures, which further diminishes their capacities.

These cerebroasthenic cases may be mistaken for cases of oligophrenia with predominance of excitation over inhibition. The history of both the cerebroasthenic and the oligophrenic cases may show some previous disease of the central nervous system, leading to the disturbance in development.

The presence of a mild diffuse residual neurological symptomatology makes cerebral asthenia resemble oligophrenia. Cerebroasthenic children, like oligophrenic children, are unsuccessful pupils in the regular schools and acquire neither skill nor knowledge. The poor performance of these children before school selection committees contributes still further to the mistakes in diagnosis. Besides the similarity between cerebroasthenic and oligophrenic children, however, there are also considerable differences. In predominantly excited oligophrenics the symptom of oligophrenic mental retardation is combined with behavioral disturbances and a diminished work capacity, in which respect they resemble asthenic children, but in contrast to oligophrenics, in asthenic states the cognitive functions are preserved. There are also differences in the character of the educational difficulties in these two groups. Oligophrenic children have difficulty mainly in understanding the meaning of any problem. Children with cerebroasthenic states find difficulty mainly with the magnitude of the problem, and cannot keep their mind on the task or remember the essential facts. In these superficially similar states, the attitude towards their difficulties is different. Although oligophrenic children of this subgroup are aware of their difficulties, their attitude is inconstant and relatively superficial in character. Cerebroasthenic children have a critical attitude towards their failures and show strong associated feelings.

The course of these two outwardly similar states also differs. In cerebroasthenic states proper medical treatment and educational measures will rapidly prove effective. But oligophrenic children of this subgroup require prolonged and specialized measures in order to bring them even to a merely relative level of compensation and, as we have shown above, their fundamental symptom, the maldevelopment of the generalizing function of speech, persists to a marked degree at later stages of their development.

In addition to the cerebroasthenic cases characterized by the predominance of excitation over inhibition, there exist forms of cerebral asthenia presenting a different picture; namely, the predominance of inhibition over excitation. The clinical picture in these children also shows a series of symptoms reflecting a diminution of cortical tone. They have headaches, vertigo, and an increased liability to fatigue and exhaustion. In their behavioral characteristics they resemble most closely those oligophrenics in whom inhibition is predominant. These children are lethargic, passive, and inhibited; they need constant stimulation and they cannot carry out a task without such additional stimulation. The predominance of inhibition in the clinical picture also leads to a disturbed work capacity.

In the process of their education, these children develop many neurotic reactions in the form of enuresis, stammering and tics. Lack of progress in their studies often leads to severe emotional crises. All these factors, taken together, still further diminish their capacity for work.

This asthenic symptom-complex in which the children show the predominance of an inhibitory state of the cerebral cortex often causes confusion with oligophrenia. In addition to their similarity, however, significant differences are also present. For instance, in spite of the low level of productivity of children in whom inhibition is predominant, experimental investigation nevertheless reveals a fair degree of development of their cognitive function. As shown above, in oligophrenic children the main difficulties arise as a result of the presence of the fundamental symptom of oligophrenic mental retardation.

The dynamics of these two conditions also differ. When provided with proper medical treatment and educational measures, inhibited cerebroasthenic children develop progressively, whereas inhibited oligophrenics require prolonged education under special conditions before showing any progress.

If the differential-diagnostic criteria enumerated above are borne in mind, it will be possible to distinguish between these outwardly similar states, and thereby avoid diagnostic mistakes when these children are being considered for special schools.

CHAPTER 7*

OLIGOPHRENIC CHILDREN WITH MARKED DEFICIENCY OF THE FRONTAL SYSTEMS

Quite different from the forms of oligophrenia which we have so far described is another form in which a diffuse lesion of the cerebral cortex is combined with a disturbance of the frontal systems. Against the background of maldevelopment of the cognitive functions these cases show an obvious and gross disturbance of the whole personality development, alterations in the system of desires and motives, combined with a considerable maldevelopment of the emotional-volitional function. The children with this defect whom we investigated usually displayed a typical maldevelopment of their motor activity. The structure of the defect in this particular form of oligophrenia was similar to the disturbances of the complex forms of human behavior and activity which have been described in lesions of the frontal divisions of the cerebral cortex in adult patients.

An extensive literature exists on the question of the role and importance of the frontal lobes in the behavior of man and animals. The findings obtained by morphologists during their studies of the development of the various regions of the human brain are also of interest in this connection.

In his paper entitled "Two centers in the human cerebral cortex," Betz (1873) wrote that the fissure of Rolando divides the surface of the brain into two parts; a) an anterior, in which large pyramidal cells occupy a predominant place, and b) a posterior (including the temporal lobe), in which the granular layers are predominant.

Polyakov (1949) pointed out the significant differences between the anterior and posterior divisions of the cortex at the time of the initial formation of the rudimentary cortex and throughout the whole course of prenatal ontogenesis, and on this basis he divided

*Besides describing the developmental history of oligophrenic children receiving their education at a special school, in this chapter we also present case reports of children under observation in the children's department of the N. N. Burdenko Institute of Neurosurgery and in the children's department of the Kashchenko Hospital, which accounts for slight differences in the character of presentation.

the neocortex into two principal parts: first, the anterior, frontal cortex, and second, the posterior (the parietal, temporal, and occipital cortex). In the anterior part the cortical anlage is appreciably wider and has a more clear-cut cellular structure, but in the posterior part it is much narrower and the cells are closely packed.

It is also known that in the early stages of ontogenesis the primitive individualization of the cortical anlage takes place much more intensively in the anterior part of the hemispheres than in the posterior. The most characteristic feature of the frontal cortex is the presence of fibers. This fibrous structure is evidently dependent on the development of interneuronal connections in the anlage of this cortex.

Careful cytoarchitectonic investigations have given clear ideas both of the different types of development of the anterior and posterior parts of the cortex and of the distinctive structure of the frontal cortex.

Kononova (1940) showed by his work that the frontal lobes of the brain undergo particularly intensive development during a child's first years. Whereas in the initial period (the first two years) growth of the frontal cortex takes place mainly by the intensive development of the cells of the fifth, afferent layer of the cortex, after two years there is a sharp increase in growth of the third layer of cells, which are mainly concerned with association. Growth of the morphological structures of the frontal cortex does not take place uniformly, but undergoes appreciable periods of intensification of tempo, occurring from the first or second to seventh year, although in some regions the increase in tempo continues until the age of 12.

The structure of the frontal cortex shows much higher degrees of differentiation and variability. The phylogenetically newer fields reach maturity later. The basal portion of the frontal cortex differs architectonically from the cortex of the convex portion of the lobe. It is phylogenetically older and is morphologically close to the limbic structures.

The orbital cortex, the gyrus cinguli and the hippocampal fissure are links of a single anatomicophysiological system. Comparative anatomical data show the frontal lobes to be the most recent structures of the brain. The higher we look on the phylogenetic tree the more we see a development of the frontal region, reaching its highest degree in man. Associative connections connect the frontal cortex with all regions of the brain. Fibers from the frontal cortex are directed not only to the other regions of the hemispheres, but also to the underlying structures. The wealth of connections of the frontal region is suggestive of its outstanding functional importance. The frontal lobes appeared last in the long evolutionary process. In man they account for as much as one third of the total mass of the brain. It thus becomes clear why the higher and specifically human forms of behavior are bound up with the functions of the frontal lobes.

Several studies on extirpation of the anterior divisions of the brain in animals have been conducted. Bianchi (1885) on the basis of his extensive experiments on dogs and monkeys, accepted the very great role of the anterior divisions of the cortex in the organization of human behavior.

Bianchi experimented on five dogs and eight monkeys. In some of the dogs he removed other areas of the brain but left the frontal lobes intact. In these cases he observed no change in the dog's behavior. Bilateral removal of the frontal regions had a considerable effect on both behavior and habits of the animals. A dog from which Bianchi extirpated both frontal lobes developed marked changes in its behavior. The external situation did not cause an appropriate response in this dog's behavior. The dog's attachments, which had previously controlled the dog's behavior, lost their hold, and the animal sometimes passed into a state of irrational excitation. Bilateral extirpation of the prefrontal ccrtex also caused a sharp change in the behavior of monkeys. For example, if an object was held out towards the monkey's open palm it would pull it towards itself, but if its palm was closed over the object it would be no longer aware of its existence. A monkey which, before the operation, had jumped up and down in the window of his cage "to call the other monkeys," continued to jump up and down in the window after the operation, but did so without any meaning or purpose.

These accounts of Bianchi were substantiated and refined by Franz (1907), who trained his animals (cats, monkeys) before and after the operation. He taught the animals to perform a number of complicated movements directed towards a certain purpose. The animal was put in a cage, which was fastened by various methods, and it was taught to open the locked door, in order to come out and take food. After extirpation of the frontal lobes these animals lost the ability to perform this type of complicated movement. Jacobsen's experiments are of particular interest for an understanding of the distinctive features of the behavioral disturbances. These experiments clearly showed that in situations in which the animal's behavior is determined by directly perceived stimuli, destruction of the frontal lobes caused no appreciable change in the behavior. If the experimenter then changed to an activity with a complex structure, however, in which the animal's activity had to be determined by motives overstepping the limits of the situation immediately seen, then resection of the frontal lobes led to a catastrophic collapse of behavior. Fulton (1935), analyzing data on the function of the frontal lobes, also came to the conclusion that this function is connected not so much with the organization of individual movements as with the organization of the animal's behavior.

Experimental research has also been undertaken by Russian workers. Rossolimo (1893) made observations on dogs after bilateral frontal lobe extirpation and found changes in the general behavior of the animals. A dog stubbornly tried to go forward, collided with objects, and only turned away when it struck an obstacle. It wandered about aimlessly, did not bark, yelp, or show fear when it saw anybody nearby, but mechanically followed the person. The dog hardly reacted at all to being called, but constantly moved about. From his observations on these dogs after operation, Rossolimo became convinced of the importance of the role of the frontal lobes in the organization of the general behavior of animals.

Animal experiments of no less interest were carried out by Zhukovskii (1897), Babkin (1909), Demidov (1909), and Saturnov (1911).

These experimental researches clearly demonstrated that bilateral resection of the frontal lobes in dogs leads to disturbance of their behavior. Pavlov was well aware of the curious behavior of an animal from which he had removed the anterior portion of the cerebral hemispheres. He wrote: "If you excise the whole posterior portion of the cerebral hemispheres of a dog (immediately posterior to the sigmoid gyrus and then along the fissure of Sylvius) you will then obtain an animal which is in general absolutely normal. It will identify you, its food, and any manner of object placed in front of it, with its nose and skin. It will wag its tail when happy. It will show you that it is happy when it recognizes you with its nose, and so on. Such an animal, however, will not react to you if you are standing far away, i.e., it does not use its eyes to the normal extent. The same may occur if you call it by name, for it will not react always to this. You may deduce that such a dog uses its eyes and ears very little, but is otherwise perfectly normal.

"If, however, you excise the anterior portion of the cerebral hemispheres to the same extent as the posterior resection, you will then obtain what is evidently a profoundly abnormal animal. He would not have an appropriate attitude toward you, nor toward his fellow dogs, nor toward his food, which he would not search for, nor, in general, toward any surrounding object. You would then have an altogether abnormal animal, in which it is evident that no trace of purposeful behavior remains. Thus there would be a vast difference between two animals, one without the anterior and one without the posterior portions of the hemispheres. You could say that one is blind or deaf, but otherwise normal, but that the other is severely disabled and a helpless idiot."*

Further experiments on animals have shown disturbances of behavior still more clearly. Experimental research by Shumilina (1949) demonstrated that the conditioned reflex activity of a dog was considerably modified after removal of the frontal lobes of the brain, as revealed by the disorganization of its motor behavior after the animal had been taught to choose between forms of unconditioned reinforcement. The behavior of such an animal shows the apparent absence of the complex process of integration which unites the separate motor acts into a single scheme of activity, in which each preceding action is to some extent an afferent factor not only for the next motor act, but also for those taking place later. Similar findings were reported by Shustin (1955).

The experiments described above thus suggest that after removal of the frontal lobes from animals at operation, general behavioral disturbances supervene. The experience of neurosurgery is of great importance in the solution of the problem of the role of the frontal lobes of the brain in the organization of the higher forms of human behavior.

Of great interest is the work of Brickner (1934). For a number of years he was attending physician to a patient from whom Dandy in 1930 had removed both prefrontal lobes as far as the premotor area because of compression by an enormous parasagittal meningioma. Observations on this patient from day to day showed that he ceased to be tactful and became euphoric, childish, lacking in initiative, uncritical, and garrulous, and made no secret of his sexual inclinations. This patient's intellectual functions changed considerably. He had obvious difficulty solving separate deliberative tasks and could not concentrate. Brickner considered that his patient was completely incapable of retaining in his memory a series of facts even for a short time or to operate with them simultaneously. As a result of these observations he concluded that the intellectual

*I. P. Pavlov, Complete Collected Works, Vol. 3, Book 1, Izd. AN SSSR, 1951, pp. 219-220.

changes accompanying lesions of the frontal lobes are primary and are due to disturbances of integrative capacity.

Penfield (1935) described two cases of meningioma of the olfactory fossa. In the first case the prefrontal region was removed on the left side, and soon after operation a number of distinctive features were observed. The patient was unable to concentrate, had difficulty counting, and lost his initiative. In the second case the right frontal lobe was removed. Immediately after the operation the patient felt quite unchanged, although subsequent observation revealed a number of curious features in her behavior: she became sluggish and lost her initiative.

Ackerly (1933) described a patient from whom the left prefrontal region was removed because of a meningioma of the olfactory fossa. Immediately after the operation the patient was euphoric, infantile, excessively garrulous, extremely egoistic, and sexually aggressive. She soon became unnaturally active. She worked at a great rate, felt quite young, and was as she described herself, always very merry, saying that it was "because all my troubles have been cut out of my head." She found it difficult, however, to concentrate on anything.

Observations of the opposite character have been made, however, by neurosurgeons. In 1925, for instance, Dandy removed a left prefrontal region and thereafter found no change in the patient. Jefferson, in 1937, described six cases of removal of the prefrontal region and also found no evident mental changes thereafter. It may be considered that the findings of these neurosurgeons may be explained by the fact that their patients were investigated by means of tests which were not capable of detecting disturbances of complex forms of behavior and activity.

Many clinical papers in the foreign literature have been devoted to the description of the psychopathology of frontal lesions. Leonora Welt (1883) described syndromes characteristic of a disturbance of the orbital cortex. These patients were restless, euphoric, and excessively talkative, or were, on the other hand, depressed. A loss of ethical standards was observed in these patients.

A case described by Zacher (1901) is not without interest. This patient became forgetful and lost all sense of time. He was lethargic, passive, indifferent, and displayed an extreme susceptibility to fatigue; at times he appeared euphoric and showed a tendency to facetiousness. He had no reactions to his illness or even to his blindness. This patient died, and necropsy revealed softening in both frontal lobes.

Poppelreiter (1918) described patients with wounds of the frontal lobe and pointed out that the most characteristic feature of these patients was their euphoric and at times almost puerile behavior. They never give the impression of suffering morally. These patients are readily distracted and their activity is disorganized. The work of Feuchtwanger (1923), based upon a large clinical material, also indicates that only a secondary weakening of the intellect is observed in frontal lesions.

Ferrier considers that loss of incentive is the main symptom of a lesion of the frontal lobes. It is because of this lack of motivation that the intellectual disturbances develop in these patients. Gruenthal reports histological findings in the case of 16 patients who died; in 12 of them he observed considerable changes in the frontal lobes. He came to the conclusion that a lesion of the orbital cortex gives rise to euphoria, disinhibition, and gross disturbances of behavior. Atrophic processes in the whole frontal system lead to loss of initiative, to lethargy and to disturbances of thought.

Rylander, in his monograph (1939), describes a pastor (under the care of Professor Olivecrona) who for a long time after removal of a tumor of the left frontal lobe showed no signs of the disease, although he jested at a friend's funeral.

With a large series of cases from World War I, Kleist (1934) studied the whole problem of cortical localization. He asserts that the lateral part of the frontal cortex is connected with psychomotor and intellectual functions, and the orbital cortex with the emotions. When he tries to tackle the interpretation of personality, however, he clearly betrays his own mechanistic and idealistic concepts. Kleist divides the personality into six "egos:" the sensual, the one of aspiration and desire, the corporal, the religious and philosophic, the personal, and the social. He localizes the personal and social "egos" in the orbital cortex.

Kleist's investigation thus combines a large series of clinically objective case studies on the problem of localization, with an obviously reactionary attempt to introduce dogma into science (the celebrated mystical "ego"). With true medieval scholasticism, he divides the human personality into six separate "egos." His clinical investigations are distorted by his attempt to mold the facts to fit his scholastic scheme.

We may now consider some of the work of Russian authors. In 1901 Korsakov wrote: "Mental diseases are, in their manifestations, essentially pathological disturbances of the personality, and by their localization they are essentially diseases of the forebrain."*

*S. S. Korsakov, Selected Works, p. 5. Moscow, Medgiz, 1954.

Korsakov expressed his views, which were progressive for the time, still more clearly in his paper "The Psychology of Microcephaly." In it he wrote that different types of ideas are formed in different divisions of the cerebral cortex — visual ideas in the occipital, auditory in the temporal, and spatial in the parietal. In the brain of the normal individual other special conditions must be present for these ideas to be combined in accordance with their meaning. These conditions are evidently found in the activity of certain divisions of the cortex. In Korsakov's opinion, these divisions are the frontal lobes. His argument in favor of the last statement was that the frontal lobes are particularly well developed in normal children and underdeveloped in microcephalics.

Bekhterev (1923) concluded from his investigations that the progressive increase in the size and weight of the frontal lobes as the phylogenetic ladder is ascended (from animals to man) is evidence of the relationship of these regions to the most important mental processes. With lesions of the frontal lobes Bekhterev believed that the leading symptom is not the intellectual impairment but the inability to concentrate.

Khoroshko (1936), challenging those workers who deny the significance of the frontal lobes in the organization and regulation of the higher mental processes, points out that careful investigations always reveal that the human brain has no silent areas, and that we are simply unable to discover their significance. From his investigations Khoroshko concludes that the most characteristic symptoms of a lesion of the frontal lobes are disturbances of behavior. These patients are impulsive and euphoric, and their behavior is inadequately motivated. It is especially common to find their power of active attention also disturbed. Following Korsakov's work on microcephalia, Khoroshko stresses that the maldevelopment of the frontal lobes in microcephalics, in association with the severe inadequacy of their mental functions, is proof of the importance of the frontal lobes in the development of the higher mental functions.

Gilyarovskii (1946) pointed out that the most characteristic symptoms of frontal lesions are childishness, lack of spontaneous activity, apathy and abulia. Gurevich (1949) reports that in traumatic lesions of the brain the following frontal syndromes may be observed: 1) apathicoabulic, 2) akinetic (absence of motive for movements), 3) affective character disturbances (irritability, fits of anger, instability of make-up, undisciplined behavior, loss of attention and memory, and feeble-mindedness as a result of the loss of frontal mechanisms). Psychopathological syndromes in lesions of the frontal lobes of the brain were also described by Yudin, Simson, Fridman, Ziman, and many others.

Clinical observations on patients with lesions of the frontal lobes of the brain have also been made by neurologists (Krol', Pines, Grinshtein, Mikheev, Sepp, Chlenov, et al.). Among the purely neurological disturbances are included the following symptoms: apraxia of movements of the trunk and limbs; weakness of the hands; nystagmus; a tendency to fall, or to past-point; disturbances of tone, sensation, and power. In all these neurological observations, however, considerable emphasis is placed on the mental disturbances.

In the Soviet literature several valuable pathopsychological investigations are reported. Attention should be drawn to the investigation of Pick's disease by Vygotskii, Birnbaum, and Samukhin (1934). From his study of a series of cases of atrophy of the cortical systems, Pick put forward the concept of a frontal type of dementia for this disease.

Under Luriya's direction, a series of investigations was carried out (Rubinshtein, Gadzhiev, Andreeva, Filipicheva, Spirin, Meshcheryakov, Ivanova) in which it was clearly shown that if a pathological lesion destroys the posterior divisions of the brain functional disturbances will appear in the clinical picture affecting visual and auditory analysis, writing, reading, and counting. Normal behavior, the ability to perform a complex, purposeful action, and a critical attitude towards the patient's own condition will however remain intact. With pathological lesions destroying the activity of the anterior divisions of the brain, however, visual and auditory analysis, speech, the technique of writing, reading, and counting are all preserved, but the behavior and purposeful activity of such patients become grossly disturbed. They are incapable of controlling their behavior and do not recognize their disability. They are easily distracted by chance stimuli and tend to forget what they are doing. Zeigarnik, who studied a large number of patients with frontal disturbances, reached the same conclusions.

All Soviet authors have given a very similar account of the psychopathological syndromes in frontal lesions; almost unanimously they accept the role and importance of the anterior divisions of the brain in the organization of the higher forms of human behavior and activity.

If we attempt to generalize the symptoms that are characteristic of frontal lesions, we shall easily be convinced that they consist mainly of three groups: 1) lethargy, akinesia, lack of spontaneous activity, a tendency towards stereotyped actions, perseveration, and a weakness of motivation; 2) disturbances in active attention and in the capacity for purposeful activity; 3) disturbances in the higher forms of human behavior, in thinking, and in the personality as a whole.

Our survey of the literature has included many facts characterizing both the changes in the behavior of animals after extirpation of the frontal cortex and the changes in all the complex forms of human behavior and activity as a result of trauma or neoplastic disease of the anterior divisions of the brain. We have been unable to find any data in the accessible literature, however, which would indicate the psychopathological features typical of maldevelopment of the anterior divisions of the cerebral cortex in children. In our view this represents a considerable handicap. A complete understanding of the role and importance of any cerebral system in the organization of complex and specifically human forms of activity is possible only by correlating lesions of the system with its functions.

We give below a few clinical observations on cases which cannot be classed as oligophrenia in the true sense of the term, but whose analysis very convincingly demonstrates the character of symptoms arising during lesions of the anterior divisions of the brain in children.

CASE 1

Borya Yu., boy aged 10 years, admitted to the children's department of the Institute of Neurosurgery on September 12, 1945. The boy suffered from sudden attacks of headache with vomiting. There were no abnormal hereditary factors.

Pregnancy and labor were normal. The child's early development was normal. His illnesses included erysipelas of the head at the age of six months, and measles complicated by otitis at three years. Until 1941 the boy was healthy and had developed normally. In November 1941 he first developed attacks of acute headache with vomiting once or twice a month, but after taking luminal he had no further attacks until 1943. One night in December of 1943 the patient had a severe attack of headache with vomiting accompanied by loss of consciousness, clonic convulsions of the left limbs and the left side of the face, and involuntary passage of urine. Except for these attacks the patient felt well, attended school and was a good student, was well disciplined, had a good grasp of situations, and was very greatly upset by the least failure in his studies. In January 1945 the patient's attacks of headache and vomiting grew worse, and he developed convulsions involving the left side, with occasional losses of consciousness. He was admitted to the Institute, where the following distinctive features were found. He had fits, usually without loss of consciousness, partial atrophy of the optic nerves from papilledema, but with well preserved vision. Skull hydrocephalic in shape, with calcification in the sellar region. Slight left-sided hemiparesis. X-ray changes and slight metabolic disturbances suggested that the pathological process was situated in the pituitary region. The appearance of focal epileptic fits, which began with spasms in the left half of the trunk, suggested that a tumor was growing upward and to the right, and was involving the wall of the lateral ventricle. The patient's mental state showed certain disturbances: he became euphoric, unrestrained, and his capacity for work decreased considerably.

On October 17, 1945, an operation was performed. An incision was made in the right frontal region. The fontanelles were not closed and the bone was thinned in places. The brain was tense, the gyri partially obliterated, and the vessels dilated. The brain tissue in the premotor area was separated by blunt dissection and a cystic cavity was found, which was filled with a xanthochromic fluid containing large numbers of cholesterol crystals and droplets of fat. The internal wall of the cavity was lined with a brownish capsule, and on the walls of the capsule were multiple white deposits. The cavity was filled with physiological saline.

The postoperative course was smooth and the patient was discharged fit and well. After discharge from the Institute he continued to attend school, but in the words of the teacher who had known the boy before operation, he was considerably changed. He had lost his ability to work, had difficulty in concentrating, and was unproductive, euphoric, and uncritical. In December 1946, while skating, the patient fell and, complaining of headache, vomiting, and inability to sleep, was readmitted to the Institute of Neurosurgery.

The patient was small in stature, dysplastic, short limbed, and underdeveloped for his age. His sexual development was that of a child of four or five. No abnormality of the internal organs was found.

In the right frontoparietal region there was a horseshoe-shaped postoperative scar. The bone flap was mobile. In the right half of the skull the posterior portion was more fully developed than on the left. Neurological examination revealed a number of special findings. Neck rigidity was present. A bilateral Kernig's sign and diffuse tenderness on percussion of the skull were elicited. Movements were full in range and uniformly diminished in power. Tests for adiadochokinesis showed greater clumsiness on the left. The tendon reflexes were diminished, especially the knee jerks. Spontaneous extension of the great toe was present, more marked on the left.

The optic disks showed considerable pallor and signs of stasis in the retinal veins. Visual acuity of the right eye 0.8, left 0.6. Slight limitation of abduction of both eyes. Otoneurological investigation revealed a disturbance of the vestibular apparatus at the level of the diencephalon with signs of increased intracranial pressure.

On December 29, 1946, cystography was carried out on the patient. Air, introduced into the cyst, filled its cavity, in the right frontal region and leaked into the posterior horn of the lateral ventricle.

The patient's mental state had appreciably deteriorated, and he appeared disinhibited, loquacious, and undisciplined. At times the patient's restlessness became marked. He would suddenly jump out of bed and laugh and joke incessantly. His remarks were accompanied by expressive gestures, mimicking movements, and laughter. The patient was uncritical, showed poor judgment, and asked a girl patient to marry him, saying that he had many fiancées. At times he would make some irrelevant statement, repeating word for word something that he had heard at home. When talking about anything he would laugh and joke and switch from one subject to another. He failed to grasp the meaning of a simple story. When doing problems he was unable to concentrate. The patient could not perform any complicated task. For instance, he was given a task consisting of two successive actions. He was quite incapable of carrying it out. Having started one operation, he lost its connection with the purpose of the task. Subsequently he began to perform random arithmetical operations, which then became completely irrational.

Gradually his mental state grew worse. He became dazed and lethargic. Against this background of lethargy, at times the patient became disinhibited. He would choose certain words, make rhymes with them, and show a tendency towards facetiousness. His restlessness increased, particularly at night.

The patient was admitted with signs of an aseptic meningitis arising as a result of rupture of a cyst of Rathke's pouch into the subarachnoid spaces. Examination of the cerebrospinal fluid confirmed the presence of large numbers of cholesterol crystals in the subarachnoid space. Gradually the pressure of the subarachnoid fluid fell and its composition returned to normal, but a marked increase in the intracranial pressure and loss of vision were observed.

A second operation was performed on the patient. An incision was made in the right frontoparietal region. The dura mater was distended and there was no pulsation of the brain. After opening the dura mater an enormous cyst was found, filling the whole anterior cranial fossa.

Whitish plaques were present on the walls of the cavity. The right frontal lobe was completely absent. The left frontal lobe was atrophied in its superomedial divisions. The posteroinferior wall of the cavity at the site of the right frontal lobe consisted of a thin, transparent membrane, separating the cavity of the cyst from the cavity of the ventricle. The region of the chiasma was inspected. A slightly thickened optic nerve was found, situated in the thickness of the membrane of the cyst. Lateral to the left optic nerve a cyst was opened, evidently situated in the residual basal divisions of the left frontal lobe. At the base of the large cyst filling the anterior cranial fossa, corresponding to the right and medial divisions of the left frontal lobe, a swollen, dark red tissue was detected, which was abundantly vascularized.

The postoperative course was serious. The patient was mentally lethargic, made spontaneous movements, did not react to his surroundings or initiate any activity. His feet were outstretched, and a flexion contracture of the ankle joints was observed. There were no active movements of the legs or of the left arm. In the right upper extremity there was only active flexion of the fingers. In the left upper extremity involuntary movements of athetoid type were present. The tone of the lower extremities was sharply increased.

The patient's condition gradually improved, and he was discharged on April 29, 1949. He was examined twice for follow-up purposes.

The patient was now amaurotic, when he turned to the side a protrusion was noted in the right frontal region, and he showed marked pituitary dwarfism. He was in high spirits, voluble in speech, and thanked everybody in a loud voice. When he was asked how he felt, he answered, "What a man I was, even if I was upset. God created suffering and it must be accepted, but whether I have sinned or not, God only knows." The patient was evidently repeating word for word what his mother had said to his grandmother about the boy's condition. He soothed his mother and told her not to worry.

"I am doing all right. I am the best boy in Zvenigorod, and my behavior has never been bad." When the doctor asked the patient a few questions to test the level of development of his thinking, the boy began to joke and make silly remarks saying, "What do you think you are doing, trying to trick me, because I am going to fool you instead and piss pure water." The patient was uncritical and showed no reaction to his blindness. He spoke volubly and eagerly. He would suddenly take it upon himself to sing and dance, which was quite out of place in the situation.

Only elementary generalization was within the boy's capacity, and he could not perform a single problem even though he grasped its meaning. For instance, he was asked to add seven to five. He could not solve this problem and answered "six," and to all similar questions he thereafter gave the same stereotyped answer. His blindness made him quite incapable of doing writing exercises. In his mother's words, the patient behaved well, nothing made him angry, and he was on the whole responsive and manageable.

Clinical Analysis of the Case

In this case we are concerned with a tumor of Rathke's pouch, with subsequent formation of cysts in the frontal region. A second operation showed almost complete absence of the right frontal lobe and the atrophy of the left frontal lobe in its medial portion. Dynamic observation of the boy showed disintegration of his capacity for purposeful activity. It will be recalled that before the onset of the disease the patient was a successful pupil in regular school. With no less clarity this case also demonstrates the disintegration of complex forms of behavior, which had reached an adequate level of development in this boy before the onset of the disease.

The gradual disintegration and deterioration of the specifically human, complex forms of activity and behavior thus correlated with the increase in the atrophic processes in the frontal divisions of the cerebral cortex.

CASE 2

Patient Yulya M., a girl aged 13 years. She was admitted to the Institute of Neurosurgery in 1938, complaining of headache attacks, accompanied by vomiting and convulsions. The girl was born at term and developed normally. Before reaching school age, she grew into a lively, active, and disciplined child. She was well developed intellectually. From eight years of age she began to attend school, where she was a well behaved and responsive student. Before the onset of her illness the girl took good care of her brother and sister, was diligent, and well organized.

At nine years of age the girl began to have attacks of headache with vomiting, but these did not interfere with her studies. At the age of 13 years the attacks became more frequent and began to be accompanied by profuse vomiting and convulsions. Two months before her admission to the Institute of Neurosurgery the girl developed increased thirst and periodically increased appetite.

During observation of the patient in the Institute incontinence of urine was found. She was disorientated, saying that she was in Noginsk and mistaking the doctor for her school teacher. Examination of the nervous system showed facial asymmetry, partial obliteration of the right nasolabial fold and exophthalmos on the left side. Severe bilateral papilledema was present, with hemorrhages on the left side. Visual acuity of the right eye 0.4, left 0.5. The limb muscles showed a diffuse lowering of tone. Left knee jerk diminished. Oppenheim's sign constant on the left, and Babinski's sign positive on both sides.

Taking all these findings into consideration, it seemed likely that a tumor was present in the diencephalic region, close to the third ventricle. On May 17, 1938, operation was performed. A flap of muscle and bone was formed in the region of the left frontal lobe. The exposed dura mater was not tense. The dura was opened, the brain was not pulsating, but was soft, and deep fluctuation was present. As a result of a puncture in the region of the pole of the frontal lobe, at a depth of 4-5 cm a turbid greenish fluid was found by aspiration. A transverse incision, 3 cm long, was then made across the pole, By blunt dissection of the brain substance, at a depth of 4-5 cm an accumulation of greenish-yellow fluid was found, contained in a transparent jelly-like capsule. The contents of the cyst were removed. The operation was then concluded.

The postoperative course was uncomplicated. The patient was discharged in a satisfactory condition. In her mother's words, soon after the operation the girl gradually began to change: from being diligent and able to work, she became absentminded, unstable, and impatient in her work, and she would never finish what she was doing. She became rude; she would start a fight for no reason; she could not control herself; she ceased to be shy and would go out into the street wearing only a petticoat. Her mother did not recognize her daughter.

The patient's headaches became more severe and were accompanied by vomiting. Bilateral choked disks were observed, changing to atrophy. An associated bitemporal hemianopsia and metabolic disturbances were attributed to the accumulation of fluid in the left frontal lobe and to the growth of the tumor itself.

The girl could remember many poems and songs, and could solve simple arithmetical problems without much difficulty. She could not concentrate for long on her school work, because she was distracted by everything going on around her, and she introduced into her conversation words which she chanced to hear. She was disinhibited, euphoric, and garrulous, and at times sarcastic and aggressive. She was uncritical of herself and considered that life was very jolly. The girl was high spirited and inclined to joking and facetiousness.

In a second operation on this patient a multilocular cyst was found in the left frontal lobe, the walls of which consisted of a mass of felt-like material, in some places white and in others brown. At a site corresponding to the third ventricle there was a massive tumor the size of a hen's egg. Biopsy showed that this was an epidermoid cyst with keratinization and calcification. The postoperative course was smooth and the patient was discharged feeling well.

Three months later the patient was admitted for the third time to the Institute of Neurosurgery, with severe mental changes. She exhibited incontinence of urine, impulsive actions, and complete loss of her ability to work.

The patient was retarded in her physical development. The internal organs showed no abnormality. Examination of the nervous system showed: the pupillary reaction to light was diminished, to convergence brisk. Bilateral papilledema, changing to atrophy, was present. Visual acuity of the right eye 0.5, left 0.1. A uniform, general and diffuse lowering of muscle power was present. Kernig's sign was slightly positive on both sides. During Romberg's test, the patient swayed to both sides. Tendon reflexes could be elicited. Pathological reflexes observed included a positive Babinski, Oppenheim, and Gordon sign on both sides. A spontaneous Babinski was often observed in this patient.

Otoneurological examination of this patient showed a dissociated diminution of hearing. A disturbance of otokinetic nystagmus was present, with a tendency for this to lapse in an upward direction. Diadochokinesis was present on both sides and caloric excitability was absent bilaterally. The above-mentioned findings indicate that the lesion was localized in the region of the third ventricle.

At times the patient was drowsy, lethargic and indifferent.

Sometimes she fell into a semicomatose state, when she would wet her bed, saying that she was completely unaware of what was happening to her. At other times she was euphoric, uncritical, and merry, quite forgetting the severity of her condition. Her purposeful activity was severely deranged and her capacity for thinking was markedly impaired.

On March 2, 1939, a third operation was performed on the patient. A tumor was found in the depth of the pole of the left frontal lobe. Resection of the cavity of the left frontal lobe was performed. In the frontal bone itself there was a thin-walled cyst filled with a greenish fluid. The tumor occupied the base of the whole frontal lobe, the whole of the middle cranial fossa on the left side and the region of the sella turcica, spreading to the right. During mobilization of the brain substance over the tumor, a fluid resembling pus was found.

After aspiration of the fluid the cavity of the dilated right lateral ventricle was found, at the bottom of which could be seen the upper wall of the optic thalamus. The part of the tumor occupying the base of the frontal lobe was removed. The area of the tumor in the region of the sella turcica, leading to the left posterior cranial fossa, was left in situ. The postoperative course was severe. On March 18, following a rise of temperature, generalized convulsions, and cardiac failure, the patient died.

The postmortem findings showed a tumor of the base of the brain of the type of a tumor of Rathke's pouch, which had spread into the third ventricle and both frontal lobes. The tumor contained numerous cysts. The right hemisphere was enlarged. The cerebral gyri were flattened. An abscess was present in the region of the pole of the left frontal lobe. Suppurative ependymitis and serous cerebrospinal meningitis were present. The pituitary was atrophic.

Clinical Analysis of the Case

This case which has just been described has much in common with the preceding case. It concerns a tumor of Rathke's pouch with subsequent cyst formation in the frontal lobes. The Rathke's pouch tumor is known to be a congenital tumor, which for a certain period in its course gives rise to no symptoms, particularly so far as psychopathological manifestations are concerned. In both cases the children were making good progress at school.

The first symptoms in both cases consisted of attacks of headache accompanied by vomiting. Their capacity for work then began to be affected; for example Yulya M., hitherto a diligent and attentive girl, became absent-minded and inattentive, and made mistakes in her writing, arithmetic, and reading.

The pattern was similar in many other cases under our observation. Disturbance of the capacity for work is a general symptom and is associated with the growth of the tumor and its situation, with the disturbances of the cerebrospinal fluid circulation, and the vascular changes. The deterioration in the patients' capacity for work was sufficiently well marked. They could not concentrate on anything, they were extremely absent-minded, and they introduced into their conversation whatever they heard from people around them. The power of thought, the regulation of behavior, and purposeful activity were all subsequently affected.

These clinical cases convincingly demonstrate that the dynamic functional derangements affecting thought, behavior and activity resulted from the growth of a tumor, with subsequent cyst formation, in the frontal region. Evidence that the frontal system was the one most affected was verified.

* * *

Having indicated the role and importance of the frontal systems in the organization of complex forms of behavior and activity, let us now turn to a description of oligophrenic children with a defect of their frontal systems.

CASE 1

Gera D., a boy of 16 years, under our observation since 1937. He was admitted to the children's department of the Institute of Neurosurgery with a complaint of mental backwardness and paresis of the whole of the right half of his trunk. There were no abnormal hereditary factors.

History. The patient's mother sustained a fall during the fifth month of pregnancy and injured her abdomen, as a result of which she developed hemorrhage for several days. The patient's birth weight was 7.4 pounds, and he was born with atrophy of the right upper extremity, in a state of flexion. His subsequent development was slow. From the age of six months he began to have spasms of the right upper limb. Until the age of nine months he did not recognize anybody. He took toys with his left hand, but did so aimlessly and without purpose and then only when the toys were held out to him; he never reached for them himself. At the age of nine months the boy was sent to the N. N. Burdenko Surgical Clinic. Burdenko himself performed an operation in the course of which a cyst of considerable size was found in the depth of the left frontal lobe. Its position was such that the surgeon had to resect the entire pole of the left frontal lobe. The operation was carried out when the boy was nine months old. After the operation the mother observed a distinct improvement in the child's condition: the convulsions ceased, the child became more active, and he made attempts to grasp objects situated at at distance from him.

He began to walk at 18 months and to talk at two years, but he stammered badly. At three or four years of age it became clear that the boy differed in his development from normal children of his age. For instance, on the one hand, his memory was good, and his speech developed relatively rapidly, he could appreciate musical themes and learn poetry, and subsequently he memorized individual letters. On the other hand, he took no part in games. When he played all he did was to take any toy or simple piece of string and trail it behind him for hours from one corner of a room to the next. He often found pieces of paper, tore them into small pieces, and stuffed them into chairs and cupboards.

Once he started an activity he would stick with it: if he took a rope or duster in his hand he would let go only reluctantly. His development was characterized by a disturbance in purposeful activity, taking place in a setting in which individual operations were relatively well preserved. At nine years of age the patient was readmitted to the children's department of the Institute of Neurosurgery, where a detailed investigation was carried out.

Physical State. In the left fronto-parietal region there was a horseshoe-shaped scar. On palpation it was found that the anterior portion of the bone was fixed, but that the posterior, parietal portion showed fairly free ballottement, rising and falling with pressure. No abnormality of the internal organs was observed.

State of the Nervous System. The pupillary reactions were brisk, convergence was stable and there was no nystagmus. The face was asymmetrical: the right half of the face was smaller, and the tone of the muscles of facial expression was much weaker on the right. All the muscles of the right upper limb showed diffuse atrophy, slightly more marked in the distal end of the limb. Diffuse muscle atrophy was also seen in the right lower limb. Active movements in the right upper limb showed a distal type of disturbance. No movements were present in the hand and fingers. Extension of the toes was absent. The tone of the limbs was increased on the right side. Positive Babinski, Oppenheim and Gordon signs were observed on the right. On the left side flexion of the digits was observed during these tests. The patient was steady during Romberg's test and there was no impairment of sensation. The neurological investigation revealed a combination of brainstem nystagmus and vestibular nystagmus with experimental dissociation.

Ophthalmological Examination. Visual acuity in the right eye 0.6, left eye 0.6. Optic fundus normal (temporal part of the right disk paler than on the left).

Otorhinolaryngological Examination. Hearing within normal limits.

X-ray Examination of the Skull. X-ray examination indicated the presence of a postoperative defect in the left frontoparietal region. The bone flap in this situation was small in size and its edges were smooth and thinned.

Mental State. The patient was sociable and at times excited, exhibiting motor restlessness, at other times lethargic and passive. He was neat and tidy, ate unaided, was well orientated, and did not lose his way in the ward. Experiments conducted on the boy showed that he had no disturbance of visual perception. He had a good spontaneous memory, and could remember poems. The patient had no disturbance in spatial integration, and he could easily copy fairly complicated figures from a pattern shown to him. He recognized without difficulty the number of elements in a given figure. He easily understood what was said to him. The relative integrity of his mental processes stood out against the background of a considerable disturbance in his activity and behavior. The patient did not mix with other children nor take part in games, and his sociability was often limited to the operation of taking away other children's toys. His usual occupation was to run along the corridors for hours on end, and efforts to direct him into prolonged and rational play were always doomed to failure. It was discovered from a series of experiments that the boy's complex actions, when broken down into their component parts, were not joined together into a single dynamic scheme. Gera could not contain his action within the limits of an original plan; some of the links of the action became detached from the chain as a whole. He could not cope with tasks in which the individual operations were separated in time; in these cases the intermediate links were easily lost from the general plan and became independent. For instance, in a situation in which he had to fetch a broom lying at the other end of the room, and then use this broom to reach a ball, Gera would run for the broom, but would then begin to sweep the floor with it. He did not use it as a means of solving the problem which had been set.

The patient could not master reading, which demands some degree of organization and fixation. He could not count and he had no concept of numbers. His activity soon became stereotyped. Perseverations were substituted for rational actions. He was lacking in the active imagination typical of his age, and he often replaced it by verbal cliches which he had learned elsewhere. It was difficult to detach him from a mechanical activity which he had started and switch him to something new.

After his discharge from the Institute of Neurosurgery, the patient was educated at a special school. In his behavior he showed little activity. He could not understand the attitude of those around him towards himself, and he was uncritical.

From the age of 13 years the patient again developed epileptic fits. He was admitted for this symptom to a psychiatric clinic. During his period of education at the special school the boy learned elementary skills: he wrote neatly and in a good hand, he read fairly well and solved simple arithmetical problems. Outwardly he became more correct and he learned some of the rules of school conduct. It was soon found, however, that the patient was uncritical towards himself and that he could not be made to develop a proper attitude towards his failures. The patient reacted with extreme emotional instability. His purposeful activity was disturbed. When writing from dictation he would suddenly introduce something quite unconnected with the subject. He refused to motivate these unwarranted intrusions. When solving arithmetical problems he easily drifted into reciting his tables, and obviously became detached from the plan of the task.

Clinical Analysis of the Case

In this particular case the etiological factor is capable of precise definition: a traumatic cyst in the left frontal region. At the age of nine months the whole of the left frontal lobe was extirpated. The whole of the patient's subsequent development follows from this defect. The distinctive neurological features, namely the presence of a right-sided hemiparesis, with the signs of maldevelopment of the right upper limb, the character of the epileptic fit, which usually began with a spasm in the right hand, followed by turning the head to the right — all these may be accounted for by changes at the site of the operation. The onset of a series of epileptic fits is possibly connected with the presence of scarring at the same site. In this case we are concerned with the analysis of the pattern of this patient's development and of the structure of his defect, in view of the fact that from the age of nine months his left frontal lobe was removed. In this particular case, therefore, an early pathological lesion of the frontal systems led to a distinctive form of mental defect.

Our patient, for instance, learned to speak without difficulty, he showed no appreciable disturbances of elementary perception, he possessed a fairly well developed ability for memorization with help, and he mastered comparatively easily the technique of reading, writing, and elementary calculation. He did not, however, incorporate all these skills into useful, rational and purposeful activity, so that his behavior was predominantly automatic, with superfluous excursions, and not subservient to any rational, intrinsic plan.

In this case we thus have the most convincing proof that the maldevelopment of the complex and specifically human forms of mental activity and of the personality as a whole is due basically to extirpation of the left frontal region at the age of nine months.

CASE 2

Volodya Z., a boy aged 10 years. He was first admitted to the children's department of the Kashchenko Hospital on October 9, 1943 and was subsequently readmitted many times. There were no abnormal hereditary factors.

History. The boy was born, from a first pregnancy, in a state of profound asphyxia. He nursed poorly and hardly cried. Talking and walking were not delayed.

At the age of two years the boy had measles, complicated by pneumonia. The disease was accompanied by meningeal manifestations. After his illness, Volodya developed lethargy and drowsiness. At five years of age, besides his general lethargy, the boy showed a tendency to wander. He would go away from home for no reason, and was often brought back by the police. He had to be removed from kindergarten because of his peculiar behavior. He paid no attention to the organized kindergarten activities, asked silly questions, laughed for no reason, etc. In this same period he began to develop compulsive movements of the head and hands. At seven years of age the boy easily learned to read. He had a good rote memory, easily learning poetry or stories by heart, but he had a poor grasp of what he had read, and at the same time he completely failed to understand the attitude of those around him towards himself: when children laughed at him, he at first laughed with them. Volodya could not play with other children, for he could not learn the rules of the game. He carried out all his duties without question. He never took anything without asking. His mother never heard him say "I don't want," "I can't," or "I won't." At the age of seven years, the patient began to study at a special school. Because of his tendency to wander, he was admitted to the clinic.

Physical State. The boy was of medium build, with a small head (circumference of the head 45 cm). His skin was pale. The usual groups of peripheral glands were palpable. The left cervical glands were slightly enlarged and firm to the touch. The internal organs showed no abnormality.

State of the Nervous System. Eyes exophthalmic. Anisocoria (R L). Reaction to light brisk. Very slight divergent strabismus. During convergence the patient's right eye deviated to the right. In the extreme positions of the eyes, nystagmus was observed. Full range of movements of the eyes present. Face asymmetrical, the right corner of the mouth being slightly depressed. He did not bite properly, the lower jaw protruding slightly during this operation. Tendon reflexes were elicited and no pathological reflexes were present.

Ophthalmological Examination. Visual acuity of the right eye 1.0, left 0.3, as a result of myopic astigmatism. Optic fundus normal.

Otorhinolaryngological Examination. Hearing within normal limits.

Laboratory Investigations. On lumbar puncture the CSF pressure was normal. Proteins 0.165%, cells 2/3, all protein reactions negative. Wassermann reaction of the blood and cerebrospinal fluid negative. Blood and urine analyses normal.

Results of Pneumoencephalography. On January 23, 1947, 85 cm^3 of cerebrospinal fluid was withdrawn and 90 cm^3 of air injected. Pressure 420 cm. The air penetrated into the slightly dilated ventricles and into the subarachnoid spaces. The ventricles were symmetrically placed. The third ventricle was slightly widened. A small fifth ventricle was also present (a developmental anomaly). The subarachnoid spaces in the parietal region were clearly filled. The pneumoencephalographic findings indicated an ill-defined internal hydrocephalus and a developmental anomaly of the brain (a fifth ventricle).

Electroencephalography. This investigation was carried out in the physiological laboratory of the N. N. Burdenko Institute of Neurosurgery. Recordings of the action potentials of the brain showed the α-rhythm to be absent in all regions of both hemispheres. Rapid asynchronous waves were recorded, more marked in the right hemisphere. Diffuse pathological delta-waves were present, more marked in the anterior divisions of the hemispheres. The EEG indicated general cerebral functional changes in the electrical activity of the cortex, with signs of irritation, more marked in the frontal divisions (Fig. 51).

Mental State. Consciousness was clear, and elementary orientation preserved. The patient knew the month, the date, the year, and the place where his mother worked.

His motor function was of a distinctive pattern. His movements were sweeping and disorganized. Many superfluous and unnecessary movements were observed. When the patient laughed, all kinds of grimaces would spread over his face. On such occasions he would rub his hands together and jump up and down in a foolish manner. Volodya was particularly inept at carrying out purposeful actions. His hands were extremely helpless, and he dropped things. When doing organized rhythmic exercises his motor activity followed the same pattern. He was confused, often continuing out of sheer inertia movements that should have been finished earlier. His vocabulary was rich, but he spoke in memorized clichés. The character of this patient's speech was noteworthy: each word was pronounced jerkily and separately, which gave the impression of scanned speech. The patient read well and wrote correctly, could easily cope with simple arithmetic, and could solve simple problems unaided. His mechanical memory was adequately developed. The patient could continue to perform mechanical work for a long time.

Experimental psychological investigation showed a maldevelopment of cognitive functions. The boy could not find the theme running

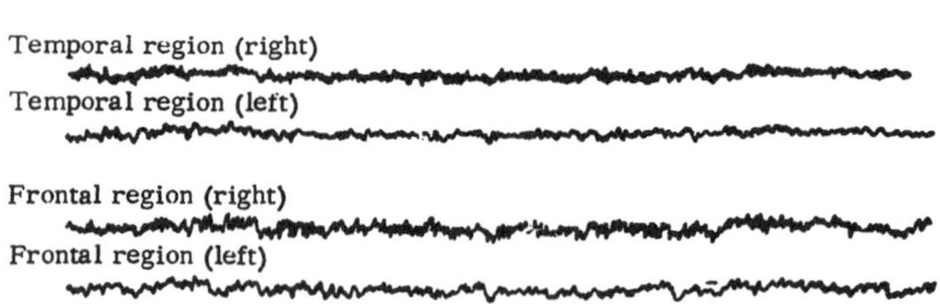

Fig. 51. Volodya Z., aged 10 years (oligophrenia, degree of feeble-mindedness). The α-rhythm is ill defined in all regions of both hemispheres. In the temporal and frontal regions of the cortex rapid asynchronous waves are recorded, indicating irritation, and these are especially well marked in the frontal divisions.

through a series of pictures, and he did not understand a story with a hidden meaning. In a picture classification experiment he revealed a maldevelopment of the generalizing function of speech. During the investigation of the individual cortical functions, the complete preservation of visual and spatial integration and of the motor and sensory aspects of speech was established.

Definite and gross disturbances were found during investigation of the motor analyzer; upon command he could not perform certain tasks involving postural and dynamic movements.

The boy was polite and considerate. He had some idea of the rules of good behavior. Before entering the doctor's office he knocked at the door, greeted the doctor courteously, and asked permission to sit, but would not actually sit down as long as somebody in the room was standing, explaining that children should not sit in the presence of adults. When he was asked a question, he immediately jumped up, raised his hand, and replied. Having given his reply he did not immediately resume his seat, but waited for permission to do so. The boy greeted the doctor repeatedly each time he entered his office.

The patient was usually lethargic and showed little spontaneous activity. He did everything he was asked. In any situation he could be made to sing, dance, or recite. He could be interrupted when engaged on any task, or he could be shunted from one form of activity to another. When this happened he did not protest, but merely submitted automatically. Volodya had no judgment towards a situation, for he did not understand it and could not make allowances for it. Feelings of fear, desire or embarrassment were alien to him. He was not offended, for he did not understand the attitude of those around him towards himself. He had exactly the same feelings towards the doctor treating him that he would have to any person who chanced to come into the department. He was indifferent towards other children. He was pleased to see his mother, but this reaction was shown only when his mother was actually in his field of vision. For instance, when the boy was summoned into the doctor's office soon after the beginning of his mother's visit, he behaved just as usual, and showed no desire whatever to go back to his mother. When left by himself he remained lethargic, inactive and disinclined to spontaneous activity. Subsequent follow-up observations on the boy did show the development of some feeling of sensitivity or anger, but these reactions were automatic and of very short duration.

Clinical Analysis of the Case

The etiology of this case is complex. The presence of a marked microcephaly, a history of backwardness from earliest childhood, together with the pneumoencephalographic findings (the presence of a fifth ventricle) suggest an intrauterine lesion of the central nervous system. A series of severe physical illnesses subsequently complicated the child's development. Before reaching school age the distinctive features of the psychopathological structure of his disability were already apparent.

His mental processes remain sufficiently well preserved, but meanwhile there is maldevelopment of all that determines the development of the personality – motives, drives, activity, purpose, and rational behavior. At school age Volodya was sent to a special school. At this time the discrepancy between the preservation of a series of skills (reading, writing, calculation) and the maldevelopment of the more complex and specifically human forms of activity became even more obvious. The foregoing findings, in conjunction with the maldevelopment of his cognitive functions, suggest that in this particular case, against a background of a lesion of the whole cortex, disturbances involving its anterior divisions stand out more prominently. This view is confirmed not only by the distinctive psychopathological picture, but also by the characteristic maldevelopment of the whole of the boy's motor activity.

It may be remembered that this boy showed no pareses nor paralyses, but at the same time he could not make use of his available motor capacities. This suggests that the lesion affects mainly the cortical end of the motor analvzer.

The electroencephalographic findings also confirm the greater degree of involvement of the anterior divisions. During the investigation of the cortical rhythm, irritation phenomena developed, and these were most obvious in the frontal divisions of the cerebral cortex.

Taken as a whole, the findings obtained support the view that this case should be classified with the variant or type of oligophrenia now being discussed.

CASE 3

Vova B., a boy aged 12 years. This boy has been under our observation for six years. He was admitted three times to the children's department of the Kashchenko Hospital because of excessive talkativeness, improper behavior, and lack of progress in his studies.

History. For 15 years his mother suffered from syphilis and she was under surveillance at the venereal disease dispensary. Her blood Wassermann reaction was strongly positive. Our patient was born during her second marriage. The father suffered from epileptic fits after sustaining a concussion. Before the concussion he had complained of persistent headaches. The father's blood Wassermann was negative, and there was no history of syphilis in the father's family. The patient's mother had seven pregnancies. From the first pregnancy a son was born who died on the ninth day. From the second pregnancy a son, now 19 years old, was born, with a strongly positive Wassermann reaction and keratitis of both eyes, which had improved considerably after specific treatment. From the third pregnancy a daughter was born, who died from sepsis at the age of 15 months. From the fourth pregnancy a daughter was born, now 15 years old, who at an early age contracted meningitis, and who was severely retarded. She had finished her studies at a special school, and was now beginning to complain of persistent headaches. Her blood Wassermann was negative. The fifth and sixth pregnancies ended in abortion. Our patient was born from the seventh pregnancy.

The course of this pregnancy was difficult: his mother had repeated hemorrhages and attacks of syncope. Labor took place at term and the child cried immediately. His birth weight was normal, the skin clear, and he took the breast well, He had to be bottle fed, however, because his mother was short of milk. He cut his first teeth at four months, began to walk at about two years and to talk during his second year. In early childhood he was alert and active. At preschool age his speech was well developed. Vova remembered everything well and his parents observed nothing abnormal in the boy's behavior. The patient had bilateral cataract, for which he had undergone four operations.

When five years old Vova was sent to a kindergarten, where his backwardness was at once recognized. Vova was completely uninterested in toys, took no part in children's games, and was unable to learn poetry or songs taught him by the teacher. At seven years of age the boy began to attend regular school, but after two months his mother suggested removing him because he seemed incapable of learning. He could not memorize a single letter because of his inability to concentrate. He did not understand the school rules. He would deliberately walk out of his classes, and would ask silly questions. At eight years of age Vova was transferred to a special school, but even there was a backward student.

Physical State. The patient was dysplastic, with some degree of retardation of general physical development. No abnormality of his internal organs was found.

State of the Nervous System. The left eyeball was smaller than the right. There was a ptosis of the left eyelid and a severe deformity of the pupils (postoperative coloboma). Pupillary reaction to light was prompt. Convergence was incomplete. No nystagmus and present. The right angle of the mouth seemed weaker when showing the teeth. The tongue was in midline. Swallowing and phonation were normal. No gross disorder of the motor sphere was found: no ataxia nor pareses. Movements of facial expression were dissociated and motor activity inadequate. Muscle tone poor. Kernig's and Lasser's signs negative. The left hand was more active. He hopped better on the left foot. Tendon reflexes were brisk. Oppenheim's sign inconstant on the right. Cutaneous and abdominal reflexes present. Cremasteric reflex absent. No sensory changes. Autonomic vasomotor reactions were brisk. Acromicria and hypoplasia of the genitalia present. Slight deposition of fat on the abdomen of hypogenital type.

X-ray Examination. No change seen in the bones of the vault of the skull and the sella turcica.

Laboratory Investigations. Examination of the cerebrospinal fluid: protein 0.132%, cells 3/3. All protein reactions negative. Ventricular CSF: cells 5/3, protein 0.165. All protein reactions negative.

Pneumoencephalography. CSF pressure 390 mm. Air penetrated into the ventricles and subarachnoid spaces. Little air in the ventricles, but there was a considerable accumulation of air in the cisterna pontis. Subarachnoid spaces wide and atrophic, more especially marked in the frontal divisions.

On account of the poor filling of the ventricles with air, it was impossible to judge the state of the ventricular system. Evidence of adhesions seen in the subarachnoid spaces.

Ophthalmological Examination. Defects of the iris in both eyes after cataract operations.

Otorhinolaryngological Examination. Hearing within normal limits.

Electroencephalography. No α -rhythm present on the electroencephalogram. In all regions of the cortex rapid waves were recorded, and these were more marked in the frontal divisions. The EEG showed gross abnormalities, with evidence of severe irritation in the anterior divisions. The presence of rapid waves in the temporal and frontal divisions suggested involvement of the diencephalofrontal systems (Fig. 52).

Investigation of the Higher Nervous Activity. During investigation of the motor reactions to a direct spoken command, superfluous movements of a perseverative character were extremely prominent. The motor conditioned reactions were very poorly stabilized.

Simple conditioned connections were easily formed (after one or two combinations), and simple differentiation was formed equally rapidly. Even after the production of differentiation, a wide generalization of stimuli was observed.

Verbal projections of the formation of simple connections were adequate, but they incorporated many irrelevant expressions. The production of more complex forms of differentiation (for example, differentiation by duration) was difficult (although such forms of differentiation were produced more rapidly at a second trial). During the establishment of these forms of differentiation, speech reactions were included. After differentiation had been established, an increase in the duration of the differential stimulus led to a marked deterioration in the quality of the differentiation. A similar deterioration was also observed when the other conditions of application of the stimuli were changed.

In verbal projections and during the establishment of complex forms of differentiation gross inertia of the old verbal connections were revealed. Projections of past experiments, collected at the beginning of each investigation, were especially defective.

During the establishment of complex forms of differentiation, no improvement in the verbal projection took place even in those cases when a new stimulus, applied to a different analyzer, was used as conditioned stimulus. In many oligophrenic children, such substitution of the conditioned stimulus leads to a considerable improvement in the verbalization of the connections. In individual cases it leads to a general refusal to answer questions.

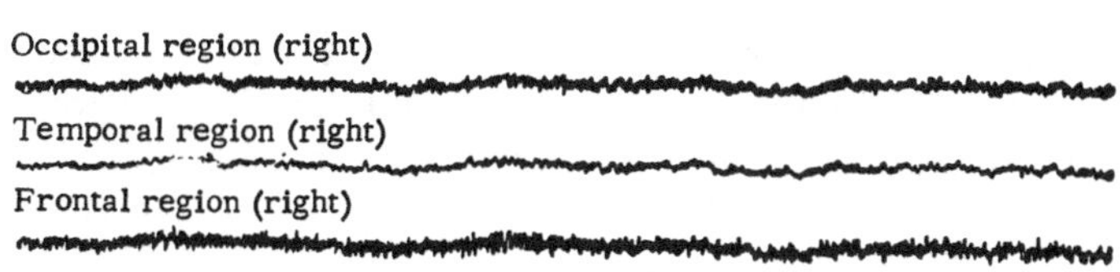

Fig. 52. Vova B., aged 12 years (oligophrenia, degree of imbecility). In all regions of the cortex rapid waves are recorded, especially marked in the frontal divisions.

After a verbal projection of the production of differentiation by duration had been obtained, the boy sometimes gave a projection which was directly opposite to the actual significance of the stimuli.

The speech reactions which were incorporated during the establishment of complex forms of differentiation were subjected to the development of inertia in the course of the experiment, as a result of which gross perseverations were observed. For instance, during the production of a conditioned reaction to every third light stimulus, the word "Don't," spoken by the child during the action of the negatively reinforced stimuli, was repeated with increasing frequency.

After a preliminary verbal instruction, simple conditioned connections were formed readily, although in these conditions the verbal projection could be imperfect. During the formation of more complicated systems of connections by verbal instruction, a very marked discrepancy was observed between the connections as they were formed, their projection, and the possibility of reproducing the instruction: connections were formed, but the boy offered a completely inadequate verbal projection of them, although he could repeat the instructions if required to do so. In many cases the instruction, when reproduced, was replaced by some previous verbal stereotype. In certain cases no differentiation could be established, although reproduction of the instruction continued to be satisfactory.

During the establishment of differential complex stimuli in accordance with the number of elements contained in them, gross disturbances of delayed inhibition were found. He had difficulty mastering conflicting instructions, such as, "Press twice if there are three signals and press three times to two signals." He could not cope with this problem: the reactions to all the signals became identical.

The findings described indicate that, besides the disturbances of higher nervous activity observed in all oligophrenics, this particular case showed gross disturbances of the dynamics of the nervous process in the motor analyzer, together with a severe defect of verbalization of the connections that were established, although speech was formally well developed. The formation of connections and the regulation of motor reactions in response to verbal instruction were severely disturbed.

Mental State. Consciousness was clear. Elementary orientation to the environment was intact. The patient's motor activity was markedly impaired, and all his movements were clumsy, awkward, and undifferentiated. His hands were especially helpless, and he frequently let things slip from them.

Investigation of the optic analyzer showed that Vova correctly recognized and named pictures shown to him both rightside up and upside down. There was no appreciable disturbance of spatial integration, as he could compose figures from specimens shown to him. The boy fully understood what was said to him, and could correctly repeat correlated phonemes. His articulation was also adequately developed.

During the investigation of individual cortical functions, gross disturbances were discovered only within the limits of the motor analyzer. Vova could not imitate positions of the hands shown to him, and he was even less able to cope with problems of dynamic movement.

Experimental psychological investigation revealed a severe maldevelopment of cognitive functions. The boy's behavior reflected an obvious distortion of personality. Vova entered the doctor's office with an air of importance, greeted the doctor politely, bowed slightly, and then folded his arms. He was outwardly clean and tidy, with a delicate skin, a fresh complexion, and shining eyes. At first glance he seemed alert and well-spoken and in fact gave the impression of being a normal child. This deceptive impression, however, was quickly dispelled. Vova correctly told his age, but when asked how old he would be in two years, he would nod his head sedately and reply with satisfaction, "Nineteen." He was not at all embarrassed when told that his answer was wrong, and he quickly switched to his usual behavior, which was imitative in character. Vova, in imitation of the departmental head, said, "I have now put out eight wall newspapers, but my work is held up by delay in getting copy. L. M. promised a paragraph, but does nothing about it, does not even think about it, and I shall not go to her on bended knees." He then took pen and paper and pretended to write, protesting when he was interrupted. He handed his scribblings to the doctor and begged him not to show them to anybody, but immediately showed them himself to the senior physician, who had just entered. The doctor tried to discourage the boy by showing him that he had been scribbling and not writing, but he did not respond to this. He just jumped up and down, tapped himself on the forehead, and continued his discourse. "Oh, sir, why am I sitting with you when I should be producing my newspaper?" With a portentous air, he then stalked out of the room.

When he was attending kindergarten, he often imitated the behavior of the superintendent of that institution, and said, "We must carry out our orders as quickly as possible. I was not satisfied with today's menu. I opened the attendance register and what do you think I found there? Instead of my name there was B. (the boy's surname). Two or three weeks passed, and still nothing happened." When imitating his father (the boy's father worked in a technical training department) Vova said: "The point was that the chief engineer thought he would go home earlier, and we had to straighten things out with the office. We criticized him, but if he doesn't want to stay then he ought to be forced to." He accompanied all these remarks with appropriate mimicry and gestures.

The nurse who came in knew something of the boy's home, and in obvious imitation of his mother, he began to say: "You don't know M. S., I have often spoken to you about her. The father is ill, and the young people won't do anything. They even couldn't visit their father on Sunday. Without me nothing will be done. I simply must be discharged home sooner. How they annoyed me, these young people Yurka and his wife Val'ka! Would you believe it, they called me to the telephone – Yurka, you see, was not at school. I realized all at once that Yurka was married. What a fool he is."

The character of the imitation always depended upon the situation. Vova sometimes was demonstrated at lectures in the large lecture theater. He saw and heard part of the lecture. Climbing up on to the rostrum, he at once began to imitate the lecturer, quite unconcerned by his surroundings. With an air of importance, folding his arms and walking about the stage, he began: "I shall now tell you about my chief engineer..."

Vova was educated in a special group at the special school, but in spite of the relative preservation of individual mental functions, he could neither read nor write. He could count up to ten on his fingers. His involuntary memory was well developed, but voluntarily he could not learn even the shortest poem by heart. He could not occupy himself at all, and would idle about for hours on end, showing no interest in anything. He did not mix with other children. Sometimes Vova would imitate one of the children misbehaving, and then through a sort of imitative aggressiveness would threaten someone, repeat gross and cynical terms of abuse, and rush on his opponent without any affect or consideration of the situation. The boy's imaginary aggression, however, caused no response on the part of the most excitable and mentally retarded children. The children laughed at him, but he did not understand their mocking. The general background of the boy's make-up was one of complacency and unconcern, with a slight touch of euphoria, and sometimes with elements of foolishness. He had a high opinion of himself. He had some sensitivities and would strive to get out of an unfavorable situation, but these attitudes were extremely unstable and they disappeared as soon as the circumstances causing them ceased to operate. All the boy's other emotions were unstable. Vova was incapable of delayed emotional reactions. He warmly greeted his mother when she came, but did not think of her in her absence. During his stay at the clinic he formed no attachment to anybody.

The boy was completely incapable of making allowances for a situation. With adults he behaved as an equal. The following example will illustrate this point. Occasionally, when going to the place where his mother worked, Vova would say to the manager, without any embarrassment, "How much longer will you be keeping my mother at work. I'm terribly upset about her!" In his mother's words, the boy never showed fear nor embarrassment, and was far too outspoken. Nobody could dare say anything in front of Vova that he did not want repeated to the person concerned. Vova showed no interest in games. The patient's entire conduct was determined by his imitativeness, for he readily retained the words, gestures, and facial expressions of those around him, and mimicked them. He was incapable of any independent activity, and moreover felt no urge to carry out any form of activity. If he could be compelled to do some elementary task, his work showed an obvious tendency towards stereotyped activity and perseveration.

Clinical Analysis of the Case

The etiology of this particular case was clear. The boy had an intrauterine lesion of the central nervous system, specific in character. This was confirmed by the presence of active syphilis in his mother, brother, and sister.

A comprehensive investigation of this patient gave grounds for making a series of assumptions regarding the pathogenesis. The EEG findings indicated not only a gross lesion, diffuse in character, but also severe irritative foci in the anterior divisions of the brain, suggesting that the frontal divisions of the cerebral cortex were especially involved.

The motor function in this case was characterized by the fact that, in the absence of paralyses and pareses, the boy could not utilize the movements of which he was capable, and the marked apraxia of his movements suggested gross maldevelopment of the cortical centers of the motor analyzer.

Investigation of the higher nervous activity in this case showed gross inertia within the motor analyzer and an incapacity to recognize his own movements.

The backwardness of the boy's development was noticed from early childhood. He was not attracted by toys, nor did he show interest in his surrounding. At first, however, this backwardness was hardly noticed by those around him. In kindergarten the boy's disability was more obvious. He did not take part in communal games; he was not interested in toys; he was indifferent to other children; and although his speech and memory were good, he was incapable of learning even the shortest piece of poetry. He remained incapable of spontaneous activity, was passive and indifferent toward his surroundings. At this age his imitative tendencies became particularly obvious.

The structure of the mental deficiency in this case was determined by the integrity of the elementary functions, by the severe maldevelopment of all the specifically human forms of activity, and of the personality as a whole. The patient subsequently learned to read, write, and carry out elementary arithmetical operations, but even at later stages of his development the maldevelopment of the specifically human forms of activity and of the personality was still obvious.

In consideration of the above facts, we are justified in classifying this case as a variant of oligophrenia of the type now under discussion.

ANALYSIS OF ALL THE RESULTS OBTAINED

In regard to etiology, this group of oligophrenic cases is extremely varied. In every case without exception, however, we are concerned with an external exogenic noxious factor — some intrauterine or early postnatal lesion of the central nervous system. In isolated cases the etiology is uncertain.

Neurological Investigation. Against the background of a residual neurological symptomatology, mainly cortical in character, gross disturbances of the motor activity stood out very clearly in the neurological pattern of our patient.

Investigation of the Electrical Activity of the Brain. Electroencephalographic investigation of children with this variant of oligophrenia revealed not only the characteristic oligophrenic changes, but also, in certain cases, a series of features specific for this particular form. By way of example we present the electroencephalogram of Gera M., a boy aged 15 years, a pupil in the imbecile class (Fig. 53).

It will be seen from Fig. 53 that in all regions of the cortex

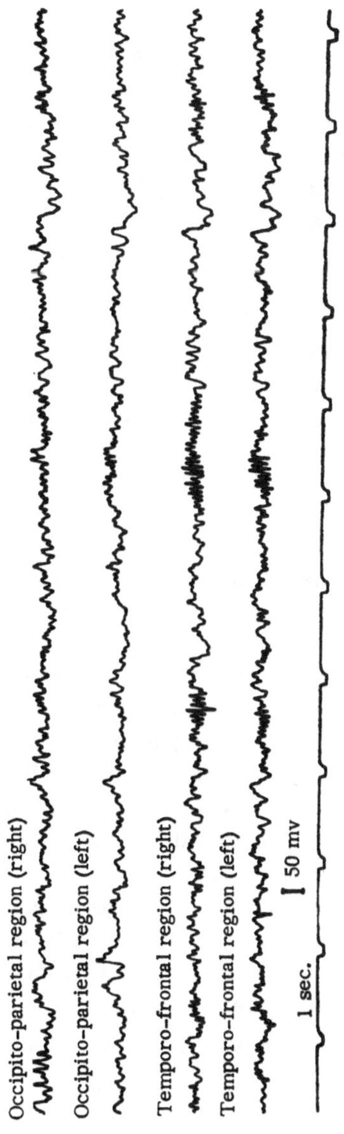

Fig. 53. Gera M., aged 15 years, (oligophrenia, degree of imbecility). In all regions of the cortex slow pathological waves and rapid waves are recorded. In the frontal regions of the cortex characteristic waves with a frequency of 22 per second appear, increasing in amplitude during light stimulation.

slow pathological waves and rapid waves are recorded. At the same time, in the frontal regions of the cortex, characteristic waves having a frequency of 22 per second develop and increase in magnitude during application of light stimuli.

A paradoxical reaction of increased amplitude of these waves indicates that the frontal regions of the brain are mainly affected. The electroencephalographic investigation thus shows not only that a diffuse cortical lesion is present, but also that the frontal systems are mainly involved. From all these facts it may be concluded that the specific feature of these children with this particular variant of oligophrenia is a combination of a diffuse lesion of the cerebral cortex with marked local disturbances in the anterior divisions of the brain.

Special Features of the Higher Nervous Activity. The children of this group are characterized by a considerable disturbance in the regulation of their conditioned motor reactions.* These disturbances may be found in the simplest conditions during the testing of the motor reactions in response to a direct verbal command. It was found that reproductive movements and superfluous movements of a perseverative character were displayed very prominently in these children, and were inhibited with difficulty. The presence of a large number of intersignal reactions and of grosser disturbances of stabilization of movement was also observed. The conditioned reactions were not stabilized through the whole series of subsequent re-examinations. Intersignal reactions were especially numerous in the younger of these children.

Simple positive conditioned connections and simple differentiation were easily produced in them. Only in children with the most severe degree of disability (and especially in the youngest of these) was difficulty encountered in establishing simple differentiation and even in forming simple positive conditioned connections. In the latter case positive reactions often failed to appear due to strong distracting action of external stimuli; moreover their appearance was masked by the frequent intersignal reactions.

The verbal projection of the production of simple conditioned connections in these oligophrenic children and in those with a mild degree of defect was adequate. Only the verbalization of the connection between the conditioned reactions and the reinforcement became much more difficult.†

*A disturbance of the verbal projection and of the connection of the conditioned reactions with reinforcement was observed even in children with a defect of the frontal systems who did not belong to the oligophrenic group.

†In these concluding remarks we summarize the results of a study of the higher nervous activity of children investigated mainly in the period 1955 to 1956.

The projection in the older children included irrelevant verbal connections formed in previous experiments, and bore no relation to the immediate conditions. In these experiments all the children showed many speech reactions which often replaced motor reactions. However, this apparently active use of speech did not improve the awareness of the conditions of the experiment.

In spite of the rapid and easy formation of differentiation, these children showed disturbances of differential inhibition, as indicated by the disinhibition of differentiation during repeated application of the differential stimulus alone. These children also revealed a weakness of active inhibition as shown by a peculiar form of multiple reaction to a single stimulus, which occurred when the action of the conditioned stimulus was prolonged, or when the child became fatigued during the experiment. In the younger children these repeated reactions were more strongly elicited. The production of delayed reactions was made much more difficult, which testified to the weakness of delayed inhibition.

During the production of more complex connections the very gross inertia of the old verbal connections was revealed. In many cases the projection completely lost its connection with the specific experiment, and was converted into a discourse on irrelevant matters. Under these circumstances the children tried to avoid answering questions.

Old connections were intruded even in the more adequate verbal projections obtained during repeated examinations involving the use of leading questions. During modification, preservation of the old projection was observed, even in cases when the motor reactions now began to correspond to the signal value of the new stimulus. Disturbances in the verbal projection sometimes even caused a complete contradiction in conditioned motor reactions: it was possible not only to have preservation of an inadequate projection in the presence of an already consummated complex system of connections, but also, on the other hand, the projection could be adequate to the task, but the action did not correspond to it. The existing verbal connection thus did not regulate the action. Nonperformance of an action in the presence of adequate verbal connections was a unique characteristic of this group of children.

The formation of conditioned connections with preliminary instruction was grossly deranged. In the children with the severest form of this defect, the formation of even the simplest connections was disturbed, and these remained unstable in spite of the frequent repetition of the instruction. Meanwhile these children were able to reproduce the instruction relatively easily. In children with a less severe form of the defect, the formation of connections in accordance with an instruction was possible, but when asked what they were doing, such children gave an inadequate verbal account, although they would correctly and completely reproduce the instruction if required to do so.

During the formation of motor differentiation, the motor analyzer exhibited a well-defined stereotypy.

Thus the most characteristic features of this group of children were the manifestations of inertia in the motor analyzer, gross disturbances of recognition of their own reactions, and also disturbances in the verbal regulation of these reactions. Gross disturbances in the cortical end of the motor analyzer were clearly revealed in the psychopathological state of these oligophrenic children in the form of characteristic changes in their psychomotor activity, so that we consider it necessary to give a detailed description of the motor activity of children with this variant of oligophrenia.*

Special Features of the Motor Activity. The views of Homburger (1926) are of exceptional relevance to an understanding of the motor activity of children with the variant of oligophrenia which we have delineated. This authority showed that until the age of one year extrapyramidal components of motor activity predominate in the child. Only at the beginning of the second year of life is there a gradual replacement of the extrapyramidal motor mechanism by the pyramidal, evidence of which is given by the disappearance of Babinski's and Rossolimo's sign. It is from this time onward that new myostatic functions begin to develop in the child, as a result of which he is able to maintain static equilibrium and to control the tone of the musculature as a whole when performing individual movements.

It is only during the subsequent development of the motor activity that a fundamental role is played by the cortical mechanisms. On this basis many researchers use the term "psychomotor activity." This stage in the development of the child is characterized by the fact that he learns to make use of his movements. This cortical mechanism of the motor activity in this group of oligophrenic children is imperfectly developed. The maldevelopment of the motor activity in the children of this group is shown above all by the disturbance of the integration of complex motor acts. While elementary movements are preserved, it is quite apparent that all those movements are disturbed which the child has to perform voluntarily. Such a child

*In this section particular attention is paid to the analysis of the motor activity, speech and purposeful activity, which accounts for the slightly different mode of presentation.

may perform a particular movement relatively well if done spontaneously or in imitation of somebody. But he is found to be absolutely incapable of carrying out this movement in response to a verbal command.

The degree of abnormality shown by the motor activity varies. In the more severe cases a complex motor act can only be performed with difficulty. It is sufficient to ask the subject to stand up, sit down or take something from the table, for him to develop a motor "storm." The child shakes his head and his body, straightens his stockings, frequently touches his coat, takes deep breaths, and makes yawning movements. All these movements appear to be compulsive. These children cannot actively carry out a specific movement, even though they understand what is required of them. For example, if the child is taken by the hand and the required movement is started, this helps him to do it. Such children can run more easily if somebody runs beside them, pulls, or pushes them. After a certain amount of training a motor complex is formed, which then terminates with difficulty. The children are unable to make the transition from one movement to another, and apparently stick to the previous movement. In the performance of the movement it is not the whole group of muscles required for the proper fluent performance of this movement that becomes involved. For instance, in these cases a ball is grasped, primarily with the hand and forearm, i.e., those divisions of the mobile system which are immediately next to the object to be grasped. The upper arm muscles take part in the movement to a lesser degree. The back and trunk muscles take no part whatever in this act. Complex movements are carried out not as complete entities but as parts. When such a child picks up a ball from the floor he first makes several squatting movements, then flexes the trunk forward a little, while simultaneously squatting. Then follows a series of grasping movements in conjunction with the preceding movements, and only then does he succeed in grasping the ball. Even during the performance of movements previously mastered, he first experiences difficulty. For example, when fastening a button, after a short period of general disorientation, expressed as absent-mindedness and fussiness, such a child makes sweeping and imprecise movements with his hands and knees, changing into wriggling movements of the trunk, while shaking backward and forward; he then will bring his hands near the button, make a few glancing movements, find the loop, grasp it tenaciously, and hold it in one hand. With the free hand he would make approximately the same movements around the button and then grasp it.

These children cannot fasten a button in a single operation.

The child's performance of a task is considerably improved if the teacher restrains his superfluous movements. Involuntary movements are performed far better by these children. Movements carried out in an affective state are done freely and correctly.

The motor disturbances in this group of children are of distinctive character. In the absence of paralyses and pareses each movement which these children are required to carry out upon instruction causes a general motor "storm," whereas involuntary movements are effected smoothly. An increase in the emotional tone improves their movements. It can be assumed from these facts that the distinctive motor disorders, outwardly resembling subcortical hyperkineses, are in fact cortical disturbances. All voluntary movements are distorted by a mass of compulsive, forced movements which tend to induce the opposite motor act. The laws governing the derangement of the motor act in this case may be explained by Pavlov's teaching on the relationships of induction. Pavlov pointed out that if a focus of excitation develops in the cerebral cortex inhibition will develop around it, and vice versa. Any positive cortical reaction, as a result of negative induction, will inhibit the negative reaction, that is, the opposite reaction, inappropriate to this stimulus. On the other hand, a negative reaction will normally inhibit a positive reaction. When cortical induction is deficient, reactions of contradictory tendency may exist simultaneously in the cortical centers of the motor analyzer. A deficiency of cortical induction of the same character lies at the basis of the disturbance of these children's movements. This pattern of motor activity was observed in children with the most marked disability. Even in less severe forms of this varient of oligophrenia, however, specific disturbances of motor activity occurred. In particular, their ability to perform imitative movements is relatively easy to demonstrate. Since the study of the motor activity in this particular form of oligophrenia is of great importance to an understanding of the structure of the defect, we shall describe the motor activity of a few of the patients whom we observed.

In the case of Borya, the motor activity was characterized by extraordinary passivity. In each of his movements his main feeling was one of helplessness. The boy was tall, with long lower limbs half flexed at the knees and with upper limbs hanging passively in front of his trunk. He was also round shouldered and his head protruded forward. He walked with his lower limbs in semiflexion, leaning forward, and with his hands pendant in front. With every step his body bounced upward, as if he were mounted on springs. He gave the impression he was moving on all fours, lightly touching the ground with his limbs. The boy ran by springing from one foot to the other, shaking still more violently, leaning forward, with his hands dangling in front of his body. When running he seemed more reminiscent of an animal. The boy was exceptionally inactive and helpless. Only now and again, when protecting himself against other children, did he raise his arms in front of him. He was incapable of self care, or of dressing or washing himself. Borya did not know how to handle the most ordinary articles. For example, he would take an article in his hands and hold it, muttering, "A towel, I must wipe my hands, I must be a good boy and wipe my hands well." Whenever the boy failed to complete a task, he usually compensated with words. The content of such statements corresponded exactly to what had been said to him by adults. He rarely displayed any spontaneous interest in objects. Often he had to have an article forcibly thrust into his hands. The boy often turned his body as if away from something strange. This led to an inability to control even his simplest movements. If you said to him, "Give me your hand," he would at first remain immobile, and would then only after a short time hesitatingly take your hand in his and hold it out like some strange object.

The boy was also extremely helpless when doing rhythm exercises. His spatial orientation was weak and he moved about haphazardly. He could not perform the simplest tasks. "Look how the wolf walks," you might say to him. "I see, I am looking now," he would say, thrusting his head forward. "Now do the same," requested the teacher. "I am doing what you want me to do now, and doing it well," he would reply, stepping into some spot.

Dima's motor activity was stereotyped. His movements were slow. He walked haphazardly, waddling from one foot to the other, making sweeping gestures with his hands and shaking his head. He would constantly mutter and threaten somebody with his finger. In his movements he imitated some particular adult. He stood with a wide stance, began to stroke his chest with wide, sweeping gestures, or, lifting his head high, he would again threaten somebody with his finger. Sometimes he flung open his arms, and throwing out his chest and stomach, with a hint of reproach he would shake his arms, or try goodnaturedly to grab somebody.

When imitating the movements of an adult person, he repeated grown-up or sophisticated expressions (Dima was brought up by his old grandfather, whom he imitated). For instance, sometimes during a rhythm lesson, instead of performing the required action, he curled up, kicked the floor, and exclaimed, "I am showing you where crabs spend the winter." It was not known how this sentence had been instigated, nor to whom it was addressed.

When he was given a certain movement to carry out to a spoken command, he became absolutely helpless and lethargic. He performed successive movements with great difficulty. He did not combine a series of movements logically, because it was all the same to him where he started the movement, at the end or the beginning. For example, he was given the following task, "Go to the door, come back again, sit on the chair, and read a book." He first took the book, then, turning it over in his hands, went to the door and closed it, and then he went to the toy cupboard, quite forgetting his task. During the performance of more complicated tasks, this patient was still more helpless. He either made use of his stereotyped, imitative gestures or shuffled about in his place in a foolish fashion.

Nelli's motor activity was static and inhibited in character. She had difficulty placing one foot in front of the other when walking. The girl made many superfluous movements of the hands and trunk, which interfered still more with her progress. Her running was still more poorly performed. Her legs were like wood, and she waddled from one foot to the other, quite unable to speed up the tempo of her movements. She could not look after herself properly. She could not dress nor wash herself, nor make her bed. Her hands were weak and her movements awkward, and her fingers had no elasticity, so that she often either gripped an object too tightly, or she was unable to grip the object tightly enough. Her movements were poorly organized. For example, when carrying a chair to the table, she held it around all its legs with both arms, and lifting it high into the air, carried it with difficulty. She could not collect a few books from the table and transfer them to another place. They fell from her hands, and she had to make repeated attempts to accomplish this task. The girl was quite unable to use her energies purposefully. She recognized new forms of movements with great difficulty. Often she could not jump over a rope. She would decompose a complete movement into its component parts: she would lift up a rope with her hands, then step or jump over the rope while it was lying on the floor. As she did this, she would be quite unaware that her actions had lost their integrity and meaning. When she had to carry out a series of consecutive actions, the girl experienced considerable difficulties. When performing involuntary movements, she was more organized, but when asked to perform the same actions in response to a spoken command, she became helpless, and her actions became silly. Characteristically this girl would accompany her movements with words such as, "I am clumsy and stupid, my hands are weak, everything drops from them, I haven't learned to do anything. What a way to grow up." She accompanied her speech with an unnecessary sweep of the hand and a nodding of the head. In her words and movements the girl imitated her grandmother, with whom she spent the greater part of her time at home.

These gestures became habitual and stereotyped for her. She often used them irrationally: "I shall be an actress, I shall sing and dance and read poetry," accompanying these words by unnecessary gestures. She performed her expressive movements purely schematically. At play the girl usually imitated only the external movements of the other children.

Specific disturbances of motor activity were also found in those children in whom a frontal deficiency arose as an isolated systemic disturbance, the other divisions of the cerebral cortex being relatively well preserved. These children were clumsy and awkward in their movements and they could not look after themselves, and in many of them motor acts were poorly performed. Specific changes of gait were observed in some of them. In nearly all these children, even simple postural movements were carried out with uncertainty, after many trials, and in the form of mirror-images of the task. Tests of synthesis were particularly difficult for them if the simultaneous participation of both hands was required. Their movements were poorly automatized. Another characteristic feature was that a movement, once developed, became indirect and could only be modified with difficulty. Phenomena of perseveration of motor acts took place. The coordination of movements was severely deranged in these children, and they had great difficulty carrying out complex simultaneous and consecutive motor acts.

Disturbances of motor activity also showed themselves in experiments conducted in accordance with the motor-speech technique. The movements of such children often bore a tonic character. Once a movement had begun, the subject could not stop it. The movements were very varied in strength, duration and number, and in the course of the experiment they were very poorly stabilized (Fig. 54).

Differentiation was formed in the effector with great difficulty; in spite of the large number of stimuli presented, with constant speech reinforcement, these subjects could not give motor reactions of different intensity in response to different stimuli.

The subjects of this group often gave unreliable projections of their movements. They estimated the number of their own reactions incorrectly. On presentation of the stimulus they pressed three or four times, but they stated that they had pressed only once. They also completely failed to estimate the strength of their own reactions. When the experimenter asked, "How did you press now?", immediately after the reaction, the subjects usually gave quite irrelevant answers.

Besides the features described above, in this group of oligophrenic children there were characteristic and marked changes in gait. In the absence of pareses or paralyses, their gait was clumsy, they often fell, they stumbled when running, they hopped from one foot to the other, leaning over almost into a horizontal position, their hands hung down in front of their body, and their running resembled that of a four-legged animal. Krol' (1933) discussed this problem of the disturbance of gait in frontal lesions. He drew attention to what he termed apraxia of gait, i.e., the inability to control the lower limbs purposefully in the absence of pareses, and he concluded that the frontal lobes play an important role in the development of gait in the erect position. He believed the frontal lobes regulated the conditions which permitted the undifferentiated functions of the four limbs to be converted into the differentiated functions of walking or standing, or into the still more highly differentiated function of the upper limbs.

Besides this imperfect development of gait, all the children whom we observed showed a severe maldevelopment of the differentiated movements of the upper limbs. The specifically human

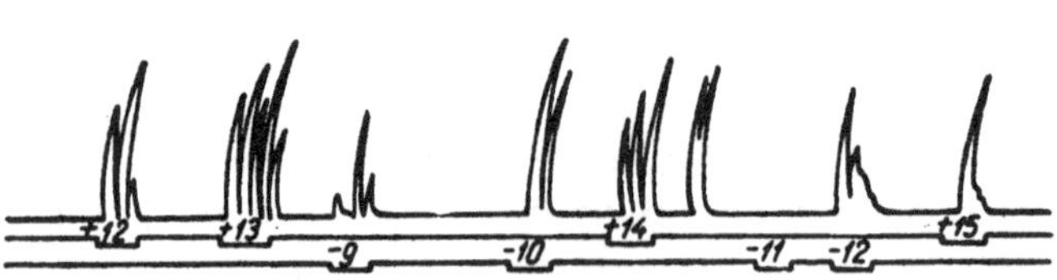

Fig. 54. Subject O., aged 13 years. Absence of stabilization of motor reactions in the course of the experiment. Top line—motor reactions; second line—positive stimuli (red light); third—inhibiting stimuli (white light). In spite of correct repetition of the instruction "When the red appears press once, but when the white light appears do not press," he reacts to nearly all the stimuli by pressing frequently, varying the intensity and duration of the pressure.

ability to use the upper limbs is imperfectly developed in this group of oligophrenic children. It may hence be concluded that the purposeful motor act is deranged in the children of this group in its motor execution.

Kleist (1908-1910) called this disturbance of a single scheme of movement the "kinetic apraxia of the organ." Research by Foerster (1920, 1936), Gurevich (1930), and Bernshtein (1940) led to the development of these concepts and to the elucidation of the role of the frontal cortex in the organization of movement. The frontal cortex, situated in front of the motor area and over the subcortical motor ganglia, transfers the organization of movements to a higher functional level, i.e., it raises it to the level of subjective action. It is these higher specific forms of motor behavior which are disturbed in the oligophrenic children of this group, while their elementary motor functions remain intact.

Special Features of Speech. The speech of the oligophrenic children of this group also shows a number of distinctive features. Some of these children have a considerable store of words and turns of phrase, and their sentences are properly constructed. For instance the boy Z., when first admitted to the hospital in 1943, spoke unceasingly about the war, knew when it had begun, against whom it was being fought, and that "we must finish off the wild animal in his own lair." His expressions were embellished with extracts from broadcasts, which he reproduced word for word.

In the doctor's office patient L. exclaimed, "Oh, I came to you to be cured and of course you will put me in the proper class now that I have come to the capital city."

In several cases the children accompanied all their actions by statements, but these statements were nothing but verbatim repetitions of what adults had told them. One of our patients whom we have mentioned already often imitated his father, who was in charge of a training department. He said: "At night, you understand, you can rest for a while, but here you must work. Who do you suppose is here to encourage you and give you orders? I, Vladimir Efremovich. I work at my own bench. Hello, I am speaking, I can hear you, comrade manager, what are your instructions? And I think to myself, 'What is he going to jump on me for this time; have patience! I am giving orders for your dismissal to-day.' I bring the key, open the box and tell Ira [Ira is the patient's sister], 'Hide it in back, let him jump; I have evidence against him, for he stayed away from work ten times.' "

Patient N. said, "I am a smart girl and I can do everything." Or, rummaging in her belongings, she would suddenly exclaim, "Oh, how I knock things around, I have lost them all," or, evidently repeating a sentence which her grandmother often used: "Oh Lord, it's like looking for a needle in a haystack," or "This letter has come out looking like a lopsided aunt."

L., the grandson of a gynecologist, often used gynecological terms in his speech. In another case, on her first day at the hospital, a girl of 13 years of age, having learned that the name and patronymic of her doctor were Mina Adol'fovna, at once exclaimed, "Mina Adol'fovna, you know, that is terrible. Mina, that is a mine used in war, and Adol'fovna means she must be related to Adolf Hitler, that wild animal who tortured some of my relatives." Next, glancing at the old ward nurse, she exclaimed, "The most remarkable part about your face is that wart on the bridge of your nose, and it has found a place where it can be sheltered." Looking at the doctor, the patient exclaimed, "Be more economical with your writing, or you will use up your paper supply. I can hear the rustling of your letter," and so on.

Dima S. often repeated some of her grandfather's expressions at the most inappropriate times, such as, "I will show you where crabs spend the winter." Sometimes his expressions were to the point and created an impression. "Oh, Krylov, what an old rascal you are, brother," he exclaimed about his classmate, a mischievous boy.

The speech of patient M. was echolalic. Often he answered a question by repeating the question. For example, the doctor asked, "What is your name?" The boy replied, "What is your name?" His speech was constructed of dialogues: "Oh I am a good boy! I am a good boy and I will behave well. I was a bit of a nuisance but I won't be any more."

These children often used expressions and words the meaning of which they did not understand. One of them, for instance, used the expression "don't count your chickens before they are hatched," but did not know what it meant. In another case the patient rushed to the doctor's office and said, "I flew in like a meteor." He was quite unaware of the meaning of this sentence.

These findings suggest that these children have a distinctive form of maldevelopment of the function of speech. In oligophrenic children of this variant there is no disturbance of the articulatory aspect of speech. As we demonstrated above, these children began to speak almost at the proper time, and easily pronounced difficult words and phrases. Their tendency to imitate adults also demonstrated the absence of any difficulty in pronunciation, for they easily reproduced complicated expressions which they had heard from adults.

It can be concluded from the clinical findings described above that in this variant of oligophrenia there were no disturbances of the sensory aspect of speech. These children understand what is said to them, and at the beginning of their attendance at school they learn analysis of sounds and letters. This by no means exhausts the distinctive features of speech development in this group of oligophrenic children.

Vygotskii (1934) put forward the view that the development of the higher mental functions takes place under the influence of speech. In a series of experimental investigations, Vygotskii and his pupils showed that the development of the generalizing function of speech led to the mediation of the process of analysis and integration by means of speech. He went on to say that through speech the necessary symbol is distinguished, so that it is possible to relate an object perceived to a definite category.

Maldevelopment of the generalizing function of speech stands out very clearly in oligophrenic children with this variant of the defect. This also lies at the basis of the maldevelopment of their cognitive functions, which is the fundamental symptom of oligophrenic mental deficiency.

The investigations started by Vygotskii and continued by his pupils showed that the development of the function of speech plays an essential part in the construction of rational action, in the development of volitional behavior, and above all in the differentiation of the motives of activity. In 1929 Vygotskii showed that children of the age of four or five years accompany their activity with expressions in which they describe the difficulties they encounter. This conversation helps the child to solve a difficult problem; it is also a manifestation of the regulating function of speech. Gradually in the process of the child's development this external speech develops, then diminishes, and is converted into internal speech. This continues to play a part in the solution of difficult problems, and it also occupies a leading role in the creation of complex intermediate forms of human behavior.

Luriya and several of his pupils (Khomskaya, Paramonova, Martsinovskaya, Lubovskii, Meshcheryakov) demonstrated experimentally the decisive role of speech in the organization of motor acts. The experiments of Paramonova showed that the regulating function of speech appears only at a definite stage of the child's development and plays a leading role in the formation of voluntary movements. Khomskaya's experiments revealed that the disturbance of voluntary movements could be compensated by means of the speech reactions of the subjects themselves.

In children with this particular variant of oligophrenia, while both the motor and sensory aspects of speech are preserved, an especially gross maldevelopment of the regulating function of speech was demonstrated. These children were incapable of formulating plans, and still less capable of making their action conform to a verbal task. Often they accompanied their activity by expressions of speech, but these expressions were usually of an irrelevant character.

The distinguishing feature of the children of this group was that even when they retained a very simple instruction they could not subordinate their activity to it. When specific demands were made of them, these children could not carry out tasks which were quite within their capacity.

Numerous clinical observations confirm the presence of a gross disturbance of the regulating function of speech in these children. For example, the girl L. was given the task of constructing a pyramid from different colored rings. Despite the fact that the instruction was repeated many times by the experimenter, the girl did not even start to solve the problem, but obsessively repeated, "Can I talk to you? Is this your room?" After persistent and frequent repetition of the instruction the girl began to manipulate the rings, but she did not accomplish her task; she uttered expressions unconnected with the actions, "May I do some work? What time tomorrow?"

The boy S. was asked to make several plasticene balls just like some samples. The boy repeated the instruction correctly, but no sooner had he taken the plasticene in his hand than the regulating role of the instruction disappeared and he began to apply the plasticene foolishly to his cheek, nose, and mouth, to throw it on the floor, and to walk on it.

The girl A. was asked to count the sticks on a table. As she handled them she accompanied her actions with inappropriate expressions such as, "When mother washes a lot of clothes she collects rags until late in the evening." When asked by the experimenter why she had remembered this, she replied, "I want to work. Give me the big picture 'The wolf and the seven kids.' I want to smash the glass. I love watermelon."

The boy S. was asked to make a pattern out of tiles. He stood the tiles in a row and accompanied his activity with completely unconnected expressions: "We have a big bedroom. I saw the television at Elena Petrovna's. Now we go to the cemetery, where we have a fine grave. Tat'yana Semenovna Skvarskaya, it says. I have lost three teeth and one is broken and hurts. Write to Tat'yana Mikhailovna, she is so fat, the day after tomorrow if you can."

From our clinical study of the oligophrenic children of this group, as from the experimental investigation of their higher nervous activity, we are justified in assuming that the specific feature of this variant of the defect is the maldevelopment of the regulating function of speech. But analysis of the clinical facts suggests that in oligophrenic mental deficiency no direct relationship can be established between the degree of preservation of the generalizing, and the degree of perservation of the regulating functions of speech. For instance, in oligophrenics of the first group, i.e., in those oligophrenic children whose clinical picture is characterized by maldevelopment of the generalizing function of speech, the regulating function of speech is relatively better preserved. We also found the regulating function of speech to be relatively well preserved in the other variants of the disability in oligophrenia.

As proof of this statement, that the maldevelopment of the regulating function of speech is more conspicuous in deficiencies of development of the frontal systems, we studied a control group of children in whom the deficiency of the frontal cortex developed only as a systemic disturbance in association with a higher degree of preservation of the general cortical activity.

Children with a systemic deficiency of the frontal cortex are able to repeat even a relatively complicated instruction (for example: "Press twice in response to one stimulus and once in response to the other"), but compliance with this instruction was attended with great difficulty. Instead of differentiated motor responses these children produced reactions which were uniform in strength and number. Either the instruction had to be repeated several times or constant speech reinforcement had to be introduced for this system of reactions to be produced.

Such a system of motor reactions could only be effected in stereotyped or in simplified experimental conditions. The slightest change in the experimental conditions (increase in frequency, introduction of extra-stimuli or shortening of the stimuli) led to a disturbance of these motor reactions. For example, in subject O. strong and weak motor reactions were supposed to be established in response to different light stimuli in accordance with a preliminary verbal instruction. But in spite of the correct repetition of the instruction, subject O. reacted to all the stimuli with reactions of equal strength (Fig. 55).

Separation of the speech reactions ("strongly"—"weakly") accompanying the motor responses had no positive influence on the course of the latter. Subject O. continued to react to the stimuli by pressures of equal strength.

In subject S. single and double motor reactions were to be established (Fig. 56). Instead of giving the reactions required subject S. at first reacted to nearly all the stimuli with a single press reaction. Later he began to press twice, but a tendency to perseverate was observed. He tended to stick to the previous form of movement. The addition of a speech accompaniment in this subject not only did not improve performance level, but even made it worse. While he verbally reacted correctly to all stimuli ("once, once, twice"), subject S. gave only single motor responses. When the experimental conditions were made more complicated, mistakes in speech also appeared. Thus in the subjects of this group the motor reactions were not subordinated to the verbal instruction of the experimenter. The child's own spoken remarks had no compensating action on his movements.

It is essential to point out that in such children a single functional system was not formed by the combination of speech and movement. The speech reactions either preceded the movements or followed them. In other words, speech was not a regulating factor in respect of the movements, as it was in the children of the other groups, and in essence it even disorganized their motor reactions.

Whereas the generalizing function of speech lies at the basis of cognitive activity, it must not be imagined that the regulating function of speech is more connected with the emotional-volitional features of the personality. It is for that reason that in oligophrenics with marked frontal deficiency the disturbance of the regulating function of speech also stands out clearly. In this group of cases speech on the one hand has no relationship to activity, and on the other hand its regulatory function is disturbed. This shows that both these factors are closely connected, internally interrelated, and mutually interdependent.

The disturbance of the regulating function of speech showed itself very clearly also during investigation of the higher nervous activity of these children. The disparity between speech and action in this subgroup leads not only to maldevelopment of the regulatory

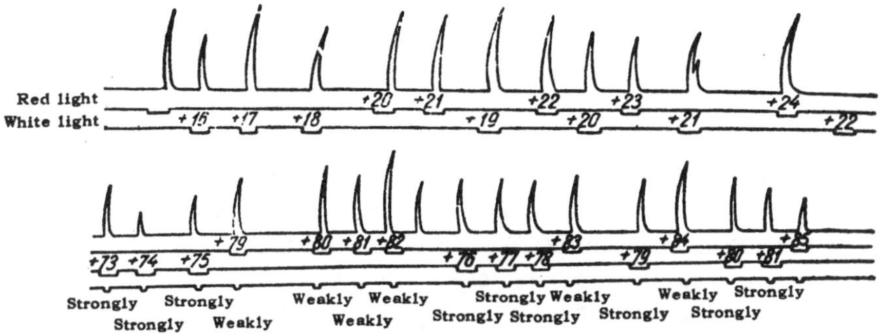

Fig. 55. Subject O. Effector differentiation (strong and weak pressure) in the same subject. Top line—motor reactions; second line—stimuli which should be followed by weak pressure reactions (red light); third line—stimuli which should be followed by strong pressure reactions (while light); fourth line—speech reactions. It may be seen from the figure that the strength of the pressure exerted by this subject does not correspond to the instruction, either with (A) or with (B) a speech accompaniment.

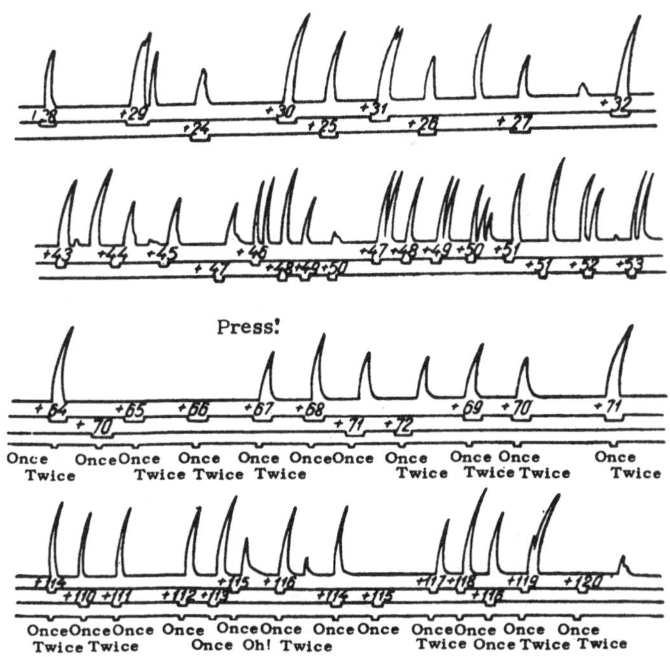

Fig. 56. Subject S., aged 12 years. Effector differentiation (one and two pressures). Top line—motor reactions; second line—stimuli which should be followed by pressing twice (red light); third line—stimuli which should be followed by pressing once (white light); fourth line—speech reactions.

speech function, but also to an inhibition of the development of other aspects of speech. The speech of these children, though it may seem superficially mature, is in fact an imitation of the speech of the adults around them. If the child is given a task requiring some speech activity of his own, he is helpless. When the child, who possesses an adequate stock of words, is asked to make up a short story in which he must use three words suggested to him, he is usually unable to accomplish the task. Instead of creating new verbal connections he reproduces ready-made clichés and expressions taken from the speech of those around him. The speech of these children does not serve the function of social intercourse, and does not organize their activity and behavior.

The Disturbance of Purposeful Activity In the children of this group the lack of any definite attitude towards a task assigned to them stands out clearly. For instance, Yu. did not react at all to a task given to her. In spite of the assignment of a task to him, M. would for a long time maintain precisely the same attitude. Other children were euphoric, disinhibited, and unable to concentrate.

The boy S. was asked to make an elementary picture from cut-out tiles, and he barely reacted to the task. The first time he received the instruction he showed no reaction, but when it was repeated he did make a number of remarks, although these were quite unconnected with the task. The third time he was instructed the child began to handle the tiles, sort them out, and toss them around. Thus these children do not show those elementary forms of relationship to a task which usually arise in children of three or four.

As shown by a series of experimental tests, these children understand words, sentences and the content of an explanation as a whole, but they cannot carry out a task because of the absence of any reaction to it. Purposeful activity, i.e., activity determined by motives, desires, or elementary emotional interest, was severely disturbed in all these children. Only when such a child was given special training did he develop a few elementary attitudes towards an assigned task.

Even when these children learned reading, writing, and arithmetic, the purposeful activity of most of them remained impaired. For example, patient N., educated in a group for severely retarded children, showed no interest in anything. While the other children attentively listened to the teacher, N. would direct irrelevant questions to the teacher, indicating that she was not listening at all. In class N. did not work, but talked to herself or to anyone who cared to listen. Sometimes she jumped up and down, walked about the classroom, and chatted to all the children, distracting them. Her writing was untidy. She could not write along the lines, she left pages blank, and sometimes wrote diagonally. The girl showed well marked perseverations, sometimes filling her entire exercise books with the repetition of one letter. For several days the girl wrote 3+ 3 = 6, no matter what task was given to her, which converted her writing into an absolutely irrational act. Thus these children exhibited perseverations during the performance of elementary arithmetical operations.

In several other cases the character of the disturbances of their activity bore a slightly different tone. The children were euphoric, disinhibited, and completely incapable of concentrating upon anything. They mixed up neighboring words, letters, and syllables in a reading exercise. They would readily join the end of one word to the beginning of the next, and they would repeat the same syllable several times.

Even in the less severe cases the disturbance of purposeful activity was plain to see. For example, the boy Z., when he began to read a book, read everything written on the cover from the top, the side, and the bottom. If he was interrupted and then given the same book again, the patient repeated the whole performance, and only then did he start to read the text of the book. When interrupted a second time the same result was obtained. At the suggestion of the experimenter, this child would read a text backwards for an hour or more, this of course being an irrational activity. He made no protest about having to read in this way, however, nor did he refuse to do so. The irrational actions were carried out by these children in just the same manner as rational acts, i.e., with no interest shown in the task.

In response to the instruction to draw a man, the children would draw a whole series of men, and when asked to draw a square, they would fill the page with squares. The actions of these children were not subordinated to an internal plan, but were determined by external factors. In talking these children interspersed odd words they had picked up or names of objects which they saw. For example, in the course of conversation with the girl N., various pictures were arranged on the table, among them being pictures of a cock, a train, an apple, a streetcar, a cucumber, a carrot, etc. The doctor asked her: "Have you been to a cinema?" She replied, "I went with my mother." "What did you see there?" asked the doctor. "Cocks," replied the girl, mixing up with her answer the name of the picture lying on the table. The girl was next asked, "What have you been studying in class to-day?" She replied, "We ate apples and cucumbers."

In less severe cases, too, the same disturbance of purposeful activity was clearly seen. These children typically made many superfluous movements, betrayed their lack of organization, and their inability to concentrate on their work, so that they never finished a task which they started, were constantly distracted by extraneous stimuli and never listened to their instructions.

Behavioral Disturbances. The children of this group showed behavioral features which distinguish them from all the oligophrenic children we have previously described. In accordance with their behavioral features these children may be divided into two subgroups.

In the children of the first subgroup, lethargy and passivity are combined with complete submissiveness. Such children can be made to sing, play, and dance in any situation. They carry out all orders without question. These children readily subordinate their behavior to established rules, even though they are unable to understand them. The child knows that before he goes into the doctor's office he must knock and await permission to enter, and that he must greet his elders first. These rules of behavior, however, remain incomprehensible to him, and he learns them mechanically. Such a child may therefore go in and out of the doctor's office several times in succession and greet the doctor again each time.

In the children of the other subgroup the external forms of behavior bear a somewhat different character. The behavior of these children is disorganized, chaotic, and impulsive. This is shown in particular when they are left to themselves. During recess, for instance, they would ask the teacher, the other children, or their parents foolish questions, would grab the other children by the clothes or hand, and rush aimlessly from one to the other.

The most specifically characteristic feature of the behavior of both subgroups is its absence of motivation. These children have no appropriate judgment or appreciation of a situation, so that they behave in the same way regardless of circumstances. Feelings of fear, desire or embarrassment are unknown to them.

These children also display inappropriate attitudes towards people around them. For example, patient V. often offended patient K. and even tried to take away his toys and candy. Nevertheless, when asked about this by the doctor, he replied that of all the children the one whom he liked best was K. This reply showed the absence of an appropriate attitude towards the offended person, and it was determined only by the fact that K. happened to meet his eye more often.

The manifestations of their emotional life also exhibit certain distinctive features. Spontaneous affective reactions are observed in these children. For instance, they are lively during visits from members of the family, hugging and kissing them. If at the climax of the visit, however, the child is called away to the doctor's office, he makes no protest. The children do not cry and they apparently forget that their father or mother is sitting in the ante-room, i.e., they have no delayed affective reactions. If an emotionally tinged reaction does arise in such a child (they may cry out or weep), it is often unrelated to a particular person. For example, a boy knocked a girl down with a ball during play. In retaliation she did not knock the boy down, but another girl. The affective discharge was misdirected.

Active forms of behavior in the children of this group are replaced by a tendency to imitate. We observed this tendency during the analysis of the special features of their motor activity and speech. The question naturally arises how this tendency to imitate can be explained. The power of imitation is extraordinarily well developed in the first years of life of any child, when he imitates gestures and facial expressions and speech. During the course of development, however, this feature gives way to the development of his individuality (his motives, desires, interests and purposes). In oligophrenic children with marked frontal deficiency, the tendency to imitate persists through much later stages of their development than in the normal child.

To understand the distinctive features of the behavior of our oligophrenic children, it is interesting to consider some experiments carried out in Pavlov's laboratory. In Urinson's experiments the anterior frontal lobes were removed from a dog, after which complete motor inactivity was observed in the animal. No sooner was a normal dog brought to this animal, however, which jumped about from one corner to another and sniffed all over everything, than the dog from which the frontal lobes had been removed copied all that the normal dog did. When the normal dog was taken away, the operated dog once more became lethargic and abandoned all spontaneous activity. These experiments were interpreted by Urinson as showing that the frontal lobes suppress the tendency to imitate.

Special Features of the Cognitive Activity. In oligophrenic children with marked frontal deficiency, difficulties in the performance of tasks requiring thought arise not only because it is difficult for them to appreciate the abstract meaning of speech and to interpret complex abstract relationships, but—it is important to remember—also because of the severe impairment of their purposeful activity. Even when they solve simple problems, well within their grasp, besides giving correct answers they will give foolish and inadequate answers, because they lack self-discrimination and do not really understand why one answer is right and another wrong.

During the solution of problems by these oligophrenic children, the controlling motive soon drops out of sight, their actions then begin to be subordinated to random impressions, and then are produced automatically. The specific features of the cognitive activity of the children with this variant of the disability are revealed during investigation of the level of development of the generalizing function of speech by means of picture classification. In the early stages of education the task of classification remains beyond tive form and the pictures are grouped together either according to superficial visible signs or the grouping is limited to identical pictures. In the later stages of their education these children arrange the pictures by the categories which they have learned by heart. Thinking in terms of situations (which develops in all the other variants of oligophrenia), does not develop at all in the children of this particular group.

Maldevelopment of situational forms of thinking is responsible for the distinctive structure of the defect in the children of this group.

As we have shown above, in the course of their anomalous development, speech in these children does not serve to plan their action nor to organize it, but is often detached and separated from action, becoming empty and meaningless. Nor does the presence of visual concrete material excite them to activity: the material does not serve to organize their past experience but rather excites a series of irrelevant associations unrelated to their concrete activity. During the analysis of the distinctive features of the cognitive activity of these children, the maldevelopment of the regulating function of speech thus is again clearly demonstrated.

SPECIAL FEATURES OF THE STRUCTURE OF THE DEFECT AS A WHOLE

In oligophrenic children with this particular variant of the disability, against the background of maldevelopment of the cognitive activity, the specific characteristics of their emotional-volitional functions, the characteristics of their purposeful activity and of their motor functions, i.e., the gross maldevelopment of the personality as a whole, stand out very clearly. In the process of their development complex forms of voluntary behavior, conscious awareness of situations or awareness of their own behavior do not appear. These children do not form differential emotional attitudes to their surroundings, and the structure of their activity is grossly disturbed.

It may be deduced from the distinctive character of the structure of their defect that in children with this form of oligophrenia we are concerned not only with a diffuse lesion of the cerebral cortex, but also with a combination of this diffuse lesion with a marked disturbance of the frontal systems. The results of neurological and electroencephalographic examination indicate that it is in this variant of oligophrenia that disturbances in the anterior divisions of the cerebral cortex stand out clearly against the background of a disturbance of cortical activity.

While still at the preschool age these children do not reveal an adequate reaction to environmental stimuli. Visual materials (toys) do not excite them to activity, and objective activity (i.e., activity related to objectives) as such does not arise. The distinctive maldevelopment of their motor activity makes it even less likely that objective activity will develop.

Vygotskii has shown that the regulating function of speech develops in the process of purposeful activity and is revealed in the form of difficulties in the performance of individual tasks. Since object-oriented activity develops inadequately in these children. the regulating function of speech is also maldeveloped.

The defective development of these children, taking place outside concrete objective activity, leads not only to the maldevelopment of the regulating function of speech, but also to the fact that speech as a whole develops unproductively. Their speech shows a tendency towards mere mechanical imitation.

The almost complete absence of objective activity, especially during play, makes the structure of the defect in the children of this group easier to understand. Nevertheless, this analysis still does not reveal the whole unique character of the defect in this particular form of oligophrenia. The structure of the defect is determined not only by the maldevelopment of the cognitive activity, but also by the distinctive behavioral pattern of these children, namely its impulsivity. The impulsivity of behavior of oligophrenic children with marked frontal deficiency is manifested against the background of intact elementary emotions. The impulsivity of their behavior is the result of their inability to recognize their behavior and to interpret it critically. This makes it essential to understand what it is that lies at the basis of this impulsive behavior.

We know that in the course of objective activity, social activity, or play, the child develops complex reactions to activity going on around him, mediated through internal speech, and differential emotional attachments to those around him. It is only later that all aspects of his personality developed. The complex forms of mediated behavior are determined not only by the fact that the child becomes aware of the impressions of activity around him, but also by the fact that he evaluates what he perceives, and on the basis of his evaluation develops a particular mode of action.

The group of oligophrenics at present being described has retained only the ability to perceive impressions of surrounding activity, and in the course of their anomalous development they do not learn to evaluate what they perceive nor to plan their actions accordingly. Patient L., the day of her arrival in hospital, examining the face of the ward nurse, exclaimed, "You have a wart and it has found a place that suits it." The entire clinical staff was surprised by her remark, never having noticed the wart for the many years they worked with the sister. Another patient exclaimed to his examining doctor, "How ugly you are! What plain eyes you have. What a big nose, and big teeth!"

When in these cases perception of the surroundings was correct, it was followed immediately by thoughtless expressions; in other words, there was neither an evaluation nor comprehension of what was perceived nor any choice of a mode of action based on such an evaluation. It is the loss of these links which explains the spontaneity of their behavior, and which leads to the inability to understand and assess a situation, the inability to interpret their own behavior critically.

In oligophrenic children of this group, complex consecutive forms of behavior are replaced either by isolated fragmentary acts (i.e., by spontaneous reactions to each fragment of the situation), or by imitative forms of behavior, which have the character of irrelevant stereotypes.

Let us try to understand what pathophysiological features are responsible for the spontaneity of the reactions observed in the children of this particular group. Some progress in this direction is made by the experimental research of Shumilina (1949), undertaken on dogs for the purpose of studying the functional importance of the frontal regions of the cerebral cortex. This worker showed that, after removal of the frontal cortex, the conditioned secretion in a dog appeared just as it did before the operation, but the conditioned motor reaction developed as soon as the animal was placed on the apparatus. The removal of the frontal cortex thus lead to the loss of the animal's ability to integrate its motor reactions into a complex situation and resulted in the development of partial reactions to individual components of this situation, i.e., the animal's behavior lost its strict dependence on a large complex of external stimuli and disintegrated into its individual component parts.

The ability of the animal to integrate its various afferent influences is due to the prerelease (i.e., prior release) of the afferent impulses. In man, this prerelease of afferent impulses is evidently achieved by means of internal speech. It is precisely this internal speech which enables man to evaluate what he perceives, to formulate plans and to develop his modes of action. If it is considered that the prerelease of afferent impulses in man is due to internal speech, it becomes clear that maldevelopment of internal speech in the children of this group is also responsible for the disturbance of their purposeful activity and for the distinctive pattern of their behavior.

Let us attempt to prove the same point by starting from an analysis of the restoration of the capacity for purposeful activity in children with this variant of the defect. In the course of their education these children went through a number of preliminary stages before they were able to organize their activity. Above all it was necessary to inhibit their impulsiveness. Even when this had been accomplished, however, they were still unable to carry out the simplest task by themselves.

In the process of play, it was possible to instill in them the rudiments of appropriate attitudes towards an assigned task, although even at this stage it was found that the children could not carry out such a task in accordance with instructions. The activity of these children subsequently became organized with the aid of the speech of the teacher himself. With this aid the children carried out their task irreproachably, but when they tried to do the task by themselves they were still unable to do so and they accompanied their activity with inappropriate expressions. Only after the child had learned to regulate his activity by his own speech, i.e., after some restoration of the regulating function of the child's own speech was it possible for him to independently carry out a task in accordance with instructions. The child's own speech thus became the regulator of his actions.

The restoration of the child's purposeful activity was thus made possible only through the creation of proper attitudes towards his activity—even though rudimentary attitudes—and by the incorporation of the regulating function of speech. The organization of behavior in certain cases was to some extent achieved through the development of internal speech. Compensation by this means led in certain cases to an advance from unthinking spontaneous behavior to the simpler forms of deliberative voluntary behavior. At first what the child perceived was evaluated for him by the teacher, who formulated in speech a course of action corresponding to the evaluation. Afterwards this procedure was carried out by teacher and child together. Only then did the child commence to carry out the task independently.

The fact that the restoration of the regulating function of speech contributes to the organization of their behavior, convincingly demonstrates the important handicap the maldevelopment of internal speech constitutes in their total defect. Observation and analysis of the specific features of behavior of this type of child lead to the same conclusion.

DIFFERENTIATION BETWEEN OLIGOPHRENIC CHILDREN WITH MARKED FRONTAL DEFICIENCY AND CHILDREN WITH SIMILAR STATES

A. Differentiation between oligophrenic children with marked frontal deficiency and children in whom maldevelopment of the frontal systems is associated with relatively good preservation of cognitive activity.

The differentiation between the form of oligophrenia which we have described and similar states is exceptionally difficult. Diagnostic mistakes are particularly numerous with cases showing a disturbance of behavior and purposeful activity, associated with faulty personality development combined with relatively well preserved cognitive activity. We accordingly studied a group of children with deficiencies of the frontal systems. Only one such case will be described.

CASE 1

Patient Lyalya Sh., a girl aged $15^1/_2$ years. She was admitted to the children's department of the Kashchenko Hospital with complaints of improper behavior. She was garrulous, hyperactive, and uncritical.

History. Lyalya was born two weeks prematurely. Her birth weight was 6.5 pounds. At the age of one year people around her noticed how difficult it was to interest her in toys. From five years of age she attended a preparatory school where she was taught German. Her behavior contrasted sharply with that of the other children. She could not understand situations and could not play with others. Her parents reported that at home the girl would often act inappropriately and appeared to be nervous. From nine years of age the girl attended school, but was unable to continue her education because of her misbehavior. She had several children's infectious diseases without complications.

Physical State. The patient was dysplastic and had an excessive deposition of fat on the thighs, chest and abdomen. No abnormality of the internal organs was found. Her sexual development was complete.

Laboratory Investigations. The blood and urine were normal. Investigation of the cerebrospinal fluid by lumbar puncture: pressure 230 mm, proteins 0.26%, cells 2/3. All protein reactions negative.

Anisocoria (R > L). Full convergence not attainable: eyes could not be fully abducted, and at times strabismus was present. The pupils reacted satisfactorily to light. The right palpebral fissure was wider. The tongue was in the midline; swallowing and phonation were normal. Movements of the limbs were normal in range but extremely clumsy. Tremor of the fingers was present, more obvious on the right. Tests of motor activity showed that the left hand was stronger than the right and she hopped better on her left foot. The muscle tone in the upper and lower extremities was diminished. The tendon reflexes were increased, much more so on the right (knee and ankle jerks). The abdominal skin reflexes were diminished. The right plantar reflex was atypical and at times extensor. The skin of the face was seborrheic and bright in color, and her limbs showed excessive perspiration. The optic fundus was normal.

Electroencephalography. The α-rhythm was relatively well defined, with a frequency of 9 per second, and was recorded only in the occipital regions of the cortex. In the parietal and frontal regions the β-rhythm was absent. In the parietal regions slow waves and rapid asynchronous waves were predominant (Fig. 57).

The EEG indicates some abnormalities of the electrical activity of the brain, as indicated by the alpha dysrhythmia and the predominance of rapid activity in the frontal regions of the cortex, indicative of irritative foci in the frontal regions.

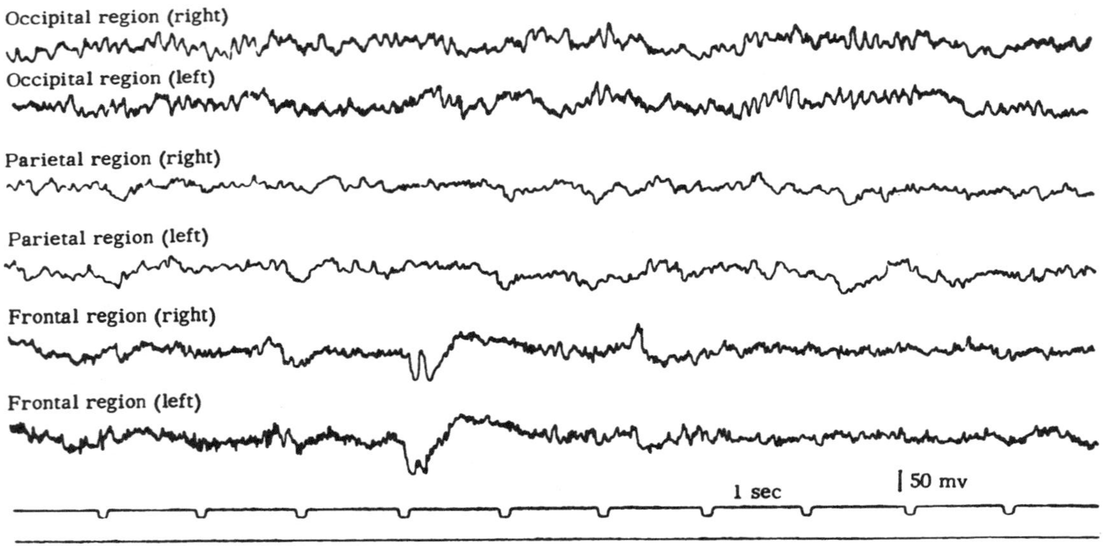

Fig. 57. Lyalya Sh., aged $15\,{}^1\!/_2$ years (gross maldevelopment of the personality as a consequence of a lesion of the anterior divisions of the brain). EEG in a state of rest. The EEG shows irritative foci in the frontal regions.

Mental State. On admission to the clinic the girl evinced no particular reaction to her unusual surroundings and readily established contact with the doctor. She was separated from her mother without any concern. She exhibited motor restlessness, her movements were clumsy, she held objects with difficulty, and she was inept and awkward. In the course of conversation she grew visibly animated, rubbed her hands, jumped up and down, and made several superfluous movements. During exercises in rhythm she was quite helpless, and could not manage to do exercises within the capabilities of much younger children. The girl could not perform two tasks simultaneously. For example, if she was asked to jump up and down in place and at the same time to clap her hands three times, she would jump up and down very clumsily, but she could not clap her hands while doing so. Her motor insufficiency was very obvious when she did any kind of work. All the children of the department took an active part in tree planting. She also set about this task eagerly, but the spade fell from her hands. On another occasion the children were given the task of collecting flower seeds, and here again the girl's complete helplessness showed itself. She gathered the seeds clumsily, but spilled them all.

Speech was well developed and her sentences properly constructed. In conversation she became more active. She spoke about the most ordinary things in a solemn tone of voice. For instance, having looked all round her and noticing dust on the inkstand, she exclaimed, "What an awful lot of dust, and how can you explain that, with so many high grade doctors in your institute." The content of her expressions as a whole was determined by stimuli reaching her at that particular moment. On seeing an ink stain she started a long discussion about how slovenly the doctors were and how the nurses did not tidy up properly. If no questions were put to the girl, she would listen to the conversation of those around her, fix her attention on individual words, and then begin to join in the argument. For instance, having heard that patient R. had tried to run out into the corridor, with her customary pathos she began to say: "M. A. is looked upon as a good doctor, but a patient nearly escaped, which is hard to understand. In one of the best hospitals in our country the patients run away," etc. Having exhausted this theme, the girl, seeing the doctor open an envelope, immediately exclaimed, with fresh animation, "Oh, see how M. A. opens the patient's letters. She wants to know what they are writing. No, you must excuse me now, I won't mail any letters, but I shall simply give them to my mother." Next, having noticed a wart on a girl's neck, she began a long discussion on this subject. The girl's spontaneous expressions revealed obvious stereotypes. During her three months' stay in the hospital, for instance, she kept returning to the same two basic themes.

She displayed many discrepancies in her intellectual functioning. For instance, L. wrote correctly, read well, and could explain the meaning of a story which she had read. Her ability to calculate was at a somewhat lower level. Processes of logical thinking were adequately developed in this patient. Her answers to questions were precise and brief, and her definitions were concise. The patient understood what was meant when she said: "a venomous person," "don't act out of line," "what you gain on the swings you lose on the merry-go-round," or "a fine cage does not fill a bird's belly," and could explain all of these when questioned by the doctor.

She understood the conventional inscriptions on pictograms, but when she had to find explanations for proverbs, she slipped into a literal interpretation, reflecting a certain incapacity to translate a thought into action. When asked to make up a story using certain suggested words, she tried for a long time to think of something, but could not compose the story.

The girl's behavior reflected a serious maldevelopment of personality. She was infantile, acted with spontaneous thoughtlessness, and was unable to take account of a situation. During class lessons she made irrelevant remarks, expressed her wishes quite impulsively, and often conversed in a loud voice. She was not susceptible to embarrassment (in class she might occasionally begin to undress). She did not understand the teasing of the other children. The girl had no true emotions; she was not homesick, and never asked about her father's health at a time her father was seriously ill. If she was asked what she missed, she replied: "The book 'Abai,' the cat Dzhul'bars, and Mother." If she was asked about her farther's illness, she would begin to discuss illnesses in general. The girl was very observant, and in conversation with any adult person, such as a doctor or teacher, she would look him over attentively and immediately pronounce her spontaneous judgment on him ("large teeth, unpleasant eyes, lots of wrinkles," etc.). In conversation with the girl, the doctor tried to suggest to her that she must not offend people, but her reply to this was that all that she said was true. The girl had no considered reactions to her environment. For example, she would meet her mother very affectionately, fling her arms around her neck, request her own discharge on May Day, cry and threaten to run away, but no sooner was she parted from her mother than all her demands were forgotten. An emotional reaction reflecting a filial attitude towards her mother arose only when she was in the girl's sight. No delayed emotional reactions were observed in the girl. L. was educated by individual instruction at home. She worked only when the teacher compelled her to carry out a particular task. During classwork in the clinic the girl was submissive and did her work, preferring routine tasks (copying, solving arithmetic problems). The patient was tense, often laughed out loud and spoke a great deal. But at other times she was lethargic and showed little spontaneous activity.

In the cases which we studied there were certain very obvious features of similarity with those forms of oligophrenia which are characterized by marked frontal deficiency. In both instances, in the presence of well-preserved optic and spatial integration, and with intact sensory and motor speech functions there are obvious disturbances at the cortical end of the motor analyzer associated with a general maldevelopment of personality. Both groups of children are unable to comprehend what they perceive and to devise the most adequate mode of action on the basis of their understanding. They are impulsive and evince no critical attitude towards their behavior. While their elementary emotions are preserved, in the process of development they do not develop any complex affective relationships to the environment. Besides these similarities, however, there are also considerable differences. These children differ from oligophrenic children with marked frontal deficiency by reason of the fact that their cognitive functions are reasonably well developed.

The study of the children of this group convinces us all the more that the specific maldevelopment of personality and the changes in motor activity are due to a maldevelopment primarily of the anterior divisions of the cerebral cortex.

B. Differentiation between oligophrenic children with marked frontal deficiency and children suffering from chronic schizophrenia in childhood.

The lack of spontaneous activity, the lethargy, the affective-volitional disorders, the motor disturbances and finally, the apparently gradual progression in the symptomatology of the defect all tend to create a similarity between oligophrenic children with a marked frontal deficiency and children in whom an insidious form of schizophrenia is present. Prolonged, dynamic observations on oligophrenic children with marked frontal deficiency enabled us to identify certain differential diagnostic signs. In early schizophrenia we have signs of degeneration. Oligophrenic children with marked deficiency of the frontal systems develop and acquire certain skills (reading, writing, counting).

Affective disturbances are observed both in oligophrenic children with marked frontal deficiency and in those with chronic schizophrenia in childhood. The character of these affective disturbances is different, however. In slowly progressive schizophrenia there is a primary disturbance of the emotional-volitional functions, whereas in this form of oligophrenia the primary emotional manifestations are fully preserved, but the secondary ones (complex constellations of emotional involvements) do not arise in development. In spite of this outward similarity, we are concerned essentially with different conditions.

C. Differentiation between oligophrenic children with marked frontal deficiency and children with temporary retardation of development.

Oligophrenic children with marked frontal deficiency are often confused with children with a temporarily retarded development. Both groups, in the initial stages of their education, do not understand the whole idea of school and they cannot therefore respond appropriately to it, they do not obey school rules and they show no interest in school activities. Since they do not appreciate the role of speech in directing action, they do not react to verbal tasks.

Besides this similarity, however, considerable differences are also observed. For instance, though children with a temporary retardation of development cannot organize their behavior responses to the complex demands of school studies, it is adequately organized and purposeful in play activity, in freehand drawing, and in listening to stories and fables. Oligophrenic children with marked frontal deficiency are incapable of carrying out any such task, including play activity.

Both groups of children are unable to carry out a task in accordance with spoken instructions, but the character of this incapacity shows considerable differences. For instance, in oligophrenic children with marked frontal deficiency, the inability to perform an individual task will lead to an irrational manipulation of objects given to them, whereas in children with temporary retardation of development the inability to perform a verbal instruction task leads to an indulgence of their own whims and fancies.

The difference between these similar conditions stands out especially clearly, however, during dynamic studies. In cases of temporarily retarded development the disturbance of purposeful activity bears a purely temporary character; in contrast to this the disturbance of motivation of activity remains a permanent symptom in oligophrenia with marked frontal deficiency.

D. Differentiation between oligophrenic children with marked frontal deficiency and that variant of oligophrenia in which the effect is characterized by gross, specific disturbances of the cortical neurodynamics.

Of all the variants of oligophrenia described above, there is one group that is especially likely to be mistaken for oligophrenic children with marked frontal deficiency. These are the children in whom disturbances of cerebrospinal fluid and cerebro-vascular dynamics are superimposed upon a general, diffuse lesion of the cerebral cortex, and in whom the clinical picture thus reveals a disturbance of purposeful activity and behavior that creates a basis for this confusion.

Besides features of similarity, however, considerable differences are also found. For instance, in oligophrenic children with marked neurodynamic disturbances in whom excitation predominates over inhibition, once some degree of compensation has been achieved, their impulsiveness overcome and their activity organized, they readily display appropriate attitudes towards their activity and develop marked personality reactions. In contrast to this, in oligophrenic children with marked frontal deficiency, even in the absence of impulsiveness and disinhibition, the disturbances of purposeful activity and the gross maldevelopment of their personality nevertheless stand out clearly.

WAYS OF COMPENSATION

The program of corrective training for oligophrenic children with marked frontal deficiency must be based upon the qualitative analysis of the structure of their defect. Accordingly, in the first place it is necessary to use teaching methods directed towards the organization of their motor behavior and purposeful activities. Since, as we have shown above, these children exhibit maldevelopment of that complex system of voluntary reaction to the environment which begins to be formed at preschool age, it is very important that compensation of the defect should start long before the child goes to school.

Special attention must be paid to the compensation of their motor activity. For this purpose efforts should be directed towards the development of the general motor activity, and especially the development of the differential movement of the fingers. The development of their motor activity must be encouraged both by the aid of special rhythmic exercises and in the course of their purposeful activity. In these oligophrenic children there is a gross disturbance of behavior, character and of the personality as a whole. At preschool age this is revealed by their abnormal attitude toward the activities going on around them. Concrete objects do not excite them to activity. For this reason one of the fundamental tasks in the compensation of their defect at an early stage is the inculcation of attitudes in these children which are appropriate to the environment, which can best be done through play activity. They must, however, be attracted to, stimulated by, and given an interest in playing. In some children, as we have shown above, there is a well-marked general disorganization of behavior, taking the form of impulsiveness and increased excitability, which makes it essential that their behavior be organized.

It is very important that the basis of a sound attitude towards didactic material should be developed in these children. They must be taught not to tear up or throw away articles which they have to use during their studies.

Only after some results have been attained in regard to the organization of their motor activity and behavior, and they have begun to develop the elements of a correct attitude towards their activity, may the teacher move on to special methods directed towards the organization of their purposeful activity.

As we have shown above, these children cannot carry out the most elementary tasks. They cannot play with toys nor take part in organized games. They play with any object placed in their hands, throwing it about, knocking it on the table, and banging it together with other objects. These children do not regard articles used for play or educational purposes as objects designed for definite purposes, and as such requiring particular respect. The development of these children by means other than goal-directed activity leads to the maldevelopment of purposeful activity and personality. They look upon any object as something which they may fiddle around with, break, or tear up. Only as a result of educational activity do they begin to develop a proper attitude towards games, toys, and teaching methods, and stop tearing things up, breaking them or damaging them. Special training in play is necessary for them: building pyramids, making simple shapes from building blocks, making pictures from tiles, and so on. During their training in simple forms of play, and later in educational activity the teacher is confronted with one fundamental obstacle which keeps these children from carrying out various forms of task: the child cannot plan and regulate his activity. Whereas it is comparatively easy for such a child to learn to do certain tasks by instruction, he cannot advance to the accomplishment of a task consisting of a group of separate actions. This becomes obvious when the child is asked to make a picture from tiles as shown by an example. The combination of the tiles and picture, and the verbal instruction does not provoke the child to activity. They move the tiles about from one place to another in a desultory way, tap them on the table and suck them. As a result of repeated demonstrations, explanations and trials, these children begin to learn to identify the parts of the picture, although they cannot combine them into a complete picture. At any time they may create random and foolish combinations: they join a dog's head to its tail, they may fit a cow's ear to its back, and so on. If each individual action is regulated by the teacher's spoken instruction, however, the children are able to accomplish the task.

At the next stage the regulating words of the teacher are replaced by her silent designation of the separate parts from the specimen picture; the child must name these parts, choose them from the complete assortment of parts, and fit them together.

At the next stage, when the child's speech can be internalized and when he can use it to regulate his actions, any external aid can be dispensed with. The child can now regulate the whole course of his work independently of external speech.

It is much more difficult for such children to change to planned activity with the aid of internal speech. Some of them remain incapable for a long time of the transfer from external to internal speech, in others this process takes place more quickly. A similar means is adopted when the children are taught elementary reading, writing, and arithmetic.

These children often acquire certain arithmetical skills: they learn to count up and down the scale, to count objects, to take a required number of objects from a total number of identical objects, to match numbers of counting sticks with suitable numbered cards, and to add and subtract a given number. They apparently have all the necessary ability to change over to the solution of the simplest arithmetical problems in addition and subtraction with the aid of counting material. Neither by demonstration nor by explanation, however, can they be taught to solve such problems. They cannot by themselves perform a group of actions which, to them, is complex. Their education must proceed by the regulation of each action.

The teacher gives separate instructions, and as these are carried out, one after the other, as a series of simple arithmetical operations, the end result is the solution of the problem.

An example is written on the blackboard. The teacher points to the first number and gives the instruction to take away the same number of counting sticks. After this part of the problem has been done, the teacher plans the subsequent course of action by pointing to the second number of the example, and gives the instruction for this to be done – the addition or subtraction of the required number. Finally, the child receives the instruction to write out the answer. At the next stage the teacher plans the child's activity by means of a silent gesture, pointing successively to each number of the example. The child himself calls out what is shown to him and determines what he must do next. Finally, at the last stage, the children themselves without any external assistance regulate their activity by their own speech.

In the cases cited the children were given tasks on an intellectual level within their grasp. Because they could not organize and direct themselves towards the accomplishment of the task, and because they could not regulate their activity by their speech, they were unable to carry out the task. The child's inability to regulate his activity was made good by the fact that the teacher planned and directed the whole course of the work by her own speech, which provided the necessary conditions for the performance of the task. The external regulator – the teacher's speech – was then replaced by the child's own speech; this created the conditions needed for the independent performance of feasible types of task.

The regulation of the child's activity, at first with the aid of the teacher's speech and later of the child's own speech, leads to some degree of compensation of their condition.

The organization of the objective activity of these children in the process of their corrective training must therefore be divided into a series of stages. The first stage is that of regulation of the whole activity of the child by the teacher's speech. Only after this has been accomplished is it possible to advance to that stage in the organization of his activity when the child learns to regulate each separate element of a task by his own speech. This stage must be prolonged, and it should be started by giving the children easy tasks which are quite within their reach. The change to more complicated tasks must be brought about gradually. The teacher's whole attention must be directed towards teaching the child to carry out a task by instruction, and thereby developing the regulating function of his speech. The transition to the next stage of independent activity by the child is only possible when some progress has been made towards the organization of his activity.

This form of defect carries with it especially abnormal and distinctive behavior. This abnormality is based upon their inability to comprehend what they perceive. The absence of comprehension leads to their inability to choose an appropriate line of action and to the development of behavioral abnormality. In the course of corrective training of these children a very complex problem arises, which needs further analysis. This is the problem of the formation of behavior: of the development of proper attitudes towards situations and towards the teacher's estimation, and of the ability to evaluate their own actions. In the course of their education these children had to be taught how to be annoyed, embarrased, or confused.

Although we know of a number of methods which may be used to teach oligophrenic children Russian and arithmetic, we can confidently state that no work has been reported which would indicate ways of encouraging development of the emotional-volitional functions, of behavior, and of character, so that the creation of such methods is essential.

This most difficult period of corrective training must be divided into a series of stages. The first stage of this work is characterized by the fact that the teacher must evaluate in his speech what the child perceives and must devise a course of action which the child must carry out; the child formulates this mode of action in his speech. In the next stage the child, with the teacher's assistance, evaluates what he sees, formulates it in his speech, and selects a mode of action corresponding to the evaluation of what is perceived, and he makes a preliminary formulation of his mode of action in speech. In the next stage the child carries out the whole of this activity unaided. This last stage of corrective training is very prolonged and as a result of it such children learn to analyze what they perceive, and thereby to develop the ability to evaluate a situation with the aid of internal speech and to develop the most adequate methods of action. They also develop to some extent the ability to regard a situation critically, although this ability is unstable, and with a change in the situation they again begin to behave inadequately. We will cite only one example from our experience of corrective training work with these children.

N. first attended the medicopedagogic advisory service of the

Institute of Special Schools and Children's Homes in 1933, at the age of $5\frac{1}{2}$ years.

In accordance with a specially planned program, individual work was undertaken with the girl, and by the time the child was eight years of age it had produced good results. It had been possible to produce considerable compensation of the motor insufficiency and to teach the girl to carry out a number of elementary tasks in caring for herself, drawing and modeling. The girl accompanied all her tasks by speech, and subsequently used it only when she met with difficulties. At nine years of age the girl began to attend a special school for her education. With the aid of additional individual tuition, entirely directed towards the further compensation of her defect, she was able to cope with the syllabus of the special school. Her behavior became much more purposeful. At 17 years of age N. left the special school and was found a job in a chemical laboratory, where she prepared the apparatus for analyses. At this age we again examined the patient, when she showed considerable compensation, which was most clearly marked in respect of her motor activity. Not only did N. perform all her duties at work, but she also helped with the housekeeping, learned to dance, and took up cycling and skating. In conversation with the girl, however, it was found that she was incapable of a sufficiently critical evaluation of a situation, and that her attitude to her environment was inadequate. Reports from her place of work showed that she was attentive and diligent, and very honest and truthful, but occasionally she spoke too candidly of her emotions and of her attitude towards her environment. Those around her were particularly upset when, at meetings, she came out with high praise of her own attainments.

Thus in this case, in which considerable compensation of the defect was achieved, a certain impulsive spontaneity nevertheless still showed itself in her behavior. The girl lived in a very cultivated circle, where she was the recipient of a great deal of attention. After a second consultation (at the age of 18 years) it was decided to continue with her individual tuition, directed towards the compensation of her defect as it affected the development of the emotional-volitional functions. Later her condition improved still further. She was transferred to more complicated work at the same laboratory, where she is still working at the present time.

This case, like many others of a similar nature, convinces us that compensation of this defect may also be attainable.

CONCLUSION

The survey of the literature has shown that much remains to be explained and studied in the etiology, pathogenesis, pathophysiology, symptomatology, and clinical classification of oligophrenia. In our present investigation, based on a dynamic study of oligophrenia in childhood, we made a number of theoretical assumptions, which were later validated by clinical and experimental findings.

With regard to the question of etiology, our findings suggest that the mental deficiency of oligophrenia may be attributed to an organic lesion of the brain, resulting from exogenic noxious influences.

Analysis of the clinical and experimental data, as well as the study of a group of children who suffered from hydrocephalus, led us to postulate that the principal pathogenetic factor in oligophrenic mental deficiency must be considered to be a diffuse (mainly superficial) lesion of the cerebral cortex. It is this pathogenetic factor which lies at the basis of the disturbance of the higher nervous activity in oligophrenic children.

Against the background of pathologic changes in the higher nervous activity, a foremost place is occupied by the pathological inertia of the nervous processes. This pathological inertia of the nervous processes lies at the basis of the difficulty of formation of complex functional systems and thereby leads to the later emergence of the fundamental symptom of oligophrenia. It is also responsible for the common feature which permits states of differing etiology to be grouped together in one single clinical form.

A series of additional pathogenetic factors, such as late hydrocephalus in a residual stage of the organic lesion, and gross local disturbances, although not specific for oligophrenic mental deficiency, may nevertheless be highly significant. The fundamental pathogenetic factor, in the form of a diffuse lesion of the cerebral cortex, in conjunction with the additional factors, determines the qualitative structural character of the disability.

Our investigations thus enabled us to make progress towards the understanding of the pathogenesis of oligophrenia and, in particular, towards the recognition of the considerable role of residual hydrocephalus.

Our purpose in this investigation was to make a more differential approach to the analysis of the distinctive pathophysiological features lying at the basis of this form of mental retardation. Much descriptive work has been published on the special features of the higher nervous activity of oligophrenic children. However, this work gives the impression that there is a uniform drop in the level of the higher nervous activity, and that the pathological changes of all the parameters of the higher nervous activity are equally important in determining the clinical picture of oligophrenia.

We have concluded from our investigation that, associated with maldevelopment of the whole higher nervous activity, the feature most specific for oligophrenia is a disturbance of the mobility or plasticity of the nervous processes. A series of special experiments, carried out on the children whom we studied, together with the analysis of the clinical facts, have shown that it is this inertia of the nervous processes which is of the greatest importance in the production of the dominant symptom of oligophrenia. It may easily be shown that inertia of the nervous processes is revealed at various levels of expression of the disability in oligophrenia. Inertia of the fundamental nervous processes is manifested irrespective of the qualitative structural pattern of the disability. In the basic form of oligophrenia, especially when some degree of compensation of the disability is present, inertia of the nervous processes is associated with an adequate equilibrium of the fundamental nervous processes. Inertia in oligophrenic children with gross neurodynamic disturbances is clearly demonstrated by clinical and experimental findings, but this type of pathological higher nervous activity is associated with a gross disturbance of the balance between the fundamental nervous processes. The disturbance of the plasticity of the nervous processes is demonstrated still more obviously in the third variant of oligophrenia, in which it is combined with a severe dissociation of the activities of the two signal systems.

Repeated experimental investigations have shown that the disturbance of the mobility of the nervous processes remains a constant pathophysiological mechanism, clearly apparent at later stages of the child's development even in cases when the disability is relatively well compensated.

Inertia of the nervous processes may be detected by various methods of investigation. Numerous clinical observations have shown that oligophrenic children can be dislodged only with great difficulty from their old stereotyped connections, which interfere with the formation of new connections.

In experimental psychological investigations of various mental processes (perception, memory, attention, thinking, imagination, etc.) the rigidity of the mental processes of oligophrenics was very clearly demonstrated. A disturbance of mobility was also disclosed during the study of the emotional-volitional functions in these children. Finally, the disturbance of mobility of the fundamental nervous processes was especially vividly manifested during the investigation of the higher nervous activity, notably in experiments on the successive formation of several systems of connections. Thus the presence of inertia in oligophrenic mental deficiency is revealed irrespective of the method of investigation used.

Until very recently the symptomatology of oligophrenia has been described without analysis of the manner in which the individual symptoms are interrelated.

Both in our analysis of the pathogenetic and pathophysiological features, as well as in our study of symptomatology, our object was to study the structure of the disability in oligophrenic mental deficiency. The whole of our analysis showed that maldevelopment of the generalizing function of speech is the fundamental symptom of oligophrenia. The study of the relationship between this fundamental symptom and the other nonspecific symptoms has facilitated the approach to the problem of the classification of oligophrenia. Let us attempt to analyze to what extent our hypothesis of this fundamental system is borne out by all the facts described above.

The conclusion from our researches could be formulated as follows: the leading symptom of oligophrenic mental deficiency is manifested in every grade of severity of the disability, although the degree of manifestation of this symptom depends on the extent of the lesion.

Proof of the leading role of maldevelopment of the generalizing function of speech in oligophrenic mental deficiency is given by the fact that this symptom may be found quite regardless of the qualitative structural nature of the disability.

In the first form of oligophrenia this symptom stands out prominently in the foreground of the clinical picture, and all the other symptoms such as, for example, the maldevelopment of the emotional-volitional functions arise in the course of the anomalous development only secondarily to the presence of the fundamental symptom.

A deviation in the child's behavior only arises when he has an inadequate understanding of the situation in which he finds himself; the misbehavior is thus bound up in the closest possible manner with the maldevelopment of the cognitive activity.

In the first form of oligophrenia the fundamental symptom determines all of the distinctive features of the clinical picture, and the additional symptoms arise secondarily.

Analysis of the second form of oligophrenia, in which the qualitative structural peculiarities of the disability are due to additional pathogenetic factors, and where the clinical picture involves specific disturbances of the cortical neurodynamics, analysis of this form also clearly reveals the fundamental symptom. In describing the clinical picture of this particular variant of the disability, the question could legitimately be asked: is the fundamental symptom of oligophrenic mental deficiency present in this particular variant? If it is present, then does it arise secondarily in connection with the sharp diminution of work capacity? Careful and prolonged clinical observations, together with control data, show very clearly, however, that in this variant of the disability also, the disturbance of the generalizing function of speech remains the leading symptom and determines the picture ot the oligophrenic mental deficiency. Even in the cases where the activity of such a child could be organized, and he could be directed in the accomplishment of a task, the fundamental symptom nevertheless remained perfectly obvious.

The presence of the fundamental symptom in a disability of this particular pattern stands out especially clearly if this variant is differentiated from the cerebroasthenic states of childhood. The resemblance between these conditions involved the presence of certain symptoms which are not specific for oligophrenia, namely a disorganization of behavior and a reduced capacity for work. The conditions differed by virtue of the presence of the fundamental symptom in oligophrenia and of its absence in the cerebroasthenic states.

The study of these children in the process of their development clearly shows that the nonspecific symptoms have a tendency to become less obvious, and some of them may disappear altogether, whereas the fundamental symptom remains more or less prominent at all stages of the child's development.

The combination of the fundamental symptom with various additional symptoms determines the qualitative structural pattern of the disability.

In the clinical study of the third form of oligophrenia, which is characterized by a distinctive and gross maldevelopment of the whole personality, which is always associated with maldevelopment of the motor activity, the detection of the fundamental symptom becomes more difficult. In this particular variant too, the question may legitimately be asked: is the fundamental symptom of oligophrenic mental deficiency present here, and if so, is it primary and fundamental, or does its appearance represent a manifestation that is secondary to the basic gross maldevelopment of personality and motor activity? In order to answer this question, in addition to oligophrenic children with this variant of disability, we also studied a control group of children, in whom a gross maldevelopment of the personality was found to be associated with a disturbance of the regulation of complex motor acts. All these disturbances arose against a background of relative integrity of the general cortical activity. When we compared these apparently similar states we found that considerable differences between them could be found.

In oligophrenics of this type, the gross maldevelopment of the personality and especially of the motor activity stands out against the background of maldevelopment of the cognitive activity, whereas in the control group these symptoms of maldevelopment of the personality and of motor activity are associated with an adequate level of development of the cognitive functions.

These findings convincingly show that the maldevelopment of the generalizing function of speech also manifests itself in this particular variant of the disability as the fundamental symptom. The association of this fundamental symptom with the maldevelopment of the personality and motor activity determines the qualitative structural pattern of the disability.

The complete analysis which we have made allows the formulation of a second conclusion which is no less important for defining the fundamental symptom of oligophrenia: this symptom is found in the different variants of the oligophrenic defect. In order to prove the hypothesis that the maldevelopment of the generalizing function of speech may be regarded as the fundamental symptom of oligophrenia, we may utilize the results of the dynamic study of the same children in the course of their education. We may remember that most of the clinical findings were made on oligophrenic children who were observed and repeatedly investigated by us over a period of six years. In all cases without exception we found this symptom at all stages of development. This does not mean that processes of abstraction and generalization did not develop in these children, but that their development was very inadequate.

For control purposes we studied children who had completed

their training at special school, had adapted themselves to working life and who showed good progress in their development. In these cases too the fundamental symptom of oligophrenia was quite obvious.

Of all the psychological methods of investigation that we used, directed toward the detection of the fundamental symptom, we attached exceptionally great diagnostic importance to the classification of objects, pictures, etc. Classification is one of the most delicate methods, because it is aimed directly at the discovery of the level at which the child reflects in his consciousness the connection between objects and phenomena he finds in his environment.

Dynamic investigation of these children by this method enabled us to detect several levels of maldevelopment of the capacity for abstraction and generalization.

The most elementary level may be considered to be that at which the task of classification itself is beyond the child's grasp, and at which each picture of an object exists only by itself.

On the next level we now see attempts at classification, but under these circumstances objects or pictures are grouped together in accordance with some unimportant sign. Immediately after this follows the next level in the development of these children as shown by classification experiments, which is associated with the appearance of thinking in terms of situations, a process which develops from very primitive beginnings and reaches ever more complex forms. Finally, a stage of development is reached at which we find both verbally acquired ideas and situational forms of thinking. In these cases the child may correctly distribute pictures into groups, but in his verbal projection he may move back to the situational connections.

Thus by means of this experimental method, just as by the use of other methods of investigation, it is clearly shown that the fundamental symptom is preserved, although it shows itself only if the tasks are made complicated.

In order to convince ourselves even more completely that the fundamental symptom is permanent, it is desirable to examine the manifestation of the symptoms which are nonspecific for oligophrenic mental deficiency. By nonspecific symptoms we mean a disturbance of analysis and integration within the limits of a given analyzer. Our investigations with our available clinical tests showed that in the initial stages of education we can find a maldevelopment of analysis and synthesis within the limits of individual analyzers. For example, within the optic analyzer this maldevelopment is characterized by the faulty perception and nonrecognition of various objects, ordinarily well known to the children, if the viewing time is shortened, or if they are shown upside down during spatial analysis and integration, when an increase in the complexity of the task made its accomplishment more difficult. With respect to the motor-speech analyzer, it must be stated that only in the initial stages of their education did these children display faults in the pronunciation of individual sounds. The same can be said about the auditory analyzer. In the initial stage of education difficulty was found in the differentiation between correlated phonemes. By the second or third years of their education, however, these difficulties were no longer found on investigation.

We may thus formulate a third hypothesis concerning the fundamental symptom of oligophrenic mental deficiency: the fundamental symptom of oligophrenic mental deficiency manifests itself at all stages of the child's development, and sometimes may be detected only when the task is made more complicated.

The symptom of maldevelopment of the capacity for abstraction and generalization is specific for oligophrenic mental deficiency. This is confirmed by the fact that, when different methods of investigation of these children were used, the difficulties in the performance of the various tasks were determined in each case by the extent to which the particular task made demands on the generalizing function of speech. For example, during the description of the picture of an object, the oligophrenic child recognizes everything represented in the picture without difficulty, but he is incapable of generalizing the material perceived with the aid of speech. The same state of affairs is repeated when the child is shown a sequence of pictures, when he can analyze the various concrete factors shown on the picture but cannot group them according to some common feature, nor draw conclusions from his store of knowledge. The same thing is found when we test their processes of comparison and discrimination, or their understanding of selections of prose, or their ability to solve arithmetical problems, or their understanding of the rules of grammar, etc.

New methods of examination developed in the laboratory of higher nervous activity of the Institute of Defectology, under the direction of A. R. Luriya, have shown that if we test the interaction between signal systems and confront the oligophrenic child with a complicated task which requires the identification of a new stimulus by means of speech, the oligophrenic child will not succeed in the task.

This fundamental symptom may thus be regarded as specific

for oligophrenic mental deficiency, for it is found in all degrees of the disability with this distinctive qualitative structural pattern, it is found at different stages of development, and when different methods of investigation are used.

During the study of the special features of the higher nervous activity it was possible to show that, against the background of maldevelopment of the entire higher nervous activity, the disturbance of the parameter of mobility is most specific for oligophrenic mental deficiency, and during the study of the symptomatology the specificity of this basic symptom also became apparent.

Both the fundamental symptom and the inertia of the nervous processes are seen with different degrees of severity of the disability, and are independent of the qualitative structural pattern of the disability, the level of its compensation, or the method of investigation. Both remain permanently established in the picture of oligophrenia, and can be found in varying degrees.

The association of the fundamental symptom of oligophrenic mental deficiency with inertia supports our view that the disturbance of mobility of the nervous processes plays a most important role in the development of the fundamental symptom of oligophrenia.

In the introductory part of our work it was pointed out that we regard oligophrenia as one form of anomalous development. In these children we are dealing, not with a progressive process, but with a true developmental anomaly. In attempting to understand this anomalous development we start from Vygotskii's theory of the mental development of the child, which is highly pertinent to the analysis of the different anomalous conditions of childhood.

The analysis of our clinical observations clearly shows a consistent pattern of anomalous development. According to our analysis of the basic form of oligophrenia, the organic lesion is diffuse and mainly cortical in character. This diffuse lesion of the cerebral cortex leads in the process of development to an insufficiency of the entire higher nervous activity, but especially to a disturbance of the mobility of the nervous processes.

The inertia which arises in the earliest stages of development of the child inhibits the formation of the complex functional systems which are the necessary foundation upon which the integrative activity of the cerebral cortex is built, and this in turn is responsible for the difficulty in the development of the generalizing function of speech. The inadequacy of development of the generalizing function of speech influences every aspect of the child's mental functions. It is as a special form of anomalous development that the distinctive pattern of the first form of oligophrenia should be regarded.

In the analysis of the second form of oligophrenia the same pattern emerges as in the first.

During the analysis of the third form of oligophrenia we observe a combination of inertia, which restrains the development of the complex systems of connections, with a primary inadequacy of the emotional-volitional functions, as a result of which the child does not develop adequate overt attitudes towards tasks assigned to him. This absence of any particular attitude to a task is combined with an inability of these children to master their movements and to use them in purposeful activity. This combination of complex pathogenetic and pathophysiological factors is the primary basis upon which this form of anomalous development rests.

This leads in time not only to the maldevelopment of the generalizing function of speech, but also to a faulty development of the specifically human forms of activity and behavior.

It can thus be seen that the systemic, causal-dynamic principle facilitated our analysis of the various forms of anomalous development in oligophrenia.

The study of the structure of the oligophrenic defect led to the identification of the fundamental symptom combined with certain additional, nonspecific symptoms. The study of the pathophysiological features of the higher nervous activity in oligophrenia, the isolation of the fundamental pathophysiological abnormality in conjunction with several other disturbances of the higher nervous activity, and finally, the study of certain aspects of the pathogenesis of oligophrenia have together provided a basis for developing a classification of oligophrenia.

We know that the problem of the classification of any given clinical form is difficult, whatever clinical investigation is undertaken. The researcher must approach the solution of this problem by first isolating a single basic principle upon which he can base his classification. It was especially tempting to construct a classification based on some common etiological factor. However, as we remarked in the survey of the literature, all such classifications have finally failed in the course of more than a century. The attempts of some workers to devise a purely etiological classification were limited to the fact that they emphatically declared that such a classification was necessary, but they were then unable to develop it on the basis of their clinical examinations and findings.

In order to tackle this problem of the classification of oligophrenic states, let us try to analyze the attempts which have been made at such an etiological classification from the study of the late sequelae of infectious diseases, toxic conditions, and trauma.

In a well-known series of clinical investigations, certain authors attempted to work on the basis of etiology. However, no sooner did an investigator begin to analyze his clinical material, than he discovered with unfailing regularity that absolutely different clinical pictures can be observed in connection with the same etiological factor. During the study of the sequelae of dysentery in children, which leads to certain mental changes in a late stage of the disease, it has been pointed out that the etiology is the decisive factor in determining the clinical picture, but this was followed by a contradiction of the authors' own declared positions, for in describing the clinical pictures they found almost every syndrome known to the pathology of childhood, from mild asthenic states, psychopathic syndromes, epileptiform reactions, gross localized lesions, to fully developed epilepsy. When the residual mental changes in tuberculous meningitis were studied the same variety of syndromes were observed, starting with mild asthenic states and ending with gross forms of dementia. In other cases the residual stage of tuberculous meningitis was characterized by changes of behavior, starting with mild forms and going on to gross psychopathic states. Finally, the same tuberculous meningitis in its residual stage could produce either mild manifestations of an episyndrome or gross forms of epilepsy (see the work of M. O. Lapides).

No more successful were those researchers who attempted to retain the principle of a single factor for the construction of a classification, but who based their classification on the localization of the lesion rather than on the etiological factor. In these investigations too, the pronouncement of a single principle of classification was merely an empty statement, and it remained completely impossible to apply this principle to the author's own clinical researches.

These failures are not all fortuitous, but tend to show a regular pattern. During classification of any particular clinical entity, the various variants of the clinical picture are not determined by any one factor in isolation, however important that factor might be. The clinical picture is determined by a variety of factors: the distinctive features of the pathogenesis, by which we mean the sum total of the factors and their interaction with each other; the etiology of the disease; the character of the pathological process itself, and of its distribution; and finally, of particular importance in pediatrics, the time at which the lesion actually appeared. The same lesion, with the same etiology and localization, may create quite a different clinical picture depending on the time at which it occurs. We demonstrated this fact in particular during the study of epidemic encephalitis in children.

On the basis of pathogenesis we distinguish four forms of oligophrenia. We may remember that in its pathogenetic aspect the first form is characterized by a diffuse lesion of the cerebral cortex, with relative preservation of the subcortical formations and without alteration of the cerebrospinal fluid dynamics. This feature of the pathogenesis is responsible for the fact that, against the background of maldevelopment of the entire higher nervous activity, there is a gross disturbance of the mobility of the fundamental nervous processes, and the distinctive features of the higher nervous activity lead, in turn, to the distinctive clinical picture, which is characterized by the presence of only the fundamental symptom of oligophrenia.

In the second form of oligophrenia we have a combination of the underlying pathogenetic factor, i.e., a diffuse lesion of the cerebral cortex, with the additional pathogenetic factor of a residual hydrocephalus. This distinctive pathogenetic feature leads to correspondingly distinctive pathophysiological features. The study of the higher nervous activity in this variant of the disability shows that the disturbance of the mobility of the nervous processes is combined with a gross, acute disturbance of the balance between excitation and inhibition. These special pathophysiological features lie at the basis of the clinical picture, in which, besides the fundamental and still dominant symptom, a series of nonspecific symptoms appear, among which we include distinctive behavioral disturbances and a sharp decline in the capacity for work.

The third form of oligophrenia is characterized by the combination of a general, diffuse lesion of the cerebral cortex with gross disturbances within the limits of the motor analyzer and in the associated subcortical formations.

These distinctive features of the pathogenesis determine the pathophysiological basis of this particular clinical form, which is characterized by a combination of marked inertia of the nervous processes with gross dissociation in the activity of the signal systems and marked disturbances of the dynamics of the nervous processes within the limits of the motor analyzer. These specific changes in the higher nervous activity themselves lead in the process of development to the characteristic features of the clinical picture, in which we have a combination of the fundamental symptom with gross disturbances in the region of the motor analyzer and changes in the emotional-volitional functions.

* * *

Let us endeavor to show what our classification of oligophrenia has to offer towards the solution of a number of practical problems. We may recall that an interesting but neglected clinical problem in oligophrenia is that of differential diagnosis. Practical workers have experienced considerable difficulties in differentiation between oligophrenia and similar conditions. The large number of diagnostic mistakes, and the consequent misdirection of children to the wrong type of establishment, has resulted mainly from the fact that states similar to oligophrenia have been taken for oligophrenia. While the problem of the classification of oligophrenia has remained unsolved, the separation of this complex and varied group of conditions from other conditions of a similar nature has presented great difficulties to us.

Our investigations have enabled us to approach the study of the problem of differential diagnosis of states similar to oligophrenia by seeking to distinguish them not from the group of oligophrenia as a whole, but from its individual variants.

For instance, the first variant of oligophrenia must be distinguished from temporary delay in development. Children with a temporary delay in development, at the beginning of their education, show a considerable outward resemblance to oligophrenic children. However, as we have shown in Chapter 2, besides the similarity between these states, considerable differences also exist.

The second variant of oligophrenia must be distinguished especially from those "pseudo-oligophrenic" states which arise in children after infectious diseases or trauma, and which are characterized by a marked lowering of the cortical tone.

The greatest difficulties in differential diagnosis are encountered in the study of the third form of oligophrenia, which, as we have shown above, must be differentiated from schizophrenic processes in children, and also from those conditions consisting merely of systemic disturbances arising in association with the integrity of the cortical activity, and from special forms of retardation of development.

It can thus be seen that the classification of oligophrenia in accordance with the structure of the disability allows a much more accurate and rational approach to be made to the problem of differential diagnosis, and thereby facilitates the practical solution of the problem regarding the placement of the child in the proper facility. All the work which we have undertaken on the study of the clinical features of oligophrenic states—careful experiments, comprehensive and thorough study, dynamic observations on the same child over a period of several years, the comparison of the individual variants and individual data at our disposal—all this is directed at two important practical tasks: to find the most effective methods of treatment of these children and to find the most suitable and effective methods of compensation for their disabilities.

Our findings facilitate a more discriminating approach to treatment. For instance, in the first variant of oligophrenia which we distinguish, it is necessary to employ therapeutic measures directed towards the stimulation of the child's development. In the second variant stimulation alone is insufficient. In addition to measures stimulating development, it is essential to employ all possible means of improving the circulation of the cerebrospinal fluid and the blood. In the third form of oligophrenia the use of general stimulation must be supplemented by the quest for other forms of treatment which would influence the motor analyzer and the subcortical ganglia.

The classification which we have described thus provides a most satisfactory basis for further research for the development of methods of selective action not on oligophrenia as a collective condition, but on its individual clinical variants. A second factor, however, is especially important at the present time, that is the necessity of creating a truly scientific basis for the corrective training work carried out with children educated at special schools. In the solution of this problem too, the variants of oligophrenia which we have distinguished also give some indication of the direction in which this work should proceed. We have worked out ways of compensation for each separate variant, but we consider it essential that the ways of compensation are planned in accordance with the qualitative structural pattern of the disability. Having concluded, for example, that in the first form of oligophrenia, in association with the fundamental symptom a series of secondary symptoms has developed, all our attention in the process of compensation must be directed to the development in these children of the ability to establish connections between isolated phenomena taking place in their environment.

It has been pointed out that this way of compensation is frankly inadequate for the second variant of the disability, and does not lead to the desired results. Besides all the various measures directed towards the stimulation of development, special measures are required in the form of treatment aimed at the organization of behavior and activity.

So far as the third form of oligophrenia is concerned, in addition to the general stimulation of development it is essential to pay special attention to the development of the motor analyzer. The child must be taught to master his movements, and then subsequently to use his movements in definite and concrete forms of activity. Particular attention must be directed towards the development of the regulating function of speech.

The study of the structure of oligophrenic mental deficiency and the identification of its fundamental symptom, the study of the distinctive features of the pathophysiological mechanisms and the identification of a fundamental parameter, and the additional data relating to the understanding of the importance of the pathogenesis of these conditions, all of these have enabled us to propose a classification of oligophrenic states in childhood. This in turn has been used to establish a system of differential diagnosis and a differential approach to treatment, and created a foundation upon which one can plan the correct organization of an educational program directed towards the compensation of the disability and adapted to suit the requirements of each individual variant of the condition.

BIBLIOGRAPHY

GLOSSARY OF RUSSIAN ABBREVIATIONS

ANM SSSR - Academy of Medical Sciences USSR
AN SSSR - Academy of Sciences USSR
APN RSFSR - Academy of Pedagogical Sciences RSFSR
Biomedgiz - State Publishing House of Biological and Medical Literature
GIZ - State Publishing House
Gospolitizdat - State Political Press
Gos. Sots. Ekonom. Izd. - State Social and Economic Press
Izd. - Press or Publishing House
Izd. Inst. Okhrany Mater. i Mladenchestva - Publishing House of the Institute for the Protection of Motherhood and Childhood.
Izd. Narkomzdrava - Publishing House of the People's Commissariat of Public Health
Medgiz - State Publishing House of Medical Literature
Novosibirsk. Oblast Izd. - Publishing House of the Novosibirsk Region
Trudy - Transactions
Uchpedgiz - State Publishing House for Educational and Pedagogical Literature
Voprosy - Problems

Periodicals:

Arkh. Biol. Nauk SSSR - Archives of Biological Sciences USSR
Arkh. Sudebnoi Med. - Archives of Legal Medicine
Doklady Akad. Nauk SSSR - Proceedings of the Academy of Sciences USSR
Eksptl. Biol. i Med. - Experimental Biology and Medicine
Fizio. Zhur. SSSR - Journal of Physiology USSR
Izvest. Akad. Nauk SSSR, Ser. Biol. Nauk - Bulletin of the Academy of Sciences USSR, Ser. of Biological Sciences
Izvest. Akad. Ped. Nauk RSFSR - Bulletin of the Academy of Pedagogical Sciences RSFSR
Moskov. Med. Zhur. - Moscow Medical Journal
Med. Obozr. - Medical Review
Nauch. Trudy Ivanovsk. Med. Inst. - Scientific Transactions of the Ivanovsk Medical Institute
Nevropatol. i Psikhiat. - Neuropathology and Psychiatry
Obozrenie Psikhiat., Nevrol. i Eksptl. Psikhol. - Review of Psychiatry, Neurology, and Experimental Psychology
Sovetsk. Nevropatol., Psikhiat. i Psikhogigiena - Soviet Neuropathology, Psychiatry, and Mental Hygiene
Trudy Fiziol. Nauch Issled. Inst. Leningrad. Gos. Univ. - Transactions of the Scientific Research Institute for Physiology of the Leningrad State University
Voprosy Defektol. - Problems in Mental Deficiency
Voprosy Detskoi Psikhonevrol. - Problems in Children's Psychoneurology
Voprosy Filosofii i Psikhol. - Problems of Philosophy and Psychology
Voprosy Izuch. i Vospit. Lichnosti - Problems in the Study and Education of Personality
Voprosy Psikhol. - Problems in Psychology
Vrach. Vestnik - Medical Bulletin
Zhur. Nevrol. i Psichiat. im. Korsakova - Korsakov Journal of Neurology and Psychiatry
Zhur. po Izuch. Rannego Dets. Vozrasta - Journal for the Study of Early Child Development
Zhur. Vysshei Nerv. Deyatel. - Journal of Higher Nervous Activity

SOVIET LITERATURE

Adrianov, O.S. The morphological features of the cortical nuclear zone of the motor analyzer in the dog. Zhur. Vysshei Nerv. Deyatel., Vol. 2 (1952).

Anokhin, P.K (ed.). Problems of Higher Nervous Activity. Medgiz, Moscow, 1949.

Arendt, A.A. Hydrocephalus and Its Surgical Treatment. Medgiz, Moscow, 1948.

Arkhangel'skii, V.M. The physiology of the motor analyzer. Arkh. Biol. Nauk SSSR., Vol. 22 (1922).

Asratyan, E.A. Motor-defensive reflexes of the dog after extirpation of the motor areas of the cerebral cortex. Doklady Akad. Nauk SSSR, Ser. Biol., Vol. 1, No. 2-3, 1935.

Azbukin, D.I. The Microcephalic Girl Mashuta. Anthropologo-Psychological and Pathologoanatomical Study. Moscow, 1911.

Bekhterev, V.M. The Basis of Knowledge of the Functions of the Brain. St. Petersburg, 1907.

Bekhterev, V.M., and M.N. Zhukovskii. Microcephalia. Obozrenie Psikhiat., Nevrol. i Eksptl. Psikhol., No. 5 (1902).

Bernshtein, N.A. The Structure of Movements. Medgiz, Moscow, 1947.

Betz, V.A. Two centers in the human cerebral cortex. Moskovsk. Vrach. Vestnik, No. 25 (1873).

Bogoroditskii, B.A. Essays on Linguistics and the Russian Language. Uchpedgiz, 1939.

Boskis, R.M. The study and training of deaf and dumb children. Izvest. Akad. Ped. Nauk RSFSR, No. 48 (1953).

Chlenov, L.G. The problem of localization in the light of recovery of function. Nevropatol. i Psikhiat., No. 11 (1945).

Davidovskii, I. V. Problems of Localization and Organopathology in the Light of the Teaching of Sechenov, Pavlov, and Vvedenskii. Medgiz, Moscow—Leningrad, 1954.

Demidov, A.A. Conditioned (Salivary) Reflexes in Dogs Without the Anterior Half of Both Hemispheres. Dissertation. St. Petersburg, 1909.

Dotsenko, M.I. L.A. Kvint's metric scale of facial psychomotor activity as used in the study of oligophrenia. Sovetsk. Nevropatol., Psikhiat. i Psikhogigiena, No. 4, 6 (1935).

Dyad'kovskii, I.E. Practical Medicine. Special Therapeutic Lectures. Moscow, 1847.

Filimonov, I.N. Comparative Anatomy of the Architectonic Formations of the Cerebral Cortex. Medgiz, Moscow, 1949.

Filimonov, I.N. Evolution of the cerebral cortex and I. P. Pavlov's teaching on higher nervous activity. Zhur. Vysshe, Nerv. Deyatel., Vol. 1, No. 4 (1951).

Filipycheva, N.A. Inertia of the Higher Cortical Processes in Local Lesions of the Cerebral Hemispheres. Author's abstract of dissertation. Moscow, 1952.

Freierov, O.E. The dynamics of oligophrenia. Nevropatol. i Psikhiat, Vol. 4, No. 2 (1954).

Freierov, O.E. The pathophysiological mechanisms of oligophrenia. Zhur. Vysshei Nerv. Deyatel., Vol. 4, No. 6 (1956).

Freze, A.U. A Short Course in Psychiatry. St. Petersburg, 1881.

Fulton, J.F., and C.F. Jacobson. The functions of the frontal lobes of the brain. Comparative investigation of the lower monkeys, the chimpanzee and man. Fiziol. Zhur. SSSR, Vol. 19, No. 1 (1935).

Fulton, J.F., and F.B. Dusser de Barenne. Functional Localization in the Cerebral Cortex [Russian translation]. Biomedgiz, 1937.

Gakkel', L.B. Comparative study of the disturbances of the higher nervous activity in patients with oligophrenia and senile dementia. Zhur. Vysshei Nerv. Deyatel., Vol. 3, No. 1 (1953).

Gartsshtein, N.G. Formation of a conditioned reflex and of conditioned inhibition in oligophrenic children. In: Systematic Investigation of the Conditioned-Reflex Activity of the Child. Moscow—Leningrad, 1930.

Gilyarovskii, V.A. Pathological Anatomy and Pathogenesis of Porencephalia. Moscow, 1914.

Gilyarovskii, V.A. Introduction to the Anatomical Study of Psychoses. Biomedgiz, 1925.

Griesinger, W. Mental Diseases [Translated from the last German edition]. St. Petersburg, 1875.

Grinshtein, A.M. Pathways and Centers of the Nervous System. Medgiz, 1941.

Gurevich, M.O. The forms of motor deficiency. Voprosy Detskoi Psikhonevrol., No. 2 (1925).

Gurevich, M.O. Textbook of Psychiatry. Medgiz. 1949.

Gur'yanov, E.V., and M.K. Shcherbak. The Psychology and Technique of Instruction in Writing at the Primer Period. Izd. APN RSFSR, Moscow, 1950.

Il'inskii, P.N. Track reflexes in mentally retarded children. Voprosy Izuch. i Vospit. Lichnosti, No. 1-2 (1927).
Ireland. Idiocy and Dementia [Translated from the English by Tomashevskii]. St. Petersburg, 1880.
Ivanov-Smolenskii, A.G. The Pathophysiology of Higher Nervous Activity. Medgiz, 1952.
Kapaev, I.I. The Study of the nervous processes during motor reactions in children. Fiziol. Zhur. SSSR, No. 1 (1954).
Kartsovnik, I.I. The Frontal Syndrome and its Clinical Variants in Penetrating Wounds of the Brain. Novosibirsk. Oblast. Izd., 1949.
Kaz'min, G.I., and V.K. Fedorov. The higher nervous activity in profound degrees of oligophrenia. Thesis of the Fourteenth Conference on Problems of Higher Nervous Activity (1951).
Khoroshko, V.K. The Relationship of the Frontal Lobes of the Brain to Psychology and Psychopathology. Moscow, 1912.
Klosovskii, B.N. and M.A. Nikitin. The present position of the problem of experimental hydrocephalus. In: Chronic Hydrocephalus in Early Childhood. Biomedgiz, Moscow, 1936.
Koni, A.F. The feeble minded and mentally afflicted. In: Reminiscences of Forensic Activity. Mayak Publishing House, Petrograd, 1922.
Kononova, E.P. The development of the poles of the frontal region and the variability in the structure of its cortex in man. Nevropatol. i Psikhiat., No. 6 (1940).
Kopylov, M.B. Fundamentals of Neurosurgical Roentgenological Diagnosis. Moscow, 1940.
Korsakov, S.S. A Course in Psychiatry. Moscow, 1901.
Korsakov, S.S. The psychology of microcephalics. Voprosy Filosofii i. Psikhol, Vols. 21 and 22 (1894).
Kovalevskii, N.I. Retarded and Abnormal Children (Idiots, Feeble-minded, Backward, Unbalanced), Their Treatment and Training. St. Petersburg, 1911.
Kraepelin, E. Introduction to Clinical Psychiatry. Izd. Narkomzdrava, Moscow, 1923.
Kramer, R.B. Localization in the Brain. Medgiz, Moscow, 1929.
Krasnogorskii, N.I. Development of Knowledge of the Physiological Activity of the Brain in Children. Biomedgiz., Moscow—Leningrad, 1939.
Kuraev, S.P. Investigation of Dogs with Disturbed Frontal Lobes of the Hemispheres in the Late Postoperative Period. Dissertation. St. Petersburg, 1912.
Leont'ev, A.N. The Development of Memory. GIZ, Moscow, 1931.
Leshli, K.S. Brain and Intellect. Gos. Sots. Ekonom. Izd., Moscow—Leningrad, 1933.
Linchenko, N.M. The pathology of chronic diseases of the brain and meninges. Zhur. Nevrol. i Psikhiat. im. Korsakova., Vol. 53, No. 2 (1903).
Lubovskii, V.I. Some aspects of the higher nervous activity of oligophrenic children. In: Problems of the Higher Nervous Activity of the Normal and Anomalous Child. Izd. APN RSFSR, 1956, Vol. 1.
Lukina, A.M. and A.L. Shnirman. Training of combined motor reflexes in oligophrenics. Advances in Reflexology and Physiology, Collection 2 (1926).
Luriya, A.R. Speech reactions of the child. In: Speech and Intellect in the Development of the Child. Moscow, 1927.
Luriya, A.R. The Regulation of Speech in Normal and Abnormal Behavior. Pergamon Press, London-New York, 1960.
Luriya, A.R. Traumatic Aphasia. Izd. AMN SSSR, Moscow, 1948.
Luriya, A.R. The role of speech in the formation of temporary connections in man. Voprosy Psikhol., No. 1 (1955).
Luriya, A.R. The Psychophysiology of Writing. Izd. APN RSFSR, 1950.
Malinovskii, P. P. Insanity as It Appears to the Practicing Doctor. St. Petersburg, 1847.
Magnan and Legrand. Degenerates [Translated from the French by Yu. V. Portugalov, with a foreword by V.M. Bekhterev]. St. Petersburg, 1903.
Margulis, M. S. The nosography and pathogenesis of acute serous meningitis. Moskov. Med. Zhur., No. 1-2 (1926).
Martsinovskaya, E.N. Disturbances of the Generalizing Function of Speech in Mentally Retarded Children. Author's abstract of dissertation. Moscow, 1955.
Mashchenko, S.M. Pathological Changes in the Cerebral Cortex in Secondary Dementia. Dissertation. St. Petersburg, 1899.
Merzheevskii, I.P. The pathological anatomy of idiocy. Nevropatol. i Psikhiat., Vol. 1 (1901).
Merzheevskii, I.P. Microcephalia. Arkh. Sudebnoi Med., No. 3 (1871).
Merzheevskii, I.P. Foreword to the translation of Ireland's book "Idiocy and Dementia." St. Petersburg, 1880.

Meshcheryakov, A. I. Disturbance of the Interaction between the Two Signal Systems in the Formation of Simple Motor Reactions in Localized Lesions of the Brain. Author's abstract of dissertation. Moscow, 1953.
Mirolyubov, N. G. Special features of the formation of reflexes to spatial relationships in severely oligophrenic children. In: Problems of Promotion of the Nervous and Mental Health of the Population. 1935.
Molotkova, I. A. Formation of conditioned reflexes to integrative stimuli in oligophrenics. Thesis given at Conference to Review Research (1953). Institute of Experimental Medicine of the Academy of Medical Sciences, 1954.
Morozov, M. S. The Anthropology, Etiology, and Psychology of Idiocy. Dissertation. St. Petersburg, 1904.
Muratov, V. A. Clinical Lectures on Nervous and Mental Diseases. 1899.
Muratov, V. A. A case of idiocy with a focal disease of the brain. Med. Obozr., Vol. 41, No. 3 (1894).
Novikova, L. A. Investigation of the electrical activity of the brain in oligophrenics. In: Problems of the Higher Nervous Activity of the Normal and Anomalous Child. Izd. APN RSFSR, 1956, Vol. 1.
Osipova, E. A. The etiology of schizophrenia. In: Problems of the Psychoneurology of Childhood. Moscow, 1925.
Ozerskii, N. I. The Psychopathology of Childhood, second edition. Ushpedgiz, Leningrad, 1938.
Panferov, G. K. The study of the reflexes in idiocy. In: Children's Diseases. Leningrad, 1927.
Paramonova, N. P. Development of the Interaction of the Two Signal Systems in the Formation of Motor Reactions in Children of Preschool Age. Dissertation. Moscow, 1953.
Pavlov, I. P. Complete Collected Works, second edition. Izd. AN SSSR, Moscow–Leningrad, 1951.
Petrova, M. K. Recognition of the physiological mechanism of voluntary movements. Trudy Fiziol. Lab. Akad. I. P. Pavlova, Vol. 10 (1941).
Pevzner, M. S. The structure of the intellectual defect in closed head injuries in children and adolescents. Transactions of the Central Institute of Psychiatry. Medgiz, Moscow, 1949, Vol. 4.
Pevzner, M. S. Development of the postencephalitic child (epidemic encephalitis). Nevropatol. i Psikhiat., No. 5 (1935).
Pevzner, M. S. Clinical characteristics of the principal variants of the disability in oligophrenia. In: Problems of the Higher Nervous Activity of the Normal and Anomalous Child. Izd. APN RSFSR, Moscow, 1956, Vol. 1.
Pevzner, M. S. Principles of Selection of Pupils for Special Schools. Izd. APN RSFSR, Moscow, 1956.
Pevzner, M. S. Disturbance of the regulating role of speech in the behavior of oligophrenics with maldevelopment of the frontal system. In: Problems of the Higher Nervous Activity of the Normal and Anomalous Child. Izd. APN RSFSR, Moscow, 1958, Vol. 2.
Polyakov, G. I. Structural organization of the human cerebral cortex from data of its development in ontogenesis. In: Cytoarchitectonics of the Human Cerebral Cortex. Medgiz, Moscow, 1949.
Pravdina-Vinarskaya, E. N. Neurological Characteristics of the Syndrome of Oligophrenia. Izd. APN RSFSR, Moscow, 1957.
Preobrazhenskaya, N. S., and I. N. Filimonov. The occipital region. In: Cytoarchitectonics of the Human Cerebral Cortex. Medgiz, Moscow, 1949.
Rabinovich, S. Ya. The classification of the oligophrenias. In: Problems of the Psychoneurology of Childhood. Medgiz, Moscow, 1946.
Rybakov, F. E. A case of microcephalia. Transactions of the Psychiatric Clinic of the Moscow University, No. 1, 1913.
Samukhin, N. V., G. V. Birnbaum, and L. S. Vygotskii. The dementia of Pick's disease. Sovetsk. Nevropatol., Psikhiat. i Psikhogig., Vol. 3, No. 6 (1934).
Saturnov, N. M. Further Investigations of Conditioned Salivary Reflexes in a Dog Lacking the Frontal Halves of Both Hemispheres. Dissertation. St. Petersburg, 1911.
Sechenov, I. M. Selected Philosophical and Psychological Works. Gospolitizdat, Moscow, 1947.
Sherrington, C. S. The Integrative Action of the Nervous System. Biomedgiz, 1935.
Shevalev, E. A. Analysis of the concept of dementia. Sovetsk. Psikhonevrol., No. 4 (1937).
Shif, Zh. I. Selection of similar light hues and naming of colors (comparative investigation of deaf-mutes, mentally retarded, and normal schoolchildren). In: L. V. Zankov and

I. I. Danyushevskii, [ed.]. Problems of the Psychology of Deaf-Mutes and Mentally Retarded Children. Uchpedgiz, 1940.
Shumilina, A. I. Functional importance of the frontal regions of the cerebral cortex in the conditioned reflex activity of the dog. In: Problems of Higher Nervous Activity. Medgiz, Moscow, 1949.
Shustin, N. Ya. Disturbance of Nervous Activity after Removal of the Frontal Lobes of the Cerebral Hemispheres in the Dog. Author's abstract of dissertation. Leningrad, 1955.
Simson, T. P. Hydrocephalus. Zhur. po Izuch. Rannego Detsk. Vozrasta Vol., 3, No. 1 (1925).
Skvortsov, M. A. The Pathological Anatomy of the More Important Diseases of Childhood. Medgiz, 1938.
Smirnov, L. I. Basis of the Morphology of the Nervous System in Normal and Pathological Conditions. Medgiz, 1935.
Solov ev, I. M. The perception of activity by mentally retarded children. In: Special Features of the Cognitive Functions of Mentally Retarded Children. Izd. APN RSFSR, 1953.
Speranskii, A. D. The role of the cerebrospinal fluid in the course of physiological and pathological processes in the brain. Eksptl. Biol. i Med., No. 7 (1926).
Sukhareva, G. E. Clinical Lectures on the Psychiatry of Childhood. Medgiz, 1955.
Tarasevich, N. N., and V. A. Tarasevich. Archicapillary forms of dementia and neuropathies in children and their causal constitutional therapy. Voprosy Defektol., No. 6 (1929).
Teplov, B. M. The concepts of weakness and inertia of the nervous system. Voprosy Psikhol., No. 6 (1955).
Tomashevskii, B. V. The Pathology of Idiocy. Dissertation. St. Petersburg, 1892.
Toporkov, N. N. Secondary dementia after amentia (results of clinical investigation with illustrations of handwriting, photographs of patients, and curves of weight, temperature, pulse, and respiration). Dissertation. St. Petersburg, 1915.
Troshin, G. Ya. The anthropological basis of training. In: Comparative Psychology of Normal and Abnormal Children, published by Dr. G. Ya. Troshin's Hospital-School, 1915.
Turetskii, M. Ya., and M. M. Model'. Chronic Hydrocephalus in Early Childhood. Izd. Inst. Okhrany Mater. i Mladenchestva, Moscow, 1936.
Ukhtomskii, A. A. Lability as a condition of the timeliness and coordination of nervous acts. Trudy Fiziol. Nauch.-Issled. Inst. Leningrad. Gos. Univ. No. 17 (1936).
Ushinskii, K. D. Man as the Object of Training. St. Petersburg, 1913.
Vasilevskaya, V. Ya., and I. M. Krasnyanskaya. Cognitive activity of pupils at a special school during work with visual material. Izvest. Akad. Ped. Nauk RSFSR, No. 68 (1955).
Veber, F. K. Pathogenesis and treatment of hydrocephalus. Minutes of the Pirogov Russian Surgical Society, 1922-1923.
Veresotskaya, K. I. Perception of depth (the third dimension) in the pictures of pupils at a special school. In: Problems of the Psychology of Deaf-mute and Mentally Retarded Children. Uchpedgiz, 1940.
Vinokurova, A. I. The 'dementia infantilis' of Heller. In: Problems of the Psychoneurology of Children and Adolescents. Biomedgiz, Moscow—Leningrad, 1936, Vol. 3.
Vlasova, T. A. The Influence of Disturbance of Hearing on the Development of the Child. Izd. APN RSFSR, Moscow, 1954.
Vogt, Karl. Microcephalus. St. Petersburg, 1873.
Voronin, L. G. Imitative powers in the lower monkeys. Fiziol. Zhur. SSSR, Vol. 33, No. 3 1947.
Voronin, L. G. Results of a comparative physiological study of the higher nervous activity. Izvest. Akad. Nauk SSSR, Ser. Biol. Nauk., No. 5 (1954).
Vygotskii, L. S. Selected Psychological Research. Izd. APN RSFSR, Moscow, 1956.
Zankov, L. V. Psychology of the Mentally Retarded Child. Uchpedgiz, 1939.
Zankov, L. V., [ed.]. Izvest. Akad. Ped. Nauk RSFSR, Vol. 57 (1954).
Zarubashvili, A. D. The profound oligophrenia of George. Collected Transactions of the Georgian Research Psychiatric Institute. Tiflis, 1945, Vol. 2.
Zernov, D. N. The Atavism of Microcephalics. Moscow, 1879.
Zhukovskii, M. N. The anatomical connections of the frontal lobes. Obozrenie Psikhiatrii, No. 12 (1897).
Zhuravleva, M. I., and A. Morgen. Formation of conditioned inhibition in oligophrenics. Thesis given at Conference to Review Research Work (1953). Institute of Experimental Medicine of the AMN SSSR, 1954.

Zislina, N. N. Electroencephalographic investigation of the functional state of the brain in oligophrenics by the method of rhythmic light stimulation. In: Problems of the Higher Nervous Activity of the Normal and Anomalous Child. Izd. APN RSFSR, 1956, Vol. 1.

Zlotnikov, M. D. The etiology and pathogenesis of primary hydrocephalus. Nauch. Trudy Ivanovsk. Med. Inst., Vol. 3 (1940).

NON-SOVIET LITERATURE

Ackerly, S. Instinctive, emotional, and mental changes following prefrontal lobe extirpation. Am. J. Psychiat., Vol. 92 (1935).

Bappert, J. Zur Berufsfähigkeit der Hilfsschüler (1927).

Bassek, W. Nachreifung bei angeborenem Schwachsinn. Z. psych. Hyg., Vol. 14 (1942). Ref.: Zentr. ges. Neurol. u. Psychiat. Halle (1942).

Benda, C. E. Microcephaly. Am. J. Psychiat., Vol. 97 (1941).

Berry, R. J. A. Brain size and mentality. Brit. Med. J., Vol. 2 (1936).

Bianchi, L. Sulle compensazioni funzionali della corteccia cerebrale. Psichiatria, Vol. 1 (1883).

Birnbaum, K. The problem of the mentally deficient child in Philadelphia. Am. J. Mental Deficiency., Vol. 49 (1945).

Bittner, von der Hecht H. Kinderpsychiatrie. Wien. med. Wochschr., Vol. 19 (1952).

Bleuler, E. Lehrbuch der Psychiatrie. Berlin, 1916

Boldt, W. H. Postnatal cerebral trauma as an etiological factor in mental deficiency. Am. J. Mental Deficiency, Vol. 53 (1948).

Bonin, G. The frontal lobe of primates: cytoarchitectural studies. In: The Frontal Lobes. Baltimore, 1948.

Bourneville, D. M. Recherches cliniques et therapeutiques sur l'hysterie et l'idiotie. Paris, 1881.

Brickner, R. M. Interpretation of frontal lobe function based upon study of case of partial bilateral frontal lobectomy. Proc. Assoc. Research Nervous Mental Disease, Vol. 13 1932.

Brugger, C. Die genetische Einheitlichkeit der klinisch unkomplizierten Schwachsinnsformen. Schweiz. Arch. Neurol. Psychiat., Vol. 45 (1940).

Bürger-Prinz., H. Die Diagnose des angeborenen Schwachsinns. Deut. med Wochschr., Vol. 1 (1936).

Burt, C. The Subnormal Mind. Oxford 1955.

Burt, C. L. Causes and Treatment of Backwardness. Philosophic Library, 1953.

Cassel, M. E., and M. M. Riggs. Comparison of three etiological groups of mentally retarded children, on Vineland Social Maturity Scale. Mental Deficiency, Vol. 58 (1953).

Clarke, Ann M. and A. D. B. Clarke, [ed.], Mental Deficiency. The Changing Outlook. London, 1958.

Cook, G. H. Consideration of the relationship of primary and secondary mental deficiencies, convulsive disorders, avitaminosis, and alteration of electroneuronal potential. Am. J. Psychiat., Vol. 101 (1944).

Denny-Brown, D. The frontal lobes and their function. In: Modern Trends in Neurology. London, 1951. Chap. 1.

Doll, E. A. The nature of mental deficiency. Psychologic. Rev. Vol. 47 (1940). Ref.: Zentr. ges. Neurol. u. Psychiat. Vol. 100 (1941).

Dollinger, A. Beiträge zur Ätiologie und Klinik der schweren Formen angeborener und fruherworbener Schwachsinnenzustände. Berlin, 1921.

Domarus, E. Zur Charakteristik des schwachsinnigen Denkens. Z. ges. Neurol. u. Psych., Vol. III (1927).

Dubitscher, F. Infantilismus, Spätentwicklung und Schwachsinn. Z. menschl. Vererbungs- u. Konstitutionslehre, Vol. 26 (1942). Ref.: Zentr. ges. Neurol. u. Psychiat., Vol. 103 (1942).

Dubitscher, F. Praktische Fragen der Schwachsinnsdiagnostik. Med. Welt, Vol. 425 (1939). Ref.: Zentr. ges. Neurol. u. Psychiat., Vol. 95 (1939-1940).

Eisenstein, I. Psychologische Untersuchungen über die verschiedenen Formen des angeborenen Schwachsinns. Dissertation. Berlin, 1929.

Esuirol, J. E. D. Les maladies mentales considerées sous les rapports médico-hygiéniques et medico-legales. Paris, 1838.

Feuchtwanger, E. Die Bedeutung von Gehirnschädigungen für die Entwicklung und die Form

intellektueller Defektzustände, insbesondere des Schwachsinns im Kindersalter. Kinderforsch., Vol. 32 (1926).
Feuchtwanger, E. Die Funktionen des Stirnhirns. Berlin, 1923.
Franceschetti, A., and C. Brugger. Über das kombinierte Auftreten von endogenem Schwachsinn und angeborenem Star. Schweiz. med. Wochschr., Vol. 10 (1944).
Franz, S. I. On the functions of the cerebrum. The frontal lobes in relation to the production and retention of simple sensory-motor habits. Am. J. Psychol., Vol. 8 (1902-1903).
Fulton, J. F., and C. F. Jacobsen. The functions of the frontal lobes: A comparative study in monkeys, chimpanzees, and man. Proc. Second International Neurological Congress. London, 1935.
Gesell. The early diagnosis of mental defect. Arch. Neurol., Vol. 22 (1929).
Geyer, H. Die angeborenen und früh erworbenen Schwachsinnzustände. Fortschr. Neurol., Vol. 10 (1938). Ref.: Zentr. ges. Neurol. u. Psychiat., Vol. 92 (1939).
Gibson, R. Differential diagnosis of oligophrenia. Am. J. Dis. Child., Vol. 83 (1952).
Goddard, H. Feeble-mindedness and heredity. J. Am. Med. Assoc. (1942).
Goht, F. Formen kindlichen Schwachsinns. Klin. Wschr., Vol. 46 (1922).
Goldstein, K., and A. Bethe. Die Lokalisation in der Grosshirnrinde. In: Handb. d. normalen und pathol. Physiol. Berlin, 1927, Vol. 10.
Götz, W. Arbeiten zur Frage des angeborenen Schwachsinns. Untersuchungen uber die eidetische Anlage bei Jugendlichen niederer Intelligenz. Arch. Psych., Vol. 88 (1929).
Gruhle, H. W. Theorie der Schizophrenie. In: Bumke, O. Handb. d. Geisteskrankh. Berlin, 1932, Vol. IX.
Heck, A. O. Education of Exceptional Children. New York-London, 1953.
Hecker, E. Klinische Beobachtung bei erworbenem Schwachsinn. Allgem. Z. Psychiat. Vol. 112 (1939).
Hell, K. Sind frühkindliche Entwicklungsstörungen (verspätetes Laufen- und Sprechenlernen, Bettnässen) verwertbar fur die Abgrenzung des exogenen vom endogenen Schwachsinn. Allgem. Z. Psychiat., Vol. 112 (1939).
Heller, T. Über infantilen Schwachsinn. Med. Klin. Vol. 34 (1938).
Heller, T. Über das Spachwerden bei einem oligophrenen Kind. Kinderpsych., Vol. 3 (1936).
Hilliard, L. T., and B. H. Kirman. Mental Deficiency. London, 1957.
Hilliard, L. T., and L. Mundy. Diagnostic Problems in the Feeble-minded. London, 1954.
Jacobsen, C., S. Wolf, and T. Jackson. Experimental analysis of functions of frontal association areas in primates. J. Nervous Mental Disease, Vol. 82 (1935).
Jefferson, G. Removal of the right or left frontal lobes in man. Brit. Med. J. (1937).
Jervis, G. A. Etiology factors in mental deficiency. Am. J. Public Health.
Jervis, G. A. Phenylpyruvic oligophrenia; introductory study of 50 cases of mental deficiency associated with excretion of phenylpyruvic acid. A.M.A. Arch. Neurol. Psychiat., Vol. 38 (1937).
Kleist, K. Gehirnpathologie, vornehmlich auf Grund der Kriegserfahrungen. Leipzig, 1934.
Kozar, Z. Toksoplazmoza. Warsaw, 1954.
Kozar, Z., L. Duzewski, A. Duzewski, and Z. Jaroszewski. Toksoplazmoza, jako przyczyna niedorozwolu umuslowego. Neurol., neurochi. Psych. Polska. Vol. 4 (1954).
Koffka, K. Die Grundlagen der psychischen Entwicklung. Eine Einführung in die Kinderpsychologie. Osterwieck am Harz, 1921.
Köhler. Les déficiences intellectuelles chez l'enfant. Paris, 1954.
Kraepelin, E. Psychiatrie. Leipzig, 1910, Vol. I-III.
Kraepelin, E. Über psychische Schwäche. Arch. Psych. (1915).
Kreezer, G. Electric potentials of the brain in certain types of mental deficiency.
Kurbitz, W. Mikrocephalie und Schwachsinn. Arch. Psychiat., Vol. 94 (1931).
Laird, A. Mental deficiency. Am. J. Diseases Children., Vol. 49 (1935).
Larsen, E. Y. A neurologic-etiologic study on 1000 mental defectives. Acta Psychiat. et Neurol., Vol. 6 (1931).
Lewin, K. Eine dynamische Theorie des Schwachsinnigen. Berlin, 1933.
Loewy, H. Training the Backward Child. Staples Press, British Bull. Service, London, 1955.
Lutz, J. Psychiatrische Probleme im Kinderhospital. Ann. Paediat., Vol. 180 (1953).
Luxenbuerger, H. Endogener Schwachsinn und geschlechtsgebundener Erbgang. Z. ges. Neurol. u. Psychiat., Vol. 140 (1932).
Maurer, H. Über encephalographische Befunde bei Schwachsinnigen (unter besonderer Berücksichtigung des erblichen Schwachsinns). Med. Welt, Vol. 13 (1939).
Mautner, H. The pathological anatomy and physiology of mental retardation. Ann. Pediat.,

Vol. 182 (1954).
Middlemiss, J. E. An analysis of 200 cases of mental defectives. J. Mental Sci., Vol. 66 (1920).
Monakow, C. von. Über Lokalisation der Hirnfunktionen. Wiesbaden, 1910.
Neustadt, R. Die Psychosen der Schwachsinnigen. Berlin, 1928.
Paddle, K. C. L. Lumbar puncture and cerebro-spinal fluid in 2000 cases of mental defiency. J. Mental Sci., Vol. 80 (1934).
Penfield, W., and Y. P. Ewans. The frontal lobe in man; clinical study of maximum removals. Brain, Vol. 58 (1935).
Penrose, L. S. Recent progress in psychiatry: Mental deficiency. J. Mental Sci., Vol. 90 (1944).
Penrose, L. S. A Clinical and Genetic Study of 1280 Cases of Mental Defect. London, 1938.
Pick, A. Zur Zerlegung der "Demenz." Monatschr. Psychiat., Vol. 54 (1923).
Pleger, W. Erblichkeitsuntersuchungen an schwachsinnigen Kindern. Z. ges. Neurol. u. Psychiat., Vol. 135 (1931).
Ponitz, K. Zur Diagnostik und sozialen Bedeutung des angeborenen Schwachsinns. Z. ges. Neurol. u. Psychiat., Vol. 153 (1935).
Probst, M. Zur Lehre von der Mikrocephalie und Makrogyrie. Arch. Psychiat., Vol. 38 (1904).
Rylander, G. Personality Changes after Operations on Frontal Lobes. A clinical study of 32 cases. Copenhagen, 1939.
Schittenhelm, E. Die Vererbung des Schwachsinns. Dissertation, Tübingen, 1938.
Schulte, W. Psychiatrie des Praktikers. Schwachsinn. Med. Klin., Vol. 29 (1956).
Schutz, E., and H. W. Muller Limmroth. Electroencephalographische Befunde bei geistig rückständigen Kindern. Nervenarzt, Vol. 12 (1952).
Schwab, E. Über das Nachzeichen von geschlossenen und Punktfiguren bei Schwachsinnigen. Berlin, 1929.
Shaffer, K. Über normale und pathologische Hirnforschung. Z. ges. Neurol. u. Psychiat., Vol. 38 (1918).
Stadler, H. E., and R. L. Dryer. Phenylpyruvic oligophrenia. Arch. Pediatr., Vol. 70 (1953).
Stefan, H. Angeborene und erworbene Schwachsinnszustande. Med. Klin., Vol. 33 (1937).
Stertz, G. Störungen der Intelligenz. In: Bumke, O. Handb. d. Geisteskrankh. Berlin, 1928, Vol. 1, Part 1.
Sterzinger, O. Begabungsuntersuchungen an Hilfsschülern. Z. Kinderforsch., Vol. 28 (1924).
Stockert, F. G. Subcorticale Demenz. Ein Beitrag zür encephalitische Denkstörung. Arch. sychiat., Vol. 97 (1932).
Strohmayer, W. Angeborene und im frühen Kindesalter erworbene Schwachsinnszustände. In: Bumke, O. Handb. d. Geisteskrankh. Berlin, 1928, Vol. 10, Part 6.
Sherlock, E. B. Prognosis in Mental Deficiency. Med. Press, 1940, p. 204.
Thelen, F. Über Erregungsformen bei schwachsinnigen Kindern. Dissertation, Bonn, 1932, p. 64.
Thiele, R. Zur Kenntnis der psychischen Residualzustände nach Encephalities epidemica bei Kindern und Jugendlichen, insbesondere der weiteren Entwicklung dieser Fälle. Berlin, 1926.
Tramer, M. Stellung der Kinderpsychiatrie zur Pädiatrie. Schweiz. med. Wochschr., Vol. 45 (1953).
Tredgold, A. P. Mental Deficiency. London, 1937.
Weygandt, W. Das Problem der Erblichkeit bei jugendlichem Schwachsinn und bei Epilepsie Z. ges. Neurol. u. Psychiat. Vol. 152 (1935).
Weygandt, W. Idiotie und Imbezilitat. Die Gruppe der Defektzustande des Kindesalters. Leipzig, 1915.
Yannet, H. Classification and etiological factors in mental retardation. J. Pediatr., Vol. 50 (1957).

FSC
www.fsc.org
MIX
Papier | Fördert gute Waldnutzung
FSC® C083411

Kolibri 360 GmbH
Ferdinand-Jühlke-Straße 7
99095 Erfurt, Deutschland
produktsicherheit@kolibri360.de